Perception beyond Inference

Perception beyond Inference

The Information Content of Visual Processes

edited by Liliana Albertazzi, Gert J. van Tonder, and Dhanraj Vishwanath

The MIT Press
Cambridge, Massachusetts
London, England

For information about special quantity discounts, please email special_sales@mitpress.mit.edu

This book was set in Stone Serif and Stone Sans on InDesign by Asco Typesetters, Hong Kong. Printed and bound in the United States of America.

Library of Congress Cataloging-in-Publication Data

Perception beyond inference : the information content of visual processes / edited by Liliana Albertazzi, Gert J. van Tonder, and Dhanraj Vishwanath.
    p. cm.
Includes bibliographical references and index.
ISBN 978-0-262-01502-8 (hardcover : alk. paper) 1. Visual perception. 2. Cognitive neurosciences. I. Albertazzi, Liliana. II. Van Tonder, Gert J. III. Vishwanath, Dhanraj
BF241.P433   2011
152.14—dc22   2010020910

10 9 8 7 6 5 4 3 2 1

Contents

Preface

The idea of producing a book such as this one owes a great deal to the fortunate encounter among researchers from different disciplinary backgrounds and driven by the same motives: a dissatisfaction with the current research paradigms for studying the mind that are formulated on the basis of standard information theory and logical analysis. Although these approaches have no doubt advanced understanding of key aspects of cognitive science, they appear unsuited for dealing with the problems and levels of complexity inherent in understanding the full scope of mental processes. Conceptual errors particularly arise when such models are taken to be constitutive of mental phenomena. The issue, which has brought together experimental psychologists, mathematicians, philosophers, linguists, computer scientists, physicists, and art scholars, has essentially been the problem of information communicated by *form* most broadly construed. The linking theme is the foundational role of perception as the origin of every potential level of signification, from the most concrete to the most abstract (Arnheim, 1969), and a particularly strong interest in the *qualitative* aspects of experience, for within these lie the clues to a richer semantic theory of information.

The book springs from a series of meetings promoted by the Mitteleuropa Foundation. The foundation's goals have been an effort to reorient international discourse and research in the cognitive and computer sciences toward a more active consideration of the ontic, epistemic, and semantic aspects in the construction and verification of theories of human mental processes, as well as the development of synthetic computational systems. In recent years, the researchers affiliated at Mitteleuropa Foundation produced a series of edited volumes connected to the leading ideas of the institution's commitment (Poli, 1997, 1998; Albertazzi, 1998, 2000, 2001a, 2002, 2003, 2006; Kecskés and Albertazzi, 2007). For the guiding idea see also Albertazzi (2001a, 2001b).

One of the outcomes of the meetings at Mitteleuropa Foundation was the creation of the Research Group on Form, many of whose members have contributed to this collection of chapters. Further factors in the constitution of the group have been mutual affinity, curiosity, attitudes toward research, intellectual friendship, and not least the breathtaking environment of the Dolomites.

More generally, the group is working on a new research paradigm for the perceptual sciences that starts from how we "experience" perception, particularly visual perception, and seeks to identify the best tools with which to model that type of complexity. In other words, the group is working on the very *origins of conscious qualitative states* as a major aspect of information theory. However ambitious, the project (experience *to* neurons and stimuli rather than the other way around) is producing stimulating ideas and innovative research, and the ideas are progressively gaining consensus among scholars in different disciplinary fields. The present volume is devoted to understanding visual appearances as the primary level of meaning in the phenomenal field.

We hope the uniqueness of this volume, both in terms of its theoretical focus and the diversity of contributions, will provide a valuable (and to date unavailable) resource for researchers looking to move beyond existing paradigms in perceptual and cognitive sciences. The range of contributions has resulted in an especially extensive and unique bibliography. The individual contributions, in addition to their own insights, provide a useful roadmap into a wide-ranging research literature, some of which we believe has been unfairly neglected in current science. We also trust that the ideas and material presented are eminently relevant to those in applied fields (e.g., design, visual media, art) that look to the perceptual and cognitive sciences for insights on the structure of the mind.

Timeline of Chapter Manuscripts

The original manuscripts from the contributing authors were submitted for review in April 2008. Revisions based on anonymous reviewer's comments were submitted in October 2009.

References

Albertazzi, L. ed. 1998. *Shapes of Form. From Gestalt Psychology to Phenomenology, Ontology and Mathematics*. Dordrecht: Kluwer.

Albertazzi, L. ed. 2000. *Meaning and Cognition: A Multidisciplinary Approach*. Amsterdam: Benjamins Publishing Company.

Albertazzi, L. ed. 2001a. *The Dawn of Cognitive Science. Early European Contributors*. Dordrecht: Kluwer.

Albertazzi, L. 2001b. "Back to the Origins." In *Early European Contributors to Cognitive Science 1870–1930*, edited by L. Albertazzi. Dordrecht: Kluwer. 1–27.

Albertazzi, L. ed. 2002. *Unfolding Perceptual Continua*. Amsterdam: Benjamins Publishing Company.

Albertazzi, L. ed. 2003. *The Legacy of Gaetano Kanizsa in Cognitive Science*, special issue of *Axiomathes* 13, Springer.

Albertazzi, L. ed. 2006. *Visual Thought. The Depictive Space of Perception*. Amsterdam: Benjamins Publishing Company.

Arnheim, R. 1969. *Visual Thinking*. Berkeley: The Regents of the University of California.

Kesckes, I., and Albertazzi, L. eds. 2007. *Cognitive Aspects in Bilingualism*. Berlin, New York: Springer.

Poli, R. ed. 1997. *In Itinere. European Cities and the Birth of Modern Scientific Philosophy*. Amsterdam: Rodopi.

Poli, R. ed. 1998. *The Brentano Puzzle*. Aldershot: Ashgate.

Acknowledgments

We would like to thank all the editors and staff at MIT Press for their infinite patience in the development of this volume, and their editorial efforts which made this volume a reality. Specifically we would like to thank Katherine Almeida, Susan Clark, Ellen Faran, Philip Laughlin, Marc Lowenthal, Gita Manaktala, Thomas Stone, and other staff with whom we did not have direct communications. We also thank two anonymous reviewers for their insightful comments which helped shape the final versions of the chapters and volume. De-Laine Cyrene and Cat Hobaiter provided their invaluable skills in proofreading, correction, and indexing. And finally we would like to thank the contributors who made this volume possible.

Introduction

Liliana Albertazzi, Gert J. van Tonder, and Dhanraj Vishwanath

The Idea

Even the simplest reflex action of a primitive organism, one that is able to mechanically "sense" a state and react to it, appears to involve some communication of information. The informational transaction in human perception, on the other hand, appears to be far more complex. It is not so much that we merely react to information, but we "see" it, and see "meaning" in it. We don't "react" to a sensory input so much as we react to the meaning of the information before us. What theory of information and communication best captures this?

The default assumption in various fields, including perception, has been the classical theory of information codified in Shannon and Weaver (1949); a theory that has been very effective in the construction of engineered communication systems that regulate the transmission of signals from source to target. Under this conception, the informational transaction operates in a closed domain where meaning is relegated to a locus outside the communicative process. In other words, the communicative act does not create meaning but merely transposes "tokens" whose semantic relevance is external to the communicative machinery. It is a concept that privileges metric quantities, follows the unidirectional parameters of stimulus–reaction, and is most effectively expressed in statistical and logical analyses.

However, in recent years, there has been increasing consensus that phenomena belonging to open systems, such as biological, psychological, social, and artistic ones, remain excluded and/or difficult to analyze in terms of this concept of information. Such phenomena are not easily computed and exhibit a sort of hypercomplexity characterized by predictive structures, internal semantics, and adaptability to surroundings. This problem has become particularly evident in attempts to model human perceptual and cognitive structure and capacities. Despite an awareness of the problem, both historically and beyond the artificial intelligence (AI) revolution, no general theory or approach has been put forward to supplant the essentially Galilean paradigm underlying Shannon's theory of information. In other words, no satisfying semantic theory of information exists; one that can capture the complex internal semantic structure underlying perception, natural language, cognition, and other aspects such as aesthetics. Among the key issues to be considered for such a theory are the distinctions between the "data-driven" and "concept-driven" nature of information processing, the role and nature of the "phases" of mental processing, and, critically, whether the construction of the world goes "from the outside to the inside" or vice versa (Albertazzi, 2001c; Hoffman, 2008a, 2008b).

Many researchers in perception have voiced the need for new conceptualizations and computational frameworks for analyzing mental processes. Yet there have been no systematic attempts to bring together researchers across a diverse research spectrum who share these concerns.

This book puts forward ideas toward the development of a semantic theory of information in the domain of perception, tackling specifically the ontological and epistemological issues of theories of visual perception. The aims are to generate a forum to highlight the challenges facing traditional information-theoretic approaches in perceptual sciences, as well as sketch out potential avenues for new synthesis.

The Brentanian Legacy

The volume's underlying theme follows the psychological and philosophical lineage exemplified by Brentano, Mach, Hering, Husserl, and the Gestalt school, a mode of discourse and analysis mostly neglected after the dramatic events connected with the Second World War. This lineage has historically stood in distinction to the more empiricist and behaviorist tradition exemplified by Wundt, Fechner, Helmholtz, Russell, Skinner, and, more recently, Gibson, Marr, and Dennett. The difference between the two approaches to psychology, exemplified originally by Wundt and Brentano, has been vividly described by Tichener (1929):

The year 1874 saw the publication of two books which, as the events have shown, were of first rate importance for the development of modern psychology. Their authors, already in the full maturity of life, were men of settled reputation, fired as investigators with the zeal of research, endowed as teachers with a quite exceptional power to influence the younger minds, ready as polemicists to cross swords with a Zeller or a Helmholtz. Yet one would look in vain for any sign of closer intellectual kinship between them; hardly, indeed, one could find a greater divergence either of tendency or of training. Psychology, seeing how much their work and example have done to assure her place among the sciences, may gladly confess her debt to both. The student of psychology, though his personal indebtedness may be also twofold, must still make his choice for the one or the other. There is no middle way between Brentano and Wundt. (p. 80)

Both traditions, quite markedly, shared a common abiding interest in psychophysics, although one group was most interested in its external side (stimulus-sensory outcome), whereas the other was focused on its internal side (physiological elaboration of the stimulus-percept) (Albertazzi, 2005). In fact, although the term "psychophysics" can only be properly applied to inquiry conducted after the publication of Fechner's *Elemente der Psychophysik* in 1860, the term also covers the work by Herbart, Müller, Lotze, Mach, Hering, and Helmholtz (Albertazzi, 2001c). A critical feature of this historical work is that it interweaves science, ontology, and phenomenological description (Albertazzi, 2001a).

Since Müller, the psychophysical account of the relationship between *interior* and *exterior* in perceptual representation has assumed that perceptual *determinations* manifest features of their underlying somatic processes; such an idea has, under various guises, been understood as interaction or parallelism.

After Fechner, psychophysics was distinguished by two main parameters: (i) the attempt to make *mathematical measurement* of psychic phenomena, and (ii) the assumption of *physics* as the underlying model so that the psychophysical correlates reflected spatial relations in a system of Cartesian coordinates, or psychological magnitudes reflected (under some transformation) physical magnitudes. In his criticism of Fechner's law, however, Brentano (1995a) had already noticed a weak point of psychophysics, for example, with respect to the idea of the psychological unit of the just noticeable difference. Brentano questioned the validity of assuming the psychological equivalence of just noticeable differences at different levels of stimulation, suggesting that:

In reality, it is by no means self-evident that each barely noticeable increase in sensation is *equal*, but only that it is *equally noticeable* . . . the quantitative relationship between equally noticeable increases in sensation remains to be examined. (pp. 67–68)

The approaches of Brentano, Mach, Stumpf, Ehrenfels, Meinong, and Husserl highlighted important phenomenological/ontological distinctions, particularly with regard to how unitary phenomenal objects are not reducible to mere sensory phenomena, for example, in the identification of complex acoustic patterns such as a chord (a distinction also recognized by Helmholtz). Moreover, as soon as such phenomenological objects appear, they become subject to intervening cognitive integrations and intellectual constructions turning them into what Meinong referred to as "higher order objects" (see Albertazzi, 2001a).

Perception as an Intentional Act

In recent decades, the ideas and tradition that started from Brentano's immanent realism has often fallen victim to an unjust and reductive form of mentalism within the cognitive sciences and, particularly, philosophy of mind. What is usually obscured by this widespread criticism is that this tradition has never been mentalistic as its critics claim, a point raised previously by others (Lorenz, 1976; Uexküll, 1982; Weizsäcker, 1968). In fact, the Brentanian legacy has been instrumental in putting forward a pioneering and sophisticated *embedded theory of perception and meaning* based on both classical psychophysics and a theory of qualitative forms. These pioneering theses, which constituted the conceptual nucleus of a semantic theory of information, can be summarized in the words of Köhler (1913), recalling Brentano's idea:

The immediately present perceptual datum is acknowledged as such and is described as exactly and as appropriately as possible . . . the endeavor is no longer to obtain an understanding of the perceptions from the sensations, but to obtain an understanding of sensations from perceptions. (p. 136)

The most concrete example of such a considered approach to perception that has now been largely verified by modern science was conducted several decades before the previously mentioned quote. Hering's (1920/1964) theory of light perception, and specifically the opponent theory of color, went against the dominant physicalist trichromacy theory of Young, Maxwell, and Helmholtz. It was based primarily on a careful descriptive analysis of phenomenal aspects of color perception, asking questions such as why yellow appears to be as phenomenally unique a hue as red or green. Despite the decades-long resistance to Hering's idea, both psychophysical and neurophysiological work eventually vindicated the central aspects of what came to be developed as the opponent process theory of color (de Valois et al., 1966; Hurvich and Jameson, 1957).

Perhaps the most crucial idea that came out of the Brentano school, and the one that has been progressively obscured (despite its subsequent development and assimilation within Gestalt theory) is that of the *act* of intentional reference; that is, that the structure of a process of seeing, thinking, judging, and so on is that of a *dynamic whole endowed with parts* in which the parts are nonindependent items, and that this act can give rise to relatively different outputs based on *subjective completions* (Brentano, 1995b; Ehrenfels, 1890; Wertheimer, 1923). In other words, the referents of the phenomenal domain are not located in the external world but are the subjective objects produced by the intentional act of perceiving. All the information that we receive from the environment surrounding us is therefore subjectively integrated (Kanizsa, 1991), and it is characterized by secondary, tertiary, expressive, and dispositional properties (Albertazzi, chapter 11, this volume), which must be explicable within any comprehensive theory of information underlying perception.

The intentional aspect of perception is vividly demonstrated in figure I.1. These examples demonstrate—in addition to the subjective role of the observer—that information content does not inhere to the external stimulus but to the internal perceptual presentation (e.g., seeing the rows of dots [lower left] as grouped in a particular way entails information that is not given in the stimulus set; similarly with the "pointing" in the upper right image). Unfortunately, in contemporary scientific analysis, many of these effects have been taken as demonstrating the automatic, neural application of ecological "rules" that reflect the objective state of the external environment or observer-environment contingencies, rather than the more fundamental point

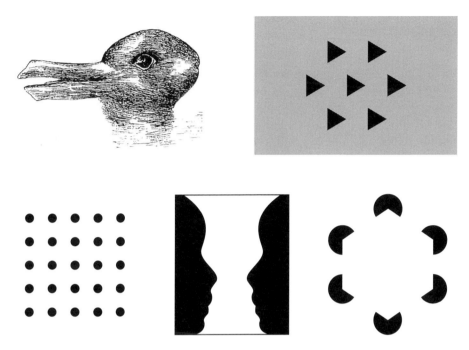

Figure I.1

Examples of multistable images where the perceived form and semantics are altered dramatically, both as a function intrinsic subjective perceptual processes and the perceptual effort of the observer. The top left image can perceptually alternate between either a "hare" or a "duck" (after Jastrow); in the top right image (after Attneave), depending on which vertex of an individual triangle is attended to, the entire configuration of triangles "points" in the direction of that vertex. In the bottom left image (a variant on the classic example by Wertheimer), the array of dots are naturally perceived to form vertical or horizontal rows, although the perceiver can perceptually "group" dots into diagonals, large or small squares. In the classic Rubin face-vase illusion, the viewer is able to perceptual alternate between the percept of face silhouettes or a vase (which can sometimes even appear volumetric). The bottom right image is a variant on the classic Kanizsa triangle illusion, where, depending on the observer, a two-dimensional (hexagon) or three-dimensional (cube) illusory figure is perceived (by van Tonder and Ohtani, 2008).

regarding subjective information content that they evince. In such an analysis, these "rules" are then used to "recover" the structure of the external world (see Vishwanath, 2005).

From the experimental point of view, the idea of the intentional act emphasizes that attention should focus on *seeing* (the visual operation) and not only on what is *seen* (the product); moreover, the latter should not be mistakenly understood as a resultant image or picture. In other words, attention should focus on the very act of referring (Albertazzi, 2003b), defined by Koenderink and van Doorn (2003) as "optically guided potential behavior." At issue is the intrinsic dynamism of perception, which does not consist of a defined, identifiable "mental state," except by abstraction. Consequently, as a complex whole, perception in its actual unfolding cannot simply be analyzed in terms of fixed immutable properties of an external reality. Rather, it must be done in terms of its true referents, which are the subjective operations and transitory objects produced by those operations. These complex operations cannot be analyzed solely on the basis of stimulus-defined "independent features," as in Marr's computational theory of vision (Marr, 1982), or in terms of the behaviorist's stimulus–response sets.

Intentionality and Presentation versus "Action" and Direct Perception
Some recent approaches to perception seem on first reading to be sympathetic to Brentanian ideas of the *act* of intentional reference, for example, Gibson's direct perception and that of the "enactive" approach to perception (Noë, 2004; O'Regan and Noë, 2001)[1]. The main reason that this mindset appears to have arisen is that the Gibsonian and enactive approaches emphasize the "action" of the observer in the construction of perceptual content (e.g., self-motion, eye movements, active exploration, etc.). Both of these approaches arise from a dissatisfaction with the static and unmotivated "representational" aspect of constructivist theories of perception (e.g., Marr, 1982) and seek instead to expose the linkage between perception and the ecological/functional aspects of the sensory field. Both approaches have been influenced by thinking originating in the Brentano School, including Gestalt Theory (Gibson) and the philosophy of Husserl (enactive theories). But in contradistinction with these original influences, both of these newer approaches implicitly hew to an empiricist-behaviorist epistemology, with the assumption of an objective information-laden reality that "makes itself available" (Noë, 2004) through the action of the observer, with the observer encoding those aspects that are of ecological relevance. Both do appear, on first reading, to avoid some of the ontological pitfalls of inferential approaches; the enactive approach also finds some sympathy in the Brentanian view insofar as mental states are considered *content-full*. Both approaches can be powerful methodological tools in behavioral and neurophysiological investigation. However, there are crucial differences.

The main differences are highlighted in the mistaken understanding of Brentano's "act" as a transaction between the mind and the external world. This view is actually more aptly applied to Gibsonian and enactive approaches, in the sense that the crucial aspect of perception in these models is that it is determined by "what we do" or that perception is something "we act out" (Noë, 2004). The predominant implication of "action" here is not in the sense of the *internal* intentional act of Brentano, but rather action as a *physical thing* conducted in the external physical world (e.g., movement, sensory exploration, etc.). In such models, this physical action exposes the contingencies between the observer's functional state/needs and the information-rich external world, allowing it to capture those aspects that are ecologically relevant. The stumbling block here becomes the same one afflicting inferential approaches. Both assume the existence of objective information external to observer, sampled by the observer, who then calibrates to it in functionally relevant ways (Vishwanath, 2005). This reliance on sensorimotor contingencies for the construction of mental content inevitably reduces such theories to a naïve realist epistemology. "Representations" of the external world are replaced here by a sort of catalogue or script of possible contingencies in interacting with the world, encoding "the way sensory stimulation varies as you move" (Noë, 2004). These sorts of approaches become difficult to evaluate because they fail to be clear on their assumptions regarding the nature of informational content and their underlying epistemology. For example, in the statement "perceptual experience acquires content as a result of sensorimotor knowledge" (Noë, 2004, p. 9), it is difficult to disentangle what is the implied distinction between "content" and "knowledge" and which should come first.

Ultimately, it does not seem necessary to invoke sensorimotor contingencies—in the manner suggested by these theories—in order to incorporate the functional (motor) relevance of perception. For example, in the visual domain, the general linkage between motor relevance and visual perception is captured by the phrase "potential behavior" (Koenderink, chapter 1, this volume), computationally more precisely in proposals where *shape* is seen as a causally nested machine of successively more symmetric states (Leyton, 1992), or where a perceptual *surface* can be considered, to a first approximation, as a *motor plan* (Vishwanath, chapter 7, this volume). None of these notions is inconsistent with sensorimotor contingencies playing a role in the *calibration* of the underlying perceptual encoding, but more important, they do not need to rely on some objective definition of structure external to perception.

Perception in Brentanian terms is neither the re-presentation of an objective external reality (the inferential approach) nor is it simply a direct or indirect resonance of such a reality due to action (Gibsonian and enactive approaches). Rather, perception is the *presentation* of a unitary occurring event of which the perceiver's subjective structure is a nonindependent part. *Content* inheres to this internal presentation, which is a subjective act of the observer, and not to an external reality or a sensorimotor calibration to that reality. The central idea in Brentano's work, that of *perception as presentation*[2], has been entirely missing from cognitive science and has only recently been reintroduced into contemporary dialogue (Albertazzi, 1998), as have efforts to evaluate and further develop the broader ideas of the Brentano school in the context of contemporary cognitive science (perception, language, and beyond) (Albertazzi, 2000, 2001a, 2002a, 2006a, 2006c, 2008b).

In starting out as a general framework, this idea of perception as a unitary occurring event with its own internal spatiotemporal "objects of reference" allows for a proper analysis of the content of perception in terms of higher and lower order terms, qualitative and quantitative aspects, and intermodal and amodal aspects. This is in distinction to most contemporary approaches that start with highly constricted domains such as sensorimotor contingencies (e.g., Gibson, enactive perception) and then try to address the totality of perceptual experience from that perspective.

The classical conception of information theory is wholly unsuitable as a conceptual framework and instrument with which to model the previously mentioned aspects. The characterization of the visual field in terms of optics is, in fact, irreducible to either the physiological or perceptual components, in that the latter have little to do with the optics of the eye and with computational primitives understood in the sense of cues and pictures (Mausfeld, 2002; Vishwanath, 2005). Perceptions are not computed from cues; rather, the intentional acts of the perceiver enable the generation of perceptions in terms of what appear as cues and/or subjective choices (Albertazzi, 2005; Brentano, 1995a; Koenderink, chapter 1, this volume). Perception is, therefore, the product of anticipatory structures that are, to a large extent, subjective or subjectively integrated rather than simply a result of inference, probabilistic or otherwise. This is because, strictly speaking, bodies or physical objects do not exist in the visual field, but rather are qualitative appearances that often do not have corresponding stimuli (Albertazzi, 2008a). More than cues, therefore, acting in the deployment of visual perception, are visual operations directed at perceptual entities and *qualities* of various kinds. The Brentanian legacy provides a clearer framework to address this aspect that is central to perceptual experience: *quality*; and provides a more meaningful way to link it to what has essentially been the sole emphasis of contemporary approaches to perception: *quantitative judgment*.

Quantity and Quality

In perceptual experience, the fact that quality is not reducible to quantity is a matter of common sense. The recognition of the problem is important because almost nothing of phenomenal perception as such is "quantitative" in nature. We perceive a natural scene in terms of sky, roads, trees, passers-by, and so on; whose components are color, shape, brightness, shade, and qualities of different type—not as terms in a description of the "stimuli"—but as genuine psychological things. The color of the lawn, a house, or clothes that we perceive does not reside in corresponding wavelengths. Similarly, perceived brightness is a phenomenon much more complex than the physical luminance of surfaces (Gilchrist, 2002, 2006; Hering, 1920/1964; Katz ,1935; Koffka, 1935).

Current perceptual science, however, even when it deals with qualitative aspects of experience, almost exclusively reasons in quantitative terms (i.e., in terms of primary properties or stimuli). Perceptual quality is typically considered to be an outcome of so-called top-down influences, cognition being the domain typically considered to be the only *functionally relevant* qualitative components of mental states. However, *perceptual qualities* in the Brentanian sense are those that are, in principle, independent of so-called top-down or cognitive modifications due to the geographical, cultural, linguistic, or social environment; to emotional and aesthetic phenomena; or to subjective preferences. Instead they are the very content-bearing referents of perception.

Two important achievements of the Brentanian approach to perception concern, first, a qualitative theory of perception, specifically the qualitative nature of the correlate of perceptual operations, and, second, the description of the nature of visual space in terms of location and quality (Albertazzi, 2006b; Brentano, 1995b).

More generally, in the Brentanian approach, the structure of perceptual events exhibits spatial, temporal, and qualitative characteristics entirely dissimilar from physical properties. Space, time, and the causes of this type of information have correlates in the physical world, but they are not reducible to them because the "units of representation," like the parts of visual space or moments of time experiences, are profoundly different. Consider, for example, the space of visual phenomena (that of location, distance, and direction). Psychophysically, it is highly anisotropic and appears to comprise a plurality of nested spaces with different quantitative and qualitative characteristics, for example, personal space, action space, and vista space (Albertazzi, 2002b, 2006c; Botvinick and Cohen, 1998; Cutting and Vishton, 1995; Làvadas, 2002; Vishwanath, chapter 7, this volume). Consider the experience of duration, which has characteristics entirely irreducible to the metric partition of external time (Benussi, 1907, 1909, 1913; Fraisse, 1964, 1974; Libet, 1982; Libet et al., 1979; Michon, 1978; Pöppel, 1994; Vicario, 1999). Consider the perception of causality, which introduces qualitative saliencies and functional relations among the components that are entirely nonexistent at the physical level (Leyton, 1992, 2001; Michotte et al., 1962; Piaget, 1954/2004). At the perceptual level, in fact, it is difficult to decide whether an event is the cause of, or only the condition for, another event or whether part of an event set physically in the future does not actually determine its occurrence—as happens in the case of stroboscopic movement or the movements of intentional causality (Kanizsa and Vicario, 1968; Michotte et al., 1962). In the case of stroboscopic movement, we in fact perceive the beginning of the movement of a spot of light *before* the perception of the apparent cause of the movement, namely, the second spot of light (Vicario, 1999).

In other words, the object that is attributed the cause of the motion in stimulus terms is perceived *after* the initial perception of the motion. Although neural explanations in terms of the Reichard detector model do provide us with an understanding of how we can establish correlation between physical flux (stimulus) and neural identification of motion (change in position), there is still much to be explained computationally at the perceptual level (i.e., the level of the actual presentation of objects and motion).

That perceptual qualities and quantities are not easily identifiable with those of physics (i.e., with the stimuli) is evidenced by a large number of examples, and especially by the science of color and lightness perception. Consider, for example, the phenomena of chromatic assimilation already described by Fuchs (1923) and Bezold (1874) (see figure I.2, plate 1, top and bottom left panels). At the perceptive level, the

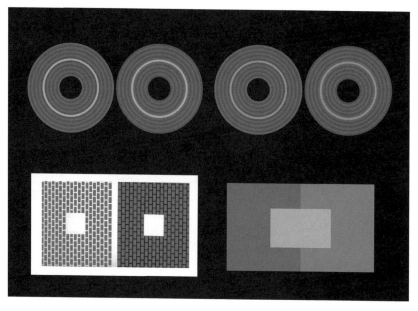

Figure I.2 (plate 1)

Top: The perceived color of the rings in the left pair appear different (pink and orange) as do the rings in the right pair (blue and green) but in each pair the physical reflectance of the rings is identical. The patterned background of purple and lime-green circles causes the illusion (Monnier and Shevell, 2003; images and permission courtesy of P. Monnier). Bottom left: Given a grid of interlaced red and black stripes, and a grid of red and white stripes, the red perceived is very different though physically identical in both cases. Bottom right: The proximal stimulus on the retina, consisting of four spatial regions, is given by light radiations specified in terms of intensity, wavelength, area, and time. Perceptually, what one sees is a transparent rectangle over two others, with the emergent property of a yellowish light spreading on the whole appearance; items that do not exist at the level of stimuli (Da Pos, 1989–1991; Metelli, 1941; see also Da Pos, Devigili, Giaggio, and Trevisan, 2007).

identity of a particular color's wavelength, in certain contexts, strictly speaking "no longer exists" because the stimuli have assumed the perceptive behavior of a related part in the general context of the phenomenal appearance as a whole, constituted by colored surfaces of different perceived lightness and opacity (Albertazzi, 2008a; Berg-ström, 2004; Da Pos, 2002; Da Pos and Albertazzi, 2010; Katz, 1935; Wertheimer, 1923). This is vividly exemplified in the bottom panels of figure I.2 (plate 1). These examples show the mereological (part-whole) relations and their interdependence in visual operations, another of Brentano's achievements (see Brentano, 1995b).

Moreover, in visual operations used to derive quantitative aspects of the perceptual presentation (such as tasks used to measure perceived slant, depth order, etc., in pictorial space.), Koenderink and van Doorn (2003) suggest that:

The act of measurement creates a novel state of affairs for the observer that yields a certain result, for instance, a number. Thus, different methods to measure it need not refer to the same [perceptual] property, at least not in principle. . . . The numbers you obtain should be labelled with the method by which they were obtained, for they are only operationally defined. (p. 261)

This aspect has been similarly expressed in the works of Köhler, Koffka, and Brunswik, who were influenced by Brentano and particularly by Stumpf's theory of *functions* (see Albertazzi, 2001c)[3].

Dispositional properties, in general, pertain to material qualities and the causal ascriptions (see Mausfeld, chapter 6, this volume); for example, how surfaces will appear under changes in their orientation and location, which haptic experiences will be elicited by them, and how they will behave under various kinds of interactions, both with an agent and other objects. Because material appearances are intrinsically transmodal in character and are also intimately embedded in internal causal analyses, traditional inferential approaches have been theoretically ill equipped to deal with them in an appropriate way.

Phenomena such as double representation, occlusion, illusory contours, apparent magnitudes, transparencies, mirror and object-like shadows, so-called subjective illusions, and so on are entirely ordinary perceptive phenomena. They gainsay both the idea of a science of perception "parasitic" on stimuli and a concept of perceptual "representation" as the processing of information already manifest at the physical level and subsequently and unidirectionally uncovered at the sensory and neuronal level (Mausfeld, 2003; Vishwanath, 2005).

A descriptive analysis brings with it the necessary recognition of the existence of an emergent qualitative level of reality. It also highlights the relative nonindependence of emergent reality from the stimuli of the physical world because of the role played by the observer and his representational system (Albertazzi, 2005; Koenderink and van Doorn, 2003). Thus, the first step consists of individuating the (so-called representational) primitives of qualitative perception, such as "surface," "dynamic structures of

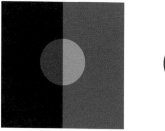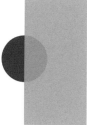

Figure I.3

The two discs are identical in physical luminance, but the perceived brightness and surface characteristics are different (image courtesy G. van Tonder).

an event," "ambient illumination," and so on; their free parameters, such as "color," "depth," "orientation," and so on; and their laws of organization. This approach to the primitives of perception, however, does not exclude at all their measurement in quantitative terms.

The understanding of perception in terms of qualities allows for a more concrete analysis of the linkage between higher order mental processes and perception; for example, the cross-modal phenomena expressed acutely in synaesthesia but more generally in linguistic communication and construction. Semantics in linguistic communication is often acknowledged as being rooted in perception, yet without a clear understanding and theory of the nature of perceptual qualities, making the meaningful linkages between language and perception remains a challenge.

The Stimulus Error and the Experience Error

From a *methodological* point of view, to develop a science of phenomenal qualities, one should avoid falling for mistakes such as the stimulus and experience errors.

The *stimulus error* consists of substituting the description of direct experience with the list of characteristics of the stimulus; in other words, what one "sees" with what one "knows" (Kanizsa, 1952; Schumann, 1904). Consider, for example, the phenomena of transparency analyzed by Metelli (1941) and revised by Da Pos (1989–1991), as in the following example (see figure I.2, color plate 1, lower right panel and figure I.3).

In perceptual situations such as motion determining color perception (Hoffman, 2003; Nijhawan, 1997) or transparency altering color, contour, and depth (Nakayama, Shimojo, and Ramachandran, 1990), Mausfeld (2003) observes that:

In many of these cases we do not know yet whether we are dealing with the problem of how the different free parameters of a *single* representational primitive are interlocked, or with the problem of how representational primitives of the same (or similar) type are interlocked. As a rough experimental diagnostic, one might conjecture that cases in which small changes in a relevant

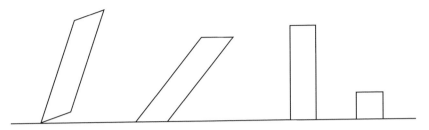

Figure I.4
Observers normally perceive the figure on the left as a tilted version of the parallelogram at "rest" with the base aligned with the supporting surface. The parallelogram at rest is in turn seen as a sheared version of the rectangle to its right. The rectangle is seen as stretched from the square. Importantly, the rectangle is never seen as an "de-sheared" parallelogram, and the square does not appear as a squashed rectangle Leyton (1992). Leyton has argued that the perception of shape reveals a nested, causal structure. For example, intrinsic to the percept of the titled parallelogram on the left is a visual understanding of its origin from a set of transformations on successively more asymmetric forms; transformations attributed to the causative action of a "second system." Thus, the symmetry states and the causal actions leading to the successively less symmetric states are simultaneously perceived (from right to left).

attribute of the input causes radical changes in other attributes indicate situations in which several representational primitives are involved. (p. 36)

Another example of the complexity of the internal representation of the stimuli in perception is given in the example of the tilted parallelepiped (Leyton, 1992), wherein one "sees" systematic causal ascriptions absent in a physical description of the stimulus (see figure I.4), and yet often we mistakenly describe the percept in terms of the same Euclidean geometry we use to describe the stimulus (Leyton, 1992).

The *experience error* operates in the opposite direction. It consists of attributing the characteristics of perceptual experience to the physical stimulus; in other words, as if the perceptual visual field (the experience) is what is affecting the retina (Koffka, 1935). This kind of error occurs when attributing components of visual behavior to the receptorial stimulation. For example, one might say that an "oriented line" is given in the stimulus, when both "orientation" and "line-ness" are, in actuality, psychological constructs. For example, one might say that a lamp emits green light when the lamp actually emits medium wavelength radiation: "green light" is a psychological construct, whereas medium wavelength radiation is a physical construct.

The Experience Error and Direct Perception
An important related issue concerns the relationship between the *direct* aspect of perception, in that we have perceptually presented before us a phenomenal visual field (alluded to by Gibson), and the *functional* aspect, which, as already mentioned,

concerns the subjective operation of the perceiver in generating the field. The two could be referred to as "external" and "internal" factors, as long as external is understood to denote the phenomenal field and not the stimuli or transcendent physical world (as is implied in Gibson's formulations). The understanding of an external reality is a cognitive configuration or categorization that transcends the perceptual operation.

The distinction between internal and external determinants is originally due to Benussi (see Albertazzi, 2001d). The lack of an understanding of this distinction, which concerns the concept of affordance (*Afforderungscharakter*), probably led Gibson to a more externalist view of the directness of perception. The *Afforderungscharakter* of the tertiary qualities also implied a specific analysis of subjective processing, as seen, for example, in Koffka (1935) and Metzger (1986). These observations led Arnheim (1980) to make the following criticism of the Gibsonian realist point of view:

> Is it not essential to distinguish the prerequisites for perception from perception itself? For example, gradients of texture, size, brightness, etc. supply, as Gibson and his disciples have shown, the data necessary to determine spatial distance and slant. But the information needed for distance and slant is one thing and the perceptual experience of depth itself is quite another. In order to explain why those data give rise to the experience of depth and slant, one must refer to principles inherent in perceptual functioning. (p. xii)

To adopt a descriptive method in perceptual science, from the very start (e.g., Hering, 1920/1964; Kanizsa, 1989; Koffka, 1935; Köhler, 1920; Metelli, 1974; Musatti, 1926), does not imply denying or avoiding quantitative methodologies or quantitative measurements in order to find descriptive laws governing the different phenomena. Rather, it suggests that before developing a mathematical model of observable data, one should develop an unbiased and detailed description of observables on which to ground the development of formal models suitable to this kind of complexity. In other words, a descriptive theory provides a preliminary taxonomy that needs to be explained on the basis of further experiments.

Moreover, descriptive and neuronal approaches to perception are not in mutual contradiction: For example, the subjective contour in amodal shapes is phenomenologically explained as a product of the structuring by the visual system that presents a triangle occluding the incomplete pattern in the stimulus. Neurophysiologically, instead, it is explained by ascribing the apparent contour to the neuronal activity in V2, which is usually activated by physically continuous lines (von der Heydt and Peterhans, 1989; Spillmann, 2009). Both are correlated analyses dependent on one another, but the phenomenological analysis is not reducible to the neuronal one as sometimes seems to be suggested by neuroscience. On the contrary, a descriptive theory of observable phenomena can be of great help for the development of neuroscience. Hering's opponent process theory, for example, based primarily on phenomenal analysis, has resulted in a framework for computational theories linking cone responses to ganglion cell responses (e.g., Conway, 2001). Kanizsa's analysis has provided an excellent basis for discovering a neurophysiological correlate of amodal contours (Baumgartner, von der Heydt, and Peterhans 1984; De Weerd, Desimone and Underleider, 1998; von der Heydt and Peterhans, 1989; Spillmann and Ehrenstein, 2004) while the Gestalt principle of figure/ground segregation has been critical in the neuronal analysis of transparency phenomena (Qiu and von der Heydt, 2007). Similarly, work on the perceptual significance of medial axis representations (Blum, 1967; Kovács and Julesz, 1994; Leyton, 1987, 1992; van Tonder, Lyons, and Ejima, 2002) suggests yet another avenue for neurophysiological investigation.

Information and Inference
The fundamental idea of the theory of perception as inference is that information is already wholly organized in the physical external environment. In other words, it is not the subjective perceptual completion of the observer that gives coherence to the various sensory elements but that sensory elements as "picked up" by the modalities are already endowed with a mutual and internal coherence of their own. Likewise, "affordances" are already given in the environment (Gibson, 1979), and they do not derive from the effect of the expressive qualities of the percept on the subject. As for visual objects, the classification made in traditional vision science refers primarily to already constituted external physical entities bounded by physical surfaces.

In particular, the basic claim of the inverse-optics approach is that an informationally impoverished *stimulus* (constituted by cues, features, measures, etc.) leads to an informationally rich *perceptual product* through some process of causal or inferential linkage (Hatfield, 2003; Marr, 1982; Rock, 1983). It is the nature of this causal linkage (the inference or inductive leap) that is considered to be the main explanandum for both computational and neurophysiological versions of inverse optics. But the essential incoherency of postulating an inferential or inductive process that *generates* information content was quite long ago pointed out in Hume's treatise. His argument pertains essentially to the informational distinction between the stimulus set used to make the inference and the perceptual product of that inference. Hume's argument correctly shows that such an informational distinction is eliminated by the very inferential process that defined it; an argument that has been validated in every possible computational rendering of "inference," whether in machine learning, AI approaches to visual perception, or probabilistic models. In all these cases, we inevitably end up with an inferential model plus some form of uniformity, regularity, or genericity assumptions that are encoded into the inferential apparatus as inductive biases, regularization, or Bayesian priors. In such inferential models of perception, the stimulus is then essentially a form of description of the perceptual presentation. The entire informational content becomes a set of metric values (Vishwanath, 2005), where there is no semantic distinction between those assigned to the stimulus and those assigned to the perceived visual field (Mausfeld, 2003). For example, depth, distance, and direction in perceptual space are all considered the same informational constructs as depth, distance, and direction in some objective external world. The result is that, even as we gain more and more sophisticated descriptions of the model, we gain little by way of understanding the complexity and richness of the actual perceptual presentation. This externalization of meaning outside the device (or observer) carries forth into the central tenets of modern analytic philosophy where content, conceptual signification, and verification are assessed in terms of *external physical reference* (see Albertazzi, 2005).

Within the inferential framework, the study of perception becomes an investigation into the *calibration* of measurement between the two domains (physical and psychological). We measure a psychological response to see how well it correlates with the corresponding physical measurements of the stimulus and then adjust our model to accommodate any deviations. This model of "calibration" is actually much more general than often appreciated, beginning with straightforward geometric calibration (space, object, surface perception) but extending naturally to the ultimate goal of perception in the inference framework: *object recognition*. Object recognition becomes the assessment of how well perceptual or cognitive judgments match a predefined taxonomy of the external world. Perceptual understanding becomes construed as "object recognition and categorization" in the same way that shape becomes a "calibration map", with perception remaining "neutral" in respect to *quality* (Vishwanath, 2005). Quality is then considered to be only a cognitive outcome arising from experience with the real world. The inverse-optics measurement-based model essentially derives from machine vision and first-generation robotics, which constitute precisely the domain where a machine's "perceptual" measures (instituted by the engineer) have no causal or informational distinction from measures used to describe the stimulus (formulated by the engineer) and where "meaning" is of no concern to device but only to the engineer. The efficacy of the device is essentially expressed in its calibration, whether it be in "reaching out" by the right amount (geometric calibration) or picking out, say, the "right" potato (object recognition), with the meaning and qualitative significance of "right-ness" defined external to the device.

Establishing the linkages between the different levels of explanation inherent in understanding the mind (stimulus measurement, perceptual judgment, neural correlate) are fairly straightforward in the inferential approach but limited in scope. Moving beyond such characterizations requires looking more carefully at the intrinsic aspects of perceptual presentation that can be computationally described (e.g., Leyton, 1992).

Perceptual Experience and Aesthetics

Finally, a reconfiguration of our approach to the study of perception has crucial implications for understanding what is usually considered in inferential approaches as higher order perceptual phenomena. Although the linkage between immediate perceptual experience and aesthetics has been a long analyzed scientific question, this question will require moving beyond simplistic models of perception, such as inference, in order to bear fruition. It will no doubt require a theory of perception that sees qualitative phenomena and the subjective operations of the observer as foundational. The last two chapters of the volume, in describing aspects of aesthetic production and experience from an art historical and design viewpoint reflect this.

Summary of Chapters

The chapters in this book argue, and lay out proposals, not so much for a search of a new model of the "causal linkage" between stimulus and mental states (as is the goal of inferential models) but rather for a clearer and more coherent effort to understand the underlying information content of perceptual presentation (and, more generally, mental states)—consistent with internal or intentional reference—which, in turn, will lead to richer and more plausible constructs for psychophysical, computational, and neural investigation. As Brentano (1995a) maintained:

Psychological reflections inform us only that there are causes, unknown in themselves, which influence the rise of subsequent psychic phenomena, as well as they are in themselves unknown effects of previous psychic phenomena. In either case psychological reflection can prove in isolated instances *that* they exist; but it can never in any way give us knowledge of *what* they are. (pp. 56–60)

The contributors in this volume express, explicitly or implicitly, tenets of a descriptive theory (Brentano, 1995b) in the different fields involved in the theme, outlining the relationships among stimuli, neuronal elaboration, and visual experience. Several chapters expose the challenges faced in establishing coherent relations among these different levels of elaboration. Some prompt further questions, for example, on how to present a precise and detailed descriptive theory of qualities as the basis for an ontology of natural perception without reducing them to neural correlates or stimulus descriptions. Several chapters clarify the necessity to formulate a new quantitative method for measurement of visual appearances, as well as the visual operations that form the basis of perception and phenomenal experience. These topics, collectively evident in the contributions, will constitute the next challenge in a theory of perception.

Koenderink (chapter 1, this volume), makes an indispensable and insightful contribution to the volume by proposing the essentials of a perception-centric theory of vision. The chapter provides an essential critique of the current mainstream theoretical approaches in vision science and the contradictions internal to it, clarifying the usage of information-theoretic terminology (e.g., information, meaning, feature, cue, clue, etc.). The remaining chapters are divided into four thematic parts: *Time and Dynamics*; *Colour, Shape, and Space*; *Language and Perception*; and *Perception in Art, Design, and Computation*.

Time and Dynamics

Ilona Kovács (chapter 2, this volume) explores a specific aspect of the stimulus-percept problem: the inherent puzzle of how discrete receptorial stimulation could give rise to stable coherent percepts. She uses as an analogy the problem of the construction of Brunelleschi's dome to demonstrate the need for an organizational framework at early stages of visual processing. The chapter demonstrates how any theory that proposes a constructive bottom-up strategy bumps into the problem of the inevitable accumulation of spatial errors in neural coding. The chapter suggests an inherent perceptual construct such as medial axis as providing the framework that counteracts the accumulation of error.

Timothy L. Hubbard (chapter 3, this volume) examines the difference between the nature of what is directly given in perceptual experience in contrast to what is descriptively available in the stimulus. The chapter argues that visual dynamics are inherently part of the structural characteristics of the perceptual experience produced through perceptual grouping. Instead of a *Prägnanz* of static objects, the chapter argues how dynamics, such as gravity, attraction, repulsion, inertia, and momentum, which capture active object transformations in the environment, are inherent parts of the percept and need to be considered in any experiential theory of perception.

Gert J. van Tonder (chapter 4, this volume) exposes the fundamental flaw involved in linking objective stimulation and perceptual experience by analyzing optical perceptual effects that cannot be explained on the basis of the stimulation alone. Using both empirical evidence and theoretical arguments, he presents a case against the common idea that the retina is a highly constrained receptive stage in a modular visual hierarchy, demonstrating that visual experience and information content are already embodied in the peculiar way that the stimulus flux is processed and encoded as early as the retina. This leads to a visual *Abtastung* (exploring shape through touch) that constitutes enriched information at the earliest stages of the visual system.

Shinsuke Shimojo (chapter 5, this volume) presents a large selection of visual phenomena that are difficult to assess solely on the basis of stimulation, demonstrating the conceptual difficultly, but necessity, in distinguishing between receptorial stimulation and visual behaviors. The examination of the neural correlates underlying them further expresses the inherent challenges in providing a coherent theory linking perceptual states, stimulus, and neural processing.

Color, Shape, and Space

Rainer Mausfeld (chapter 6, this volume) explores the fundamental aspects of material qualities. He suggests that dispositional properties, in general, pertain to material qualities and the causal ascriptions; for example, how surfaces will appear under changes in their orientation and location, which haptic experiences will be elicited by them, and how they will behave under various kinds of interactions, with both an agent and other objects. Because material appearances are intrinsically transmodal in character and also intimately embedded in internal causal analyses, the chapter explains how traditional inferential approaches have been theoretically ill equipped to deal with them in an appropriate way due to a sort of ontological self-agnosia.

Dhanraj Vishwanath (chapter 7, this volume), in examining surface and depth perception in pictures and real scenes, suggests a linkage between perceptual objects and qualities and the quantification of psychophysical judgments. He suggests that a linkage is possible as long as one is clear about epistemological and ontological assumptions. The chapter makes proposals regarding what constitutes a "perceptual surface," how the perception of three-dimensional structure may involve two distinct modes, and how such descriptions allow for a clearer understanding of quantitative results. The author proposes that, although the reliability of psychophysical judgments in depth perception is typically considered a purely *quantitative* construct, it is actually *qualitatively* expressed, giving rise to our vivid sense of immersion and reality.

Ohad Ben Shahar and Steven W. Zucker (chapter 8, this volume) aim to computationally define a fundamental aspect of perceptual organization: *continuity*. In traditional inferential approaches, continuity has been applied in a sort of "ends" analysis, in the sense that continuity (putatively given in the external world) is only relevant once the image has been segmented consistently. This chapter seeks to develop the idea of continuity in more intrinsic terms by linking it to the covariance of continuity among various aspects of the visual field, such as color and shading. The authors express these ideas in a biologically plausible computational framework, suggesting that linkages among different the levels of description (perceptual experience, computation, and neural organization) may be possible.

Baingio Pinna's (chapter 9, this volume) contribution on Petter's figures concerns all the conditions where a black homogenous irregular pattern is perceived as made up of independent surfaces separated in depth and delineated by illusory contours in the area of apparent intersection and stratification. Pinna suggests that Petter's rule is a contour formation rule due to global boundary contour interactions determining the depth organization of the visual components. This rule derives from the formation of two different kinds of contours, modal and amodal, linked together by the dynamics of the filling in of contour gaps.

Language and Perception

In their chapter, Baingio Pinna and Liliana Albertazzi (chapter 10, this volume) suggest that there is no perception without *three* forms of organization: forms of grouping, forms of shape, and forms of meaning. Through the method of experimental phenomenology, they suggest a continuum among the three, showing how perceptual meaning is an emergent result spontaneously conveyed by vision. Finally, they argue that the interplay among the three forms of organizations is the basic component of the primitive language of vision, which lays the foundations of natural language.

Liliana Albertazzi (chapter 11, this volume) proposes that true or creative metaphors are founded on structures of phenomenal perception and involve the construction of new perceptual entities. The chapter shows how a metaphorical object evokes constituent *patterns* inherent in the source domains of the metaphor but that are then subjected to a transformation and fusion in real time, giving rise to new perceptual entities. Such entities exhibit the properties of Gestalten and behave according to the laws of figural organization. Moreover, they are an exact description of some aspect of reality. The chapter explains how metaphors evidentiate aspects of the originary structure of information and therefore are crucial to understanding mental content most broadly construed.

Perception in Art, Design, and Computation

Amy Ione (chapter 12, this volume) discusses Monet's constructs of space on canvas, which is far from an accurate physical spatial layout in natural perspective. Instead of recording external space in a physical framework, the paintings seem to suit the *act* of perceptually creating space from an internal conception outward, and hence, the paintings become a rich source of perceptual meaning about the qualitative and quantitative aspects in the depicted spaces.

Ernest Edmonds (chapter 13, this volume) focuses on abstract generative art, discussing key processes through which these predominantly visual works become meaningful. Especially of interest are the boundaries between unintelligible complexity and predictable responsiveness that a viewer experiences in an art installation. At this threshold, established perception is challenged and needs to become particularly creative to invent new meaning. The chapter argues that "becoming information" at this boundary is what underlies the visual appeal of some of the most successful generative art.

Notes

1. The term "enactive" originates in earlier work by Maturana and Varela (1987), whose ideas finds more sympathy in the Brentanian approach presented here. In their work "enactivism" is more an internal that an external construct; in contrast to the more recent work that has adopted this term.

2. The term *Vorstellung* in German is connected to inner, imaginative presentations vs. external representations or *Darstellungen*. *Vorstellung* as mental presentation is a term which assumed increasingly psychological connotations from Leibniz to Tetens. In Brentano 1874, *Vorstellungen* or psychic phenomena are not contents or ideas, but *acts*.

3. Wertheimer, Koffka, Köhler, von Allesch, Lewin and Gelb were among Stumpf's close collaborators. Brunswik also acknowledges his debt to Brentano, though his position was more constructivist in flavor (see Albertazzi 2001b).

References

Albertazzi, L. ed. 1998. *Shapes of Form. From Gestalt Psychology to Phenomenology, Ontology and Mathematics*. Dordrecht: Kluwer.

Albertazzi, L. ed. 2000. *Meaning and Cognition: A Multidisciplinary Approach*. Amsterdam: Benjamins Publishing Company.

Albertazzi, L. ed. 2001a. *The Dawn of Cognitive Science. Early European Contributors*. Dordrecht: Kluwer.

Albertazzi, L. 2001b. "Back to the Origins." In *Early European Contributors to Cognitive Science 1870–1930*, edited by L. Albertazzi. Dordrecht: Kluwer. 1–27.

Albertazzi, L. 2001c. "Presentational Primitives: Parts, Wholes and Psychophysics." In *The Dawn of Cognitive Science. Early European Contributors*, edited by L. Albertazzi. Dordrecht: Kluwer. 29–60.

Albertazzi, L. 2001d. "Vittorio Benussi." In *The School of Alexius Meinong*, edited by L. Albertazzi, Dale Jacquette, and Roberto Poli. Asghate: Aldershot. 95–133.

Albertazzi, L. ed. 2002a. *Unfolding Perceptual Continua*. Amsterdam: Benjamins Publishing Company.

Albertazzi, L. 2002b. "Towards a Neo-Aristotelian Theory of Continua: Elements of an Empirical Geometry." In *Unfolding Perceptual Continua, Unfolding Perceptual Continua*, edited by L. Albertazzi. Amsterdam: Benjamins Publishing Company. 29–79.

Albertazzi, L. ed. 2003a. "The Legacy of Gaetano Kanizsa in Cognitive Science." *Axiomathes* 13 (3–4).

Albertazzi, L. 2003b. "From Kanizsa Back to Benussi: Varieties of Intentional Reference." *Axiomathes* 13 (3–4): 239–259.

Albertazzi, L. 2005. *Immanent Realism. Introduction to Brentano*. Berlin, New York: Springer.

Albertazzi, L. 2006a. "Das rein Figurale." (Pure figuration) *Gestalt Theory* 28 (1/2): 123–151.

Albertazzi, L. ed. 2006b. *Visual Thought. The Depictive Space of Perception*. Amsterdam: Benjamins Publishing Company.

Albertazzi, L. 2006c. "Introduction to Visual Spaces." In *Visual Thought. The Depictive Space of Perception*, edited by L. Albertazzi. Amsterdam: Benjamins Publishing Company. 3–34.

Albertazzi, L. 2008a. "The Ontology of Perception." In *TAO-Theory and Applications of Ontology:* Vol. 1. Philosophical Perspectives, edited by Roberto Poli and Johanna Seibt. Berlin, New York: Springer.

Albertazzi, L. 2008b. "The Perceptual Whole." In *Handbook of Mereology*, edited by Hans Burkhardt, Johanna Seibt, and Guido Imaguire. Munich: Philosophia Verlag.

Arnheim, R. 1980. "Foreword." In *The Perception of Pictures: Vol. 2. Dürer Devices: Beyond the Projective Models of Pictures*, edited by M. A. Hagen. New York: Academic Press.

Baumgartner, G., von der Heydt, R., and Peterhans, E. 1984. "Anomalous Contours: A Tool of Studying the Neurophysiology of Vision." *Experimental Brain Research* (Suppl.) 9: 413–419.

Benussi, V. 1907. "Zur experimentelle Analyse des Zeitvergleichs." (On the Experimental Analysis of Comparisons of Temporal Durations). *Archiv für die gesamte Psychologie* 9: 572–579.

Benussi, V. 1909. "Über 'Aufmerksamkeitsrichtung' beim Raum- und Zeitvergleich." (On the "Direction of Attention" in the Comparison of Spatial Extensions and Temporal Durations). *Zeitschrift für Psychologie* 51: 73–107.

Benussi, V. 1913. *Psychologie der Zeitauffassung.* (Psychology of Time Apprehension) Heidelberg: Winter.

Bergström, S. S. 2004. "The Ambegujas Phenomenon and Colour Constancy." *Perception* 33: 831–835.

Bezold, W. von. 1874. *Die Farbenlehre in Hinblick auf Kunst und Kunstgewerbe.* (The Theory of Colour from the Viewpoint of Art and Art Works) Braunschweig.

Blum, H. 1967. "A Transformation for Extracting New Descriptors of Shape." In *Models for the Perception of Speech and Visual Form*, edited by W. Whaten-Dunn. Cambridge, MA: MIT Press. 362–380.

Botvinick, M., and Cohen, J. 1998. "Rubber Hands 'Feel' Touch That the Eyes See." *Nature* 391: 756.

Brentano, F. 1995a. *Psychology from Empirical Standpoint*, edited by L. McAlister. London: Routledge.

Brentano, F. 1995b. *Descriptive Psychology*, edited by B. Müller. London: Routledge.

Conway, B. R. 2001. "Spatial Structure of Cone Inputs to Color Cells in Alert Macaque Primary Visual Cortex (V-1)." *Journal of Neuroscience* 21(8): 2768–2783.

Cutting, J. E., and Vishton, P. M. 1995. "Perceiving Layout and Knowing: The Integration, Relative Potency, and Contextual Use of Different Information About Depth." In *Handbook of Perceptual Cognition: Perception and Space Motion*, Vol. V, edited by W. Epstein and S. Rogers. New York: Academic Press. 69–117.

Da Pos, O. 1989–1991. *Trasparenze* (Transparency) Milan: Icone.

Da Pos, O. 2002. "On the Nature of Colours." In *AIC Color 2001*, edited by R. Chung. *SPIE* 4421: 42–46.

Da Pos, O. and Albertazzi, L. 2010. "It Is in the Nature of Color . . ." *Seeing and Perceiving* 23: 39–73.

Da Pos, O., Devigili, A., Giaggio, F., and Trevisan, G. 2007. "Color Contrast and Stratification of Transparent Figures." *Japanese Psychological Research* 49 (1): 68–78.

De Valois, R. L., Abramov, J., and Jacobs, G. H. 1966. "Analysis of Response Patterns of LGN Cells." *Journal of Optical Society of America A* 56: 966–977.

De Weerd, P., Desimone, R., and Underleider, L. G. 1998. "Perceptual Filling in: A Parametric Study." *Vision Research* 38: 2721–2734.

Ehrenfels, C. von. 1890. "Über Gestaltqualitäten." (On Gestalt Qualities). *Vierteljahrschrift für wissenschaftliche Philosophie* 14: 242–292.

Fechner, T. 1860. *Elemente der Psychophysik.* (Elements of Psychophysics) Leipzig: Breitkopf & Härtel.

Fraisse, P. 1964. *The Psychology of Time.* London: Eyre and Spottiswood.

Fraisse, P. 1974. *Psychologie du rythme.* (Psychology of Rhythm) Paris: Presses Universitaires de France.

Fuchs, W. 1923. "Experimentelle Untersuchungen über die Änderung von Farben unter dem Einfluss von Gestalten (Angleichungserscheinungen)." (Experimental Investigations on Colour Change under the Influence of Gestalten [appearances of similarity]). *Zeitschrift für Psychologie* 92: 249–263.

Gibson, J. J. 1979. *The Ecological Approach to Visual Perception.* Boston: Houghton-Mifflin.

Gilchrist, A. L. 2002. "Articulation effects in lightness: Historical background and theoretical implications." *Perception* 31: 141–150.

Gilchrist, A. L. 2006. *Seeing Black and White.* Oxford: Oxford University Press.

Hatfield, G. 2003. "Representation and Constraints: The Inverse Problem and the Structure of Visual Space." *Acta Psychologica* 114: 355–378.

Hering, E. E. 1920/1964. *Outlines of a Theory of the Light Sense (Zur Lehre vom Lichtsinn)*, translated by L. M. Hurvich and D. Jameson. Cambridge, MA: Harvard University Press.

Hoffman, D. D. 2003. "The Interaction of Colour and Motion." In *Colour Perception: From Light to Object*, edited by R. Mausfeld and D. Heyer. Oxford: Oxford University Press. 361–379.

Hoffman, D. D. 2008a. "Conscious Realism and the Mind-Body Problem." *Mind and Matter* (6)1: 87–121.

Hoffman, D. D. 2008b. "Ratselhafte Zeichen einer multimodalen Benutzerschnittstelle" (Sensory Experiences as Cryptic Symbols of a Multi-Modal User Interface). *Kunst und Kognition*. Munich: Verlag.

Hurvich, L. M. and Jameson, D. 1957. "An Opponent-Process Theory of Color Vision." *Psychological Review* 64 (6, Part I): 384–404.

Kanizsa, G. 1952. "Legittimità di un'analisi del processo percettivo fondata su una distinzione in fasi o stadi." (Legitimacy of an Analysis of the Perceptual Process Founded on a Distinction of Phases or Stages) *Archivio di Psicologia, Neurologia e Psichiatria* 15 (3): 251–264.

Kanizsa, G. 1989. *Grammatica del vedere*. (Grammar of Seeing) Bologna: Il Mulino.

Kanizsa, G. 1991. *Vedere e pensare*. (Seeing and Thinking) Bologna: Il Mulino.

Kanizsa, G., and Vicario, G. B. 1968. "La percezione della relazione intenzionale." (The Perception of Intentional Relation) In *Ricerche sperimentali sulla percezione*, edited by G. Kanizsa, Gaetano and Giovanni B. Vicario. Trieste: Università degli studi di Trieste. 69–126.

Katz, D. 1935. *The World of Colour*. London: Routledge.

Koenderink, J. J., and van Doorn, A. 2003. "Pictorial space." In *Looking Into Pictures*, edited by H. Hecht, R. Schwartz, and Margaret Atherton. Cambridge MA: MIT Press. 239–299.

Koffka, K. 1935. *Principles of Gestalt Psychology*. New York: Harcourt, Brace, and World.

Köhler, W. 1913. "Über unbemerkte Empfinfungen und Urteilstäuschungen." (On Unnoticed Sensations and Illusions of Judgment). *Zeitschrift für Psychologie* LXVI 66: 51–80.

Köhler, W. 1920. "Die physische Gestalten in Ruhe und im stationären Zustand" (The Physical Gesalten in Rest and in Stationary Conditions). In *A Source Book of Gestalt Psychology*, translated by W. Ellis. London: Routledge. 17–54.

Kovács, I. and Julesz, B. 1994. "Perceptual Sensitivity Maps within Globally Defined Visual Shapes." *Nature* 370: 644–646.

Làvadas, E. 2002. "Functional and Dynamic Properties of Visual Peripersonal Space." *Trends in Cognitive Sciences* 6 (1): 17–22.

Leyton, M. 1987. "Symmetry-Curvature Duality." *Computer Vision, Graphics, and Image* 38: 3.

Leyton, M. 1992. *Symmetry, Causality, Mind*. Boston: MIT Press.

Leyton, M. 2001. *A Generative Theory of Shape*. New York: Springer.

Libet, B. 1982. "Brain Stimulation in the Study of Neuronal Functions for Conscious Sensory Experience." *Human Neurobiology* 1: 235–242.

Libet, B., Wright, E. W., Feinstein, B., and Pearl, D. K. 1979. "Subjective Referral of the Timing for Aconscious Sensory Experience." *Brain* 102: 191–224.

Lipps, T. 1897. *Raumaesthetik und geometrisch-optischen Täuschungen*. (Aesthetics of Space and Geometrical-Optical Illusions). Leipzig: Barth.

Lorenz, K. 1976. *Behind the Mirror*. Methuen, London: Harcourt Brace.

Marr, D. 1982. *Vision*. San Francisco: Freeman Press.

Maturana, H. R. and Varela, F. J. 1987. *The Tree of Knowledge: The Biological Roots of Human Understanding*. Boston: New Science Library.

Mausfeld, R. 2002. "The Physicalistic Trap in Perception Theory." In *Perception and the Physical World*, edited by D. Heyer and R. Mausfeld. Chichester UK: John Wiley and Sons. 75–112.

Mausfeld, R. 2003. "Conjoint Representations and the Mental Capacity for Multiple Simultaneous Perspectives." In *Looking into Pictures*, edited by H. Hecht and R. Mausfeld. Cambridge, MA: MIT Press. 17–60.

Metelli, F. 1941. "Oggettualità, stratificazione e risalto nell'organizzazione percettiva di figura e sfondo." (Objectuality, Stratification and Salience in the Perceptual Organization of Figure and Ground) *Archivio di Psicologia, Neurologia e Psichiatria* 2: 831–841.

Metelli, F. 1974. "The Perception of Transparency." *Scientific American* 230: 91–98.

Metzger, W. 1986. *Gestaltpsychologie* (Gestalt Psychology) ed. by Michael Stadler and H. Crabus, Frankfurt a.Main: Verlag Waldemar Kramer.

Michon, J. A. 1978. "The Making of the Present: A Tutorial Review." In *Attention and Performance VII*, edited by J. Requin. Hillsdale, NJ: Erlbaum. 89–111.

Michotte, A., and collaborators. 1962. *Causalité, permanence et réalité phénoménale*. (Causality, Permanence and Phenomenal Reality) Louvain: Publications Universitaires.

Monnier, P., and Shevell, S. K. 2003. "Large Shifts in Color Appearance From Patterned Chromatic Backgrounds." *Nature Neuroscience* 6 (8): 801–802.

Musatti, C. L. 1926. *Analisi del concetto di realtà empirica*, (Analysis of the Concept of Empirical Reality) Il Solco, Città di Castello. Reprinted in 1964, as *Condizioni dell'esperienza e fondazione della psicologia*. (Conditions of Experience and Foundations of Psychology) Florence: Editrice Universitaria.

Nakayama, K., Shimojo, S., and Ramachandran, V. S. 1990. "Transparency: Relation to Depth, Subjective Contours, Luminance, and Neon Color Spreading." *Perception* 19: 497–513.

Nijhawan, R. 1997. "Visual decomposition of color through motion extrapolation." *Nature*, 386, 66–69.

Noë, A. 2004. *Action in Perception*. Cambridge, MA: MIT Press.

O'Regan, J. K., and Noë, A. 2001. "A Sensorimotor Account of Vision and Visual Consciousness." *Behavioural and Brain Sciences*, 24 (5): 939–1011.

Piaget, J. 1954/2004. *The Construction of Reality in the Child*. London: Routledge and Kegan Paul.

Pöppel, E. 1994. "Temporal Mechanism in Perception." *International Review of Neurobiology* 37: 185–202.

Qiu, F. T., and von der Heydt, R. 2007. "Neural Representation of Transparent Overlap." *Nature Neuroscience* 10: 283–284.

Richards, W. 1996. "Priors by Design." In *Perception as Bayesian Inference*, edited by D. Knill and W. Richards. Cambridge, UK: Cambridge University Press.

Rock, I. 1983. *The Logic of Perception.* Cambridge, MA: MIT Press.

Schumann, F. 1904. "Beiträge zur Analyse der Gesichtswahrnehmungen: 1. Einige Beobachtungen über die Zusammenfassung von Gesichtseindrücken zu Einheiten." (Consideration on the Analysis of Visual Perception: 1. Some Observations on the Process of Unifying Visual Impression) *Zeitschrift für Psychologie* 23: 1–32.

Shannon, C. E., and Weaver, W. 1998 (originally published in 1949). *The Mathematical Theory of Communication.* Urbana, IL: University of Illinois Press.

Spillmann, L. 2009. "Phenomenology and Neurophysiological Correlations: Two Approaches to Perception Research." *Vision Research* 49 (12): 1507–1521.

Spillmann, L., and Ehrenstein, W. 2004. "Gestalt Factors in the Visual Neurosciences?" *The Visual Neurosciences* 19: 428–434.

Tichener, E. B. 1929. *Systematic Psychology. Prolegomena.* Ithaca-London: Cornell University Press.

Uexküll, J. von. 1982 (1940). "The Theory of Meaning." *Semiotica* 42 (1): 25–82.

van Tonder, G. J., and Ohtani, Y. 2008. "Measuring Perceived Surface Facets and Internal Contours in 'Kanizsa' Cubes." *Gestalt Theory* 30 (1): 51–60.

van Tonder, G. J., Lyons, M. J., and Ejima, Y. 2002. "Visual Structure of a Japanese Zen Garden." *Nature* 419: 359–360.

Vicario, G. B. 1999. "Forms and Events." In *Shapes of Forms. From Gestalt Psychology and Phenomenology to Ontology and Mathematics*, edited by L. Albertazzi. Dodrecht: Kluwer. 89–106.

Vishwanath, D. 2005. "The Epistemological Status of Vision and Its Implications for Design." *Axiomathes* 15: 399–486.

von der Heydt, R. and Peterhans, E. 1989 "Mechanisms of contour perception in monkey visual cortex. I. Lines of pattern discontinuity" Journal of Neuroscience 9: 1731–1748.

Weizsäcker, V. von. 1968. *Der Gestaltkreis. Theorie der Einheit von Wahrnehmen und Bewegung* (The Gestalt circle: Theory of the Unity of Perception and Movement) Stuttgart: Georg Thieme Verlag.

Wertheimer, M. 1923. "Untersuchungen zur Lehre von der Gestalt." (Investigation on the Theory of Gestalt) *Psychologische Forschung* 4: 301–350.

1 Vision and Information

Jan J. Koenderink

The term "information" has a precise meaning in Shannon's "information theory" that might be paraphrased as "selective information" or "structural complexity." The concept applies to the physical and physiological level. "Information" as used in informal discourse and psychology is a categorically different concept. It has to do with *meaning* and thus applies to the mental realm. Although the two concepts are entirely unrelated, they are commonly confused in psychological and physiological contexts. In discussions concerning perception, the confusion extends to such related psychological concepts as "cue" and "data" and physiological concepts as "detector" and "representation." In Shannon's theory such terms occur in the "communication" over a "channel" between a "sender" and a "receiver" sharing a common "code." In perception an agent (observer) acts in its *Umwelt*. There is no shared code, but a diagnostic (one way) process where the meaning is intentional (derives from the receiver). The chapter analyses the perceptual process on both the physical/physiological and the experiential levels. Such an analysis suggests reinterpretations of the psychophysical relations, usually (pejoratively) denoted "controlled hallucination." It is suggested how such a view might be fleshed out.

The emphasis of this chapter is on *visual perception*. The concept of "information" pervades the literature on both theoretical and empirical visual psychophysics, yet the concept remains an elusive one. I pursue various interpretations of the term.

Suppose you are a stationary, monocular, but otherwise generic human observer. Circumstances being normal, you are likely to "see a scene in front of you" (notice that "a scene" might also appear in a dream). Although entirely effortless on your part, this scenario is commonly considered to be a major scientific problem in need of a theoretical explanation (Palmer, 1999). The mainstream scientific account of "seeing the scene in front of you" (here "the" scene is understood as real) runs roughly as follows.

You are an object in the physical world. The scene you are in has a certain geometrical layout, is composed of objects with certain material properties, and is suffused with a field of electromagnetic radiation (Gershun, 1936). For the purposes of vision, this complexity can be summarized completely through the *radiance*. This concept is standard in physics, whereas in computer vision the radiance is known as the "plenoptic function" (Adelson and Bergen, 1991). The radiance describes the "density of rays" in the language of geometrical optics. It can also be framed in terms of photon flux or electromagnetic radiant power density if you want, but this is not essential. The radiance is incident at the location of your eye from any conceivable direction. The radiance is non–negative throughout, and is such that the ray density for a certain direction is invariant with respect to displacements of the eye along that direction. Otherwise the radiance is an arbitrary function of direction that sums up "everything there is to see" at the location of your eye. This is the account of *physics*.

The account of mainstream *artificial intelligence* (McCarthy, 1959) departs from this and talks of the radiance of an "image" providing "cues." The observer is an intelligence that performs sequences of parallel computations or inferences on the bases of the image with the aim to arrive at an interpretation of the cues. The result of this computation is an "inverse optics" (Poggio, 1984) representation of the scene that caused the image.

The account of mainstream *psychology* (Palmer, 1999) (nowadays "cognitive science") again departs from this and has it that the physiological substrate is a wetware computer that exactly runs the algorithms proposed by artificial intelligence. This causes certain brain locations to be in certain states. This again makes the agent have certain experiences, the common suggestion is "causally," but at this stage perhaps the more honest term is "magically." Eventually this results in your "perception of the scene in front of you." Here "perception" is a technical term that denotes an experience "due" to some form of physical interaction going on at your sensitive body surface.

This is the current scientific view of what there is to "see the scene in front of you." Although other views are known these are not considered "scientific," although perhaps of historical interest.

To discuss the dichotomy, I refer to what I call the "Marrian" and the "Goethean" accounts of perception (to be explained later). Although of course a schematization, this serves to illustrate the dichotomy by contrast as it were. Roughly speaking, what I call the Marrian perspective regards perceptions as due to world-to-mind processes, whereas what I call the Goethean perspective treats perceptions rather as due to mind-to-world processes. Thus the two views flatly contradict each other. It is suggested that it either is—in broad outline—like this:

Marrian account   Perception is the result of standard computations on optical data (that is, the scientific account) or that the perception is due to some magic.

Goethean account   Perception is controlled hallucination.

The latter is considered unscientific because physics is evidently prior to experience. With "hallucination," I indicate a process of microgenesis (Brown, 2002) that continuously produces the next thread of perceptual experience while the current one fades, apparently beyond voluntary control. It is the vital rhythm of vision, rather than the contents of visual experiences.

The mainstream Marrian account is accepted almost unconditionally in the sciences, though usually implicitly because it is considered "self-evident." The paradigmatic author is perhaps David Marr (1982), which is why I refer to the mainstream account as the "Marrian account." The alternate account might indeed be called "Goethean" because of Goethe's remark from the didactical part of the *Farbenlehre* (1808–1810):

The eye exists due to light. From arbitrary animal organs the light calls forth an organ that will become its equal. The eye forms itself in the light for the light in order that the inner light might meet the outer.

Such a view is commonly discarded as "mystical" by the hard-core scientist.

In this chapter, I argue that the mainstream Marrian account of what it is to "see the scene in front of you" is incoherent and scientifically untenable, whereas the Goethean account is viable, thus running against the grain of the mainstream view. The most direct way to argue this theory would be through an ontological analysis of experience and science. I do not take this route, but I analyze the most salient concepts involved in terms of science and experience. These are "structure," "data," "information," "cue," "representation," "perception," "veridicality," "hallucination," "neural substrate" and so forth, which are the terms one encounters over and over again in scientific accounts of perception (Palmer, 1999). I pursue this somewhat circuitous route because I assume that my readers will mainly be from the sciences rather than philosophy. Thus, my arguments directly apply to various, often implicit, assumptions current in mainstream vision research. A certain philosophical naiveté in the exposition is inevitable, but the goal seems worth the cost.

Information

The term "information" is well known to be ambiguous (MacKay, 1969). *Informally*, it is often used to describe a fragment of semantic content; *formally*—in Shannon's sense (Shannon, 1948, see also Meyer-Eppler, 1969)—it is a precisely defined measure of structural complexity (typically of the *process* that generates the structure, thus rather "potential structural complexity" than just "structural complexity") without any semantic connotation (MacKay, 1950). The former sense is in our context synonymous with "data," or "cue," the latter sense with "structure." In this chapter, I do not use the term "information" much, but where I use "data" or "cue" you may read "information" in the former sense, whereas if I use "structure" or "selective information" you may read "information" in the latter sense. This simple distinction clears up a lot of muddy reasoning.

First let me illustrate the difference between the two concepts of "information" through a pair of examples:

Example 1   You throw up a coin, catch it and put it on the top of your left hand, placing the palm of the right hand over it. You are about to lift your right hand in order to reveal the outcome of the throw. The outcome has some trivial consequence to which you have committed yourself.

Example 2   You have been tried for murder and wait for the jury's verdict. It will be either freedom or the gallows, the odds being (to your mind) about fifty-fifty.

In both cases you are expecting one of two possible outcomes with fifty-fifty odds. In terms of Shannon's information theory these are equivalent cases. You may as well abstract from the fancy settings, you are dealing simply with a binary choice. In either case, the answer is worth exactly one bit of selective information. Notice that the value of the outcome in the two cases is not exactly equivalent to you as a person, however. Apparently the "one bit of selective information" fails to describe the situation to the appropriate level of detail—to you. What is lacking is the "meaning" of the outcome. Shannon's formalism is not designed to capture it.

In the account of physics (Young, Freedman, Sandin, and Ford, 1999) you deal only with *structure* and transformations of structures into yet other structures. The optical input, that is, the radiance, is a structure; it is transformed into the retinal irradiance, a structure, the optic nerve activity, another structure, the activity of the visual brain areas, again another structure, and so forth. All these are indeed structures and thus meaningless. Any one of these structures is obviously correlated (albeit through numerous levels of indirection) to the physical structure of the scene in front of you, although it is hard to see how this could "explain" your awareness of that scene. This would boil down to saying that the physical world (via numerous levels of indirection) explains your perception, an "explanation" that most people would probably consider self-evident, although perhaps not enlightening. It has been proposed as the "direct perception" theory in psychology, the concept being mainly due to Gibson (1950). In Gibson's view the observer simply "resonates" with the world.

Records, Pictures and Images

Various technicalities (important ones) pertain to structures to which I can spend no more discussion in this short chapter. I will use the term "record" for a collection of structural elements (think of numerical values for instance) stored in some conventional order. An example would be a photograph stored on a computer disc, say in TIF or JPEG format. I use the term "picture" for such a collection of structural elements that has a natural topological structure. A photograph displayed on a computer screen is an example. Here the topology is that of a rectangular matrix of "pixels" defined by the screen manufacturer. A record can be displayed as a picture if you add the topological structure (the program that displays the file does that); the topological structure itself has no relation to the content of the image (i.e., it may be the same for a large set of very different pictures). An "image" is a mental entity that may occur if you look at the picture displayed on the screen. It is categorically different from the "picture" in that it depends on a "beholder's share" (Gombrich, 1960). Thus, different observers have different images for the same picture simultaneously, and a single observer may have different images for the same picture successively.

Such distinctions are important in technical applications. In vision science, one typically skips such issues, however. For instance, the distinction between "records" and "pictures" or "images" has to do with *local sign*, a notion that has received scant interest since its introduction by nineteenth-century authors (Lotze, 1876; von Helmholtz, 1860). This is not to say that these issues are of minor importance. They are of fundamental interest and at some point vision science will have to face them squarely.

To "see a picture" may mean having an image of the (flat) screen or piece of paper:

Remember that a painting—before it is a battle horse, a nude model, or some anecdote—is essentially a flat surface covered with colours assembled in a certain order. (Maurice Denis, 1998)

Or it may mean having an image of a "depicted scene." In the latter case, the "beholder's share" is evidently huge. Similar things occur when you simply see the scene in front of you, however. In "seeing" the Coke can at your feet as "having been dented" (Leyton, 1992), it may not even occur to you that it may as well have been manufactured in dented form to begin with (e.g., as a "pop–art" object). You "see" the histories (and, to some extent, the futures) of objects. "Anticipation and repeal" (Pestilli, 1993) bring the image to life as it were. You experience antique Greek sculptures (mere chunks of marble or bronze from the physics perspective) as living human bodies, moving from a certain inner tension. Such examples could be multiplied *ad infinitum*. The beholder's share is always a major aspect of your images.

Perception

In the account of artificial intelligence the optical input is described as "data." This notion should be deeply troubling, because the term "data" implies a "sender" and a "receiver" "communicating" over some "channel." A "datum," then, is defined as an element of such a communication. Either the sender and receiver share the "code" for the channel, as in communication, or the receiver possesses a model of the sender and monitors the sender's state, as in diagnosis. Thus, either the world is an "agent", abhorrent to the mainstream view, or the perceiver "hallucinates." Indeed, a model, like a scientific theory, is a product of the creative imagination—equally abhorrent to the mainstream view. In the mainstream view there is only structure; data does not apply.

It may be objected that structure is sufficient to trigger efficacious behavior and that the "data" can be defined relative to this behavior. This is true, for example, for the "releasers" that abound in biology (Braitenberg, 1984; Lorenz, 1973; Riedl, 1975). However, the triggered behavior is necessarily "blind" behavior, this is obvious in the cases where the triggered actions are obviously inefficacious (as the Northern Lapwing trampling on a wet cloth on the laboratory workbench, apparently "to drive the earthworms out"). Moreover, here "data" is defined as a property of the observer in the world, rather than just of the world, the optical input say. This insight is important because, as I argue later, the scene in front of you is as much a property of you as it is a reflection of any external world. The difference between "automatic" reactions and perception proper can be operationalized as follows:

Perception is optically guided potential *behavior.*

The *actual* behavior depends on the perceiver's current goals and emotional state. The scientist studying the observer may vary the observer's goals and record behavior for a given optical structure, the perception (in terms of meaning) is invariant over the variation of goal, although the actual behavior may vary greatly. Releasers only trigger actual behavior and do not signify "perception" in this sense. Of course, one must think of a continuous spectrum rather than a dichotomy here.

"Cues" occur in ancient philosophies, but the most salient modern Western author is no doubt Bishop Berkeley (1709). It is relevant that Berkeley never tires of stressing the essentially *arbitrary* nature of the cues. Cues are structures to which you have learned—through statistically uncontradicted optically guided behavior—to associate certain properties or processes in the world. In the case of the releasers, this learning is phylogenetic; one is simply born with the cues all "wired in," but many cues are learned during childhood or even adulthood. Notice that this involves some kind of "model." You don't "compute perceptions from cues." Rather, the cues allow you to generate hallucinations and/or constrain freely generated hallucinations.

It is perhaps not superfluous to stress that "hallucination" is different from the mainstream notion of "prior." A prior—as used in Bayesian inference—is a generic, usually statistical, property of the environment (Purves et al., 2001). For example "light comes from above" is such a prior (if put in suitable formal format). It applies, on the average, for terrestrial animals that live in open spaces. Such priors package "frozen" prior experience as it were. "Hallucinations" differ by not being frozen, but being highly adaptable, applying to the *actual* situation. Hallucinations can be regarded as specific, necessarily tentative, instantiations of the observer's present "situational awareness" instead of its average past. ("Situational awareness" is to be understood in approximately the sense of Minsky's [1974] "frames": *A Frame is a collection of questions to be asked about a hypothetical situation; it specifies issues to be raised and methods to be used in dealing with them;* Cassirer's [1923–1929] "symbolic forms" are likewise a kind of "superframe," this notion derives from Kant [1968]). That "hallucination" plays an important role in perception is a notion generally eschewed in science but rather familiar in the arts. Think of Leonardo da Vinci's (1680)

... master Botticelli stated ... [that] just by throwing a sponge soaked with various colors against a wall to make a stain, one can find a beautiful landscape. If it is true that in this stain various inventions can be discerned, or rather what one wants to find in it, such as battles, reefs, seas, clouds, forests and other similar things, then surely, this is like the ringing of bells in which one can understand whatever one wants to ...

or William Shakespeare:[1]

Hamlet: Do you see yonder cloud that's almost in the shape of a camel?
Lord Polonius: By the mass, and 'tis like a camel, indeed.
Hamlet: Methinks it is like a weasel.
Lord Polonius: It is backed like a weasel.
Hamlet: Or like a whale?
Lord Polonius: *Very like a whale.*

Such observations are common and were apparently quite popular with Shakespeare's audience. The resistance from the sciences no doubt derives from the conviction that science depends on the fact that observations are objective, that is to say, independent of any observer.

Cues and Clues

"Cue" often means "signal for action"[2] (the "releaser" meaning), or "a hint or indication about how to behave in particular circumstances"[3] (often Berkeley's meaning), or "a piece of information or circumstance that aids the memory in retrieving details not recalled spontaneously."[4] The latter meaning is somewhat related to that of "*clue*" ("a piece of evidence or information used in the detection of a crime or solving of a mystery," or "a fact or idea that serves as a guide or aid in a task or problem"[5]). This meaning is of interest because it hints at the fact that *clues are selected*. This is also true of perception: somehow the observer "selects" certain cues and "ignores" others. This must clearly be just a way of speaking, though, because cues are defined with respect to the observer. Thus, an "ignored cue" is an oxymoron: Any cue is a "selected" cue. Rather, you have to rephrase the case as follows: *The observer selects structure and promotes it to cue status.* Of course, this implies that the observer is *actively involved* in the generation of cues (see figure 1.1 [Bradley and Petry, 1977]; this version of the Necker–cube may be due to Kanizsa, although I am not sure). This selection of cues has been described as "symbol formation," the creative power of the human mind, by Susanne Langer (1942).

Such an idea is quite natural. Consider the well-known Sherlock Holmes stories (Baring-Gould, 1967). Throughout the story, Sherlock Holmes collects clues, mostly apparently irrelevant trivialities. The important point here is that the world offers

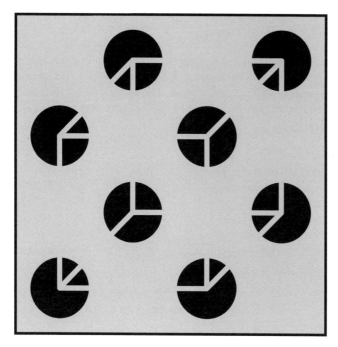

Figure 1.1

Here the "scene in front of you" is a collection of black blobs on a gray background. You are likely to "see" either one of two views of a cube, although infinitely many alternative interpretations are possible. The two views may alternate in time. You also see your location (either above or below the cube), an occluding screen with circular apertures through which you see a black space behind, gray "connecting lines" where there is no local optical structure, etc. Thus you have one of many possible presentations: What is there if you don't look? Cues you select are (among more) the junctions of three curves, collinearity and parallelity, all highly nongeneric features of 2D projections of 3D wireframe configurations. You also use the fact that the eight local patterns may form a coherent whole (an unlikely coincidence). Notice that this is actually an arrangement of gray and black. The "cube" is entirely your hallucination although there is plenty of "evidence" if you look for it, thus other agents (e.g., your friends) are not unlikely to entertain similar visions.

infinite numbers of equally trivial observations, and Sherlock Holmes selects ones that will become meaningful at the conclusion of the story. As Holmes explains the case all these apparently irrelevant trivial observations become very meaningful, whereas the infinitely many observations that could just as well have been made are never even mentioned. That would be impossible anyway and moreover boring *ad nauseam* because would be entirely meaningless (consider Searle's [1983] "Background"). It is only Holmes' explanation (truly his *perception*) of the plot that renders the clues meaningful. Thus, the clues are necessary to construct the plot, and the plot is necessary to be able to select (or rather, create) the clues.

Selecting cues is equivalent to selecting the "appropriate algorithm" to start inverse optics calculations. This is where (contemporary) computer vision (Forsyth and Ponce, 2002) essentially differs from biological vision: The selection of the "appropriate algorithm" is done in a *deus ex machina* fashion, although usually not acknowledged. This may well be called "cheating" because the "hard problem" is exactly this. The problem of *selection of cues* is central to vision, and it can only be solved by way of hallucination (computer vision would probably say "analysis by synthesis"). There is simply no way to "transform" mere structure into meaning, you—as *perceiver*—have to *supply* it. The selection of the algorithm is even more important than the calculation (various algorithms might do equally well) and requires the equivalent of "situational awareness."

Notice that a typical optical fact (e.g., a broken twig near the path, a crushed cigarette butt, etc.) is entirely meaningless; it will remain unnoticed or is bound to be forgotten the next moment. It is but a mere structure, unless it fits into your present "situational awareness"; then it is noticed and promoted to cue status.

This *modus operandi* perhaps sounds suspiciously nonscientific. In following the correct "scientific method" (VanCleave, 1997) you are not supposed to pick and choose your data! A paper submitted to a psychology journal will get rejected if you confess to have omitted an observer, or have weeded out "outliers" in the data. Yet one cannot jot down any random "observation" because there is a potential infinity of them to be had; science would soon grind to a standstill. The theories of science—even physics—have all been arrived at through the *selection* of "data" from mere "structure," not through indiscriminate crunching through the infinite riches of structure available to you. Indeed, the breakthroughs are typically related to unexpected selections (think of Newton, Einstein, etc.). Of course, the worry that one's view of nature might become biased this way is exactly why scientists are "not supposed" to pick and choose their data. Is the scientific view of nature "veridical" despite the fact that real-life scientists *do* pick and choose? The problem is very real because science is indeed the work of man and subject to the usual limitations. Although the Age of Enlightenment is usually closely linked to the arrival of the Scientific Revolution, science has some dark secrets to hide.

The Issue of the "Veridicality" of Perceptions

The *veridicality* issue often comes up in the study of perception. This is indeed exactly why the Goethean account is so unpalatable to the mainstream scientist. A hallucination, or anything imaginary, is by definition non–veridical ("an experience involving the apparent perception of something not present"[6]); only straight computations on optical data (the Marrian account) can ever hope to be veridical ("coinciding with reality"[7]). This all too common notion is misguiding, however, because it assumes that the radiance at a point completely and unambiguously specifies the scene in front of the observer; which is far from being the case. *Any radiance is compatible with an infinity of possible scenes.* Each such scene would equally well "explain" the optical structure available to the observer. Thus, the Marrian problem is hopelessly underconstrained or, as the computer vision community has it, "ill posed" (Hadamard, 1902). "Solving the problem" would at best yield an infinite set of solutions. To arrive at the "representation" of the scene in front of the observer, one needs additional tools that allow one to weed out the "wrong ones" from the "actual" one. Because such tools cannot depend on the optical input, the solution already utilized that to the fullest extent, the Marrian scheme has to be augmented with either "magic" or arbitrary choice to work as advertised. But both are equally objectionable from the mainstream perspective. The current way to handle this dilemma is the "Bayesian approach to perception" (Bayes, 1763; Knill and Richards, 1996).

Notice that only an external meta–observer would be able to decide on veridicality in the conventional sense. For the observer itself, the perception is primary; indeed, it is all there is. The perceptions simply "happen" to the observer—much like sneezing—and are "presentations" rather than "representations," there being nothing to "represent" prior to presentations. This notion is troubling to the mainstream view because one would prefer to base the judgment of "veridicality" on an empirical, operational basis. The alternate move is to identify "veridicality" with "uncontradicted (efficacious) optically guided behavior." But then one is no longer forced to prefer the Marrian account over the Goethean account. *Controlled hallucination* can very well evoke uncontradicted (efficacious) optically guided behavior as long as the hallucinations are checked against the actual optical structure. This approach mirrors Holmes' way of solving a crime. Holmes imagines a plot (a hallucination, not a perception) and checks it against the available evidence. This process effectively weeds out mere fancies and allows him to select the structure that will become evidence in a bootstrap fashion.

Parenthetically: "Presentations" only last for the specious present (less than a second) before fading and being replaced with fresh ones, their microgenesis remaining preconscious.

The stuff of higher consciousness (discursive thought; Kant's [1783] *Vernunft* as opposed to *Verstand*) is not presentations but might be called "representations," which contain remembrances of reified, consolidated and otherwise schematized presentations. Memory selects and orders, it assigns causal connections, and so forth. Presentations have many potential follow-ups and are ambiguous, whereas memories are fixed. Thus representations can be "known," whereas presentations are merely experienced. Marcel Proust (1913–1927) (and many other authors) feel that only such representations make up your conscious "reality." In this chapter I consider only presentations. They are "symbolic forms" in Cassirer's (1923–1929) sense rather than "logical forms." In other words, to *see* is an action of the *Verstand* (presentational awareness), whereas to *look at things* is an action of the *Vernunft* (discursive mind). To understand presentations, one needs to study the "Laws of Imagination," rather than the "Laws of Thought" (Langer, 1942). More on this later.

Perception: World to Mind or Mind to World?

If perception is indeed anything like this, then the Marrian causal chain is *inverted*. Instead of "data" arriving at the eye, being processed, being further processed (Neisser, 1967), and finally resulting in a "representation" of the scene in front of you, the agent explores the world in any conceivable direction until it encounters *resistance*. Thus, the action radiates out from the agent rather than converging on it. Here the "world" is anything that resists this centrifugal action, whether in the brain, the body, or the environment in which the agent's body happens to be. A "resistance" may be understood as the encounter of unexplained structure, the "explanation" being conformity to the current presentation. Most structure will be irrelevant in this respect, thus the probing actions are structured, probings for shreds of evidence. (This requires expertise and perhaps explains why even grown–ups have to "learn to see" in drawing courses, a fact that seems odd to those who never draw. "Not being able to draw" is a perceptual, rather than a motor defect.)

This very action *turns structure into data*. The potential meaning is in the question, the actual data in the answer, but without a question there can be no answer. What you see is indeed primarily *what you look for* (although "action" should not be understood as premeditated. To "see" is not different from "to beat one's heart" in that respect). A "question" presupposes at least the general nature of possible answers. Thus, "questioning" cannot arise out of the blue; rather it arises from (possibly tacit) knowing or understanding. A question presupposes an expectation of possible answers. There is an analogy with Shannon's information theory here: A "signal" as yet to be received is a structural entity known to belong to a certain set of possible structures. (As an aside: The very existence of a question presupposes an intelligence, and the horizon of possible answers is limited by that same intelligence. Posing a question to another intelligence changes the set of possible answers. This limits the applicability of Shannon's communication theory).

This is not unlike the "format" in a computer language: The format decides on the meaning of a bit pattern (i.e., *structure*), for example, whether it is a number, a string, and so on (i.e., *data*). Indeed, the format *imposes* the meaning in a willy-nilly fashion as you discover (to your chagrin) if you typed the wrong format in your program text. The program appears to be waiting for you to type an integer number say; you type "137." If the format is that of a text string, the program will crash. *You* know that you *intended* an integer number (in fact you actually *typed* it!), but the program treats anything you type as a text string and it can't treat a text string as it could a number (e.g., square it): the moment it tries it has no option but to quit or crash (excuse my use of anthropomorphic language—programs are just mindless machines). In vision "formats" are straightjackets that force mere optical structure into meaningful entities. They are conventionally known as "Gestalts." These root-level entities are already mental things. Mind stuff is meaningful from the very beginning, and the meaningless "sensations" that figure in the literature are nonentities.

Once again, this is the crux of Sherlock Holmes stories. As the reader progresses through the story, a great many irrelevant facts are encountered and right away forgotten because there appears to be no reason to hold on to them. Then, at the final showdown, Holmes uses such irrelevant facts as crucial evidence. And they indeed acquire an important meaning when regarded in terms of Holmes' explanation of the plot (the "format" the writer so cunningly hid from the reader). A cigarette butt in a flower pot (or anything arbitrary) may be enough to bring the countess to the gallows, if only the format is right.

The concept of the "centrifugal nature" of perception has been around for ages. Thus the "rays" in Euclid's optics (see the translation by Kheirandish, 1998) radiate out from the eye to probe the scene. Likewise, Goethe's (1978)

If the Eye weren't Sunlike,
It could never See the Sun;
. . .

expresses this very idea in poetic form, echoing the Neoplatonist Plotinus.[8] The "microgenetic theory" of mind of Jason Brown (2002) is a modern formulation of the same concept. For the hard-core scientist such notions are hard to swallow and when stated as bluntly as William Blake's saying *"nothing is real beyond imaginative patterns men make of reality,"* typically rejected as unacceptable. But what are scientific theories else but "imaginative patterns men make of reality"?

The Process of Perceiving

In addition, notice that the cue (resistance) can be encountered *anywhere*. If you consciously hunt for clues, Sherlock Holmes fashion, you will search the world, perhaps for footprints in the sand. Looking for "footprints" indeed turns depressions in the overall flattish surface of the sand into "footprints." Otherwise they would be mere depressions, unnoticed structure due to the effects of winds or lightning. In the generic perception of the scene in front of you, the resistance is often encountered in the brain. (You might well object that one doesn't see one's own brain. True, but neither do you see the sand "out there"! I take some short cuts in the description for the sake of easy reading here.) Indeed, any "cue" is *indirect*, the footprint is not the foot, the activity of a simple cell not an "edge." "Edge detectors" in your primary visual cortex (Tolhurst, 1972) are (logically) created at the moment that you start to look for edges; otherwise the neural activity is simply more (meaningless) structure. The mainstream notion of dedicated "edge," "line" (Hubel, 1989), "grandmother" (Barlow, 1972), etc., detectors is but a device to impose meaning on structure in a *deus ex machina* fashion. It is incoherent and does not account for the intentionality of perception. The footprint might be encountered in the brain, but that is not to say through a "footprint detector." In the context of the process of "looking for footprints," the brain is simply used as a *proxy* for the sand. The brain is used as a proxy for the sand much as a screwdriver is used as a proxy for the screw. You "turn the screw" by actually rotating the handle of the screwdriver. You operate on the screw through its proxy, that is, the screwdriver. The screwdriver *becomes* the screw; it is fully "transparent" to you, thus you "turn the screw," not the handle of the screwdriver. Likewise, the cortex is fully transparent; you "see the sand." In both perception and action there exist numerous layers of indirection and it is typically ambiguous and irrelevant what to consider as the "true" source or target. From the agent's perspective, "sources" and "targets" are intentional objects whose "ultimate natures" are entirely outside its scope.

Any such "meaning" exists strictly to the perceiving agent. An outside observer, say the physiologist registering neural activity, records only structures and of course may correlate such structures with other structures, such as the physical structure of the scene in front of the observer. Such correlations are equally meaningless as the structures, at least if the outside observer assumes a strictly scientific attitude. That is why science will never "explain" your perceptions: that is simply outside its realm. Experiential reality (for any given observer) and scientific reality cannot "mesh" because they are located in different strata of existence. (I use the notion of "strata of existence" informally in this chapter. The primary reference is Hartmann (1942, see also Poli, 2001). This deviates significantly from the mainstream view, which holds that (given time) physics will explain physiology and physiology will explain psychology. Although this cheerful view is the drive for much scientific endeavor, it is a basic category mistake.

That "meaning" is necessarily "subjective" (i.e., not available to an outside observer) is often taken as problematic. Consider some examples. How can it be that *you* can take the activity of some neuron in *your* brain into account in arriving at *your* feelings, whereas someone else can't? The question confuses ontological levels and is on par with the search for a brain center for "consciousness." Your experiences are more strongly correlated with some things or processes and less so with others. If you look someone straight in the face, you can't see the back of her head. From an optical perspective vision is only skin deep. You can indeed see a neuron in someone else's brain fire, for instance, if you attend a brain operation and watch the oscilloscope, but it won't help you much. You can at most correlate the firing with the scene in front of the other. The awareness of the scene in front of you is your current take on the world. It no doubt correlates with many physical processes as recorded by an external physicist to whom you are just another object, processes including firings of neurons in your brain, photon absorptions in your retina, and various properties of objects outside of your body. When you talk to somebody face to face, you see the other's face, but not yours. The other sees your face, but not her own. You use the edge detectors in your head, she the edge detectors in her head. There need be little mystery in all this.

Vision Science

Shannon's concept of information is perfectly suited to the needs of the honest physiologist and the hard-core behavioral psychologist (Skinner, 1945). The latter is indeed just a physiologist because he lets only structures count. Given such and so physical processes applied to a rat, so many lever presses are recorded. The physiologist controls an optical system and records times of action potential occurrences. Fine! No problem to compute information volumes and channel capacities. Moreover, the Marrian account suits the occasion perfectly. The problems only start with the "dishonest" physiologist who desires to talk of "edge detectors" and "centers for consciousness" and with the psychologist proper. Such a scientist is not satisfied with the unravelling of mappings from structures onto other structures. Then Shannon's concept of "information" becomes largely irrelevant. It needs to be replaced with talk of "meanings" of some kind. The "beholder's share (Gombrich, 1960)" is one aspect of images that cannot be computed from pictures. It eludes the Marrian scheme, and Shannon's theory simply doesn't apply.

The behaviorists were the proverbial "honest" physiologists although in the guise of psychologists. Their objective was to cleanse "behavior" from the least shred of "meaning" (e.g., "I have no sympathy with those psychologists . . . who try to introduce a concept of "meaning" ["values" is another sacred word] into behavior"; Watson, 1920, p. 103). Thus a "verbal report" is described as a complex of muscular contractions causing a certain shaking of air molecules (Hebb, 1966). This removes all meaning from the structure, causing the "verbal report" to be entirely meaningless (i.e., anything but "verbal" or "report"). The *meaning* of the verbal report is quite independent of the actual structure of air molecule movements. For instance, if one asks the person to "repeat" the report in other words, in another language, and so on, the structure of air molecule movements varies wildly, whereas the meaning is preserved. The "meaning" is not in the physical structures but is a mental entity. The behaviorists indeed removed mind and consciousness from the description and thus turned psychology into (honest) physiology. Recent mainstream "cognitive science" (Costall, 2006) is but an elaboration of this, purportedly admitting the mind but only as a hypothetical link in the "S–R" (stimulus–response) chain via the cognitivist hypotheticodeductive paradigm, which actually serves to discard the mind effectively. Science is saved, although relevance is sacrificed.

In the Goethean account the scientist (now a psychologist proper) reads intentionality in the rat's behavior. The animal presses the lever because it has some situational awareness based on prior experiences and it desires to expand its current sphere of existence ("Umwelt"[9]; see below). It is this basic urge to grow that seeks out resistance and turns structure into meaningful data. This leads the animal to impose a meaning—in the alternate sense of "information"—on selected physical structures. The rat constructs a "scene in front of me (the rat)." It will not (or only partly) coincide with the scene in front of the scientist because he/she either selects different structures and promotes them to different cues (Nagel, 1974). To "study the rat's mind" amounts to trying to predict the rat's behavior in terms of its selection of structures as cues and the role of such cues in the rat's creation of its world. It involves an understanding of the rat's *Umwelt*.

A "theory of information" as it applies to agents will be quite unlike Shannon's "information theory" and have more in common with biosemiotics. Thus Jakob von Uexküll (1940/1982) observes:

Every action, therefore, that consists of perception and operation imprints its meaning on the meaningless object and thereby makes it into a subject-related meaning-carrier in the respective Umwelt

where "Umwelt" denotes the subjective universe of the agent. This is just another way to describe the "probing for evidence" process described earlier. It is the mind that endows the world with meaning in the process of expanding its subjective universe. An interpretation in terms of Charles Pierce's (1955) "semiotics" is not unreasonable, although it is perhaps best understood as a manner of speaking. Notice that this description is thoroughly "constructivist," in the sense that the "objective world" is entirely left out of the discussion. Another way of expressing this is that the mind works in a "centrifugal" (hallucinating, probing) instead of a "centropetal" (building representation through signal processing) manner. The mind deals with proxies of its own making (Pierce's sign vehicles) and what the proxies "represent" is none of its business. Its business is efficacious action. It is indeed artificial to distinguish sharply between "action" and "perception," the semantic units are perception–action cycles (see Brentano, 1874). To perceive is to perceive meaning and meaning is what makes a difference in (perhaps future) doing. "Meaning" is your interface to the "world" as you cannot possibly know it (for all you can know is the interface)!

Presentation as Construction

Many authors have remarked that the scene in front of them looks perfectly crystal clear to them. For example, Nietzsche (1977) said:

When I go out I am always amazed to notice the wonderful definition with which everything strikes me, the forest such and the mountain so, and how there isn't the slightest confusion or hesitation in anything I see.

I completely relate to this and little wonder as I am looking at my own construct. Indeed, what could be better understood? In looking at the world you merely see an aspect of yourself. Here Giambattista Vico's (1725/2002) *Verum esse ipsum factum* hits the nail on the head. Yet some authors (Bridgman, 1959; Ruskin, 1843–1860) confess that what they see when looking at the scene in front of them is "mystery" (Ruskin's term) or even chaos. Thus John Ruskin (1843–1860, "Modern Painters") wrote,

Go to the top of Highgate Hill on a clear summer morning at five o'clock, and look at Westminster Abbey. You will receive an impression of a building enriched with multitudinous vertical lines. Try to distinguish one of those lines all the way down from the next one to it: You cannot. Try to count them: You cannot. Try to make out the beginning or end of any of them: You cannot. Look at it generally, and it is all symmetry and arrangement. Look at it in its parts, and it is all inextricable confusion.

Perhaps surprisingly, these descriptions are in no way contradictory. Presentations are like islands of articulation in oceans of mystery. That this has to be the case is evident when you consider the channel capacities of the visual system in Shannon's way. The optic nerve has a channel capacity of 10^8–10^9 bits per second, whereas estimates of the structural complexity of perceptions are generally below 100 bits per second. The many orders of magnitude gap indicates that perceptions have to be *very* selective. In some circumstances, this may suddenly strike you, as when you suddenly hear a human voice in the midst of meaningless random noises, although meaningless structures (in any modality) usually remain in the background.

The (to many) paradoxical observations that presentations are simultaneously crystal clear and yet full of mystery becomes perhaps more understandable if you compare photographs and paintings as sources of information relating to the scene in front of the camera or the artist. In photographs you might be able to find hitherto unnoticed details with the help of a magnifier (Michelangelo Antonioni's movie *"Blowup"* from 1966 (MGM) after Julio Cortazar's *"Las Babas del Diablo"* in *"Las Armas Secretas"* [Cortazar, 1959] is perhaps the paradigmatic example). But a magnifier doesn't help you to see more detail in a painting, except for the touches that is. A painting is "done" the moment the painter chooses to put his brushes down. Presentations are not "incomplete" either. They are just as complete as a painting is. Perceptions are "complete" the moment you have the presentation (on the topic of "completeness" see also Albertazzi, 2006). The optical structure contains essentially infinite structure that never shows up in a presentation, however. This is one reason that a presentation may differ from the fading one it replaces.

Reading the "Book of Nature"

What *do* you (optically) experience when confronting the scene in front of you? It seems likely that the building blocks of the experience are nested hierarchies of "symbolic forms," with irreducible "Gestalts" at the root level. Gestalts (Albertazzi, 2006; Metzger, 1953) come as complete entities; they are often textured but have no parts (think of the "rustling of leaves" or the "movement of wind" through the grass). Gestalts are meaningful entities (mental objects) similar to the "innate releaser mechanisms" identified by biologists such as Lorenz (1973) and Tinbergen (1951, 1975). The "releaser" notion is a useful one. When you experience a Gestalt (the Gestalt *is* the experience), you have found a "key" that unlocks part of the optical structure and turns it into meaning. Because you have only a (very) finite number of keys at your disposal, the key would be certain to be a "false key" if only a "true key" existed. As we all know all too well, any lock can be opened in numerous ways (e.g., by a professional burglar). Because no "true key" exists (the very notion is void), you might say that every key is a true key to the extent that it "fits the lock." A gull will roll a nearby potato to its nest (apparently experiencing it as an egg), whereas you will think this odd (wrong format silly!). No doubt the Gestalt serves the gull well, although not in this (artificial) case. Your Umwelt evidently differs from that of the gull's, and in this case, you are right in that the convex object is not likely to hatch. In other cases, it may be harder to assess whose perception is more likely to serve well in guiding future actions. Most animal species act remarkably efficaciously on the basis of their optical inputs.

Agents that score frequent efficacious transactions with the world on the basis of their optical experiences might be said to be "good perceivers." They apparently have a large bunch of keys at their disposal and have distilled from previous experiences what the various keys "unlock." Do they "perceive the world correctly" or—in the old fashioned expression that seems to apply more directly to the Shannon theory of information—do they *know* "how to read the Book of Nature?" I think not because no *a priori* agreed-on code exists. There is no "communication channel." There is not even a diagnostic channel because there is simply no "ground truth" of the matter. Such successful observers indeed have learned to avoid incapacitating harm to their bodies by pruning their behavior, using optics as means to do this especially timely. That is why they appear to "see correctly." In an important sense they do, yet each one has (or "lives") its own truth. "Truth" is not absolute (recall Susanne Langer's [1953] definition of "fact": "Fact" is not a simple notion. It is that which we conceive to be the source and context of signs to which we react successfully . . .).

Although the "Book of Nature" is never being *read*, it is constantly being "*written*." It is written in the bodies of organisms, from the molecular scale to the macro scale, where it provides "keys" to efficacious behavior on all time scales (Riedl, 1975). It is also written in individual's subjective experiences. Here Schrödinger's (1944) notion that consciousness is correlated with what I—in the context of the present discussion—would call overcoming a resistance (due to probing) by "tweaking a key" (Schrödinger refers to the "*Vegetationsspitze* of our stem") seems especially apt.

When our keys fit, we are automata; when we manage to broaden our Umwelt by tweaking a key, we experience a micro-enlightenment as it were. Conscious experience can perhaps be understood as a series—no temporal order implied (Hoyle, 1968)—of such flashes.

Topology of Space and Time

Presentations are like momentary flashes, although they are temporally "thick." In that sense, they are like Euclid's "points," which are defined as "that which has no parts," the *extension* being left undefined. Indeed, a point may have *any size* as Kandinsky illustrates (1926). A point may also have internal structure (or rather texture), although not internal geometrical relations. Only distinct points can stand in geometrical relation to each other. Thus the internal parts of points are "orderless" in the point geometry. This has many implications (e.g., for two distinct structural elements, A and B it may not be possible to say that A is located to the left or the right of B, implying that classical logic [the Law of the Excluded Third] does not apply [Bell, 1998]). It is the same with the temporality of the presentations: the temporal structure in the duration of a presentation is not necessarily successive. Unlike Euclidian points, presentations do not stand in temporal relation to each other because there is only one presentation at any one time. A "past presentation" would be a memory (i.e., not a presentation proper). Presentations are "colored" with actual, still uninterpreted optical structure, thus there is potentially "more to see." With memories, this is not the case; the memory itself being all there is. Although presentations are independent entities, both the optical structure and memories enter as possible constraints. The independence is most obvious in sudden perceptual reorganizations as when a Necker cube flips.

Perception and Cognition

Presentations are the "concrete reality" of an agent; and as such, beyond right or wrong, they cannot be "in error." Hence, Shakespeare's[10]

What's in a name? That which we call a rose
By any other name would smell as sweet,

or Joshu's "*Mu!*" (Case I of the Mumonkan [Blyth, 1966]).

Error creeps in only at the moment cognition takes over. (In writing on Bonnard's art Whitfield[11] remarks: ". . . the precision of naming takes away from the uniqueness of seeing"). Who takes a rope for a snake only commits a mistake in discursive thought, the presentation is simply concrete reality in which the rope and snake are "not two." Only poetical (i.e., imaginative) thought can approach the concreteness of presentations. Blake's "Tiger, tiger, burning bright, in the forests of the night, . . ." is either terribly real (to you, in poetic thought) or nonsense (in discursive thought). This is the topic of the XL Case of the Mumonkan, where Hyakujō (720–814 AD) (Blyth, 1966) stands a jar on the floor and commands the perplexed monks: "Don't call it a jar, but tell me what it is!" A famous case such as Picasso's "Head of a Bull" (1943, now at the Museé Picasso, Paris, France) made of a bicycle saddle and handlebars concretizes the perception of a bull's head through iconic metaphor. More mundane examples are provided by any painting, where the *touches* act as iconic metaphors: You cannot possibly "paint a scene," you can only create a concrete distribution of pigments on a planar carrier (think of Magritte's "*Ceci n'est pas une pipe*"). For a "likeness" you need a spectator, the likeness being in her presentations, rather than on the canvas.

Conscious optical experiences have been (no doubt pejoratively) called "mental paint" (Block, 2003). Indeed, they are *constructions* of the observer ("hallucinations") rather than results of "inverse optics." But "wiping off the paint" would hardly reveal a clearer view because nothing would be left! Images of the Umwelt can only be done in "mental paint." Informationally, some Umwelts are more structurally complicated than others (here the Shannon concept of information applies), but all images are equally "true." They are "true" from the inside out as it were, because there is no such a thing as the *actual* scene. At least not something you could *know* in any other way than through your interface.

Origination of Perceiving

Something that is by itself *meaningless* has to be in place to fire up the "perception action cycle" from scratch. You may well assume that there exists—at the rock bottom—nothing but a blind urge to *expand* or *grow*. This tendency is observed in all life forms, including mere proto-life forms. In an intentional sense such a goal is to "dominate the world," but at the earliest stage (molecules in the primeval soup say) such an urge still lacks a true intentionality. It is *outwardly* directed, however. Because of this goal, the agent is "active" and willy-nilly encounters *resistance*, forcing it to become *reactive*. This marks the onset of the "perception-action cycle," which implies a differentiation between the self and everything else ("the world"). Thus, changes of state become differentiated into self-initiated events (the only true "actions") and changes inflicted by the environment (which might naturally be denoted "suffering"). Thus, the mechanism that drives all this is the urge to expand the Umwelt ("Wille")

(Nietzche, 1901, 1977; Schopenhauer, 1844), which leads to resistance (a "suffering" due to an "action") and eventually to presentation ("Vorstellung") (Schopenhauer, 1844). Notice that much of this is merely turning structure into structure (the Shannon theory of information applies), but that psychogenesis arises from *action* (seeking out and encountering resistance), not *reception*. This *creative element* does not fit Shannon's theory of communication.

It is the *expectation* of a *resistance* to a self-initiated action that enables intentionality. The resistance can be understood as the "answer" of the world to the "question" posed by the probing. In essence this is not different from experimentation in the sciences:

And, irrespective of what one might assume, in the life of a science, problems do not arise by themselves. It is precisely this that marks out a problem as being of the true scientific spirit: all knowledge is in response to a question. If there were no question, there would be no scientific knowledge. Nothing proceeds from itself. Nothing is given. All is constructed. (Bachelard, 1938)

Thus it would seem that "science" fits very well into this scheme. It can be seen as the "perception" of a society of humans that attempts to broaden its Umwelt, and in the course of that grows novel sensory organs, actuators, and so forth. It puts the "Philosophy of science" (Rosenberg, 2000) in the unfortunate position of an ant trying to describe the intelligence of the ant heap.

Psychophysics

Do these reflections have a bearing on how one should conduct the study of (visual) perception? Yes, in my view they are *crucial*. In classical "psychophysics" one purports to study psychogenesis in its functional dependence on physical stimuli. This scheme assumes a centripetal process, and has to be replaced with a centrifugal one. Instead of elements of perception being "subjective correlates of physical states," they should be regarded as elements of the perceiver's Umwelt. The elements of perception may not have immediate "physical correlates," and the Umwelt need not be structured along the lines of the physical world, as described by our present mainstream science. I consider a few instances of this below. Thus, the "problem of psychophysics" (if there is one) is to find the correlates of experiential matter (qualia) in the physical world (structural elements and relations), rather than the other way around. This turns (conventional) psychophysics topsy-turvy, of course.

The study of "perception" is perhaps best differentiated in an "internal" part, in which one formally describes the structures of the various "qualities" (or Gestalts), and an "external" part, in which the internal relations are correlated with physical structures.

The internal descriptions are part of psychology proper, the external are part of what might rightfully be termed "psychophysics." From the perspective of pure phenomenology (all that is "given"), the perceiver cannot be isolated from the "world" at all, however; thus the distinction between inner and outer views has to be taken *cum grano salis*.

Qualities

No quality is an "island" (hard to say what an isolated quality might "mean"); qualities are located with respect to each other in what biologists (Riedl, 1975) denote as "homology fields." This is essentially Goethe's (1789/1790; see also d'Arcy Thompson, 1917) concept of morphology. Thus, qualities define each other, bootstrap fashion. Formally, the internal (i.e., by the perceiver itself) description would have to be based on various symmetry principles. This is similar to what happens in mathematics (e.g., projective geometry). The parts (points, lines, planes, etc.) are defined in terms of symmetry properties and relations to each other and the whole (i.e., projective geometry) is due to the parts and their relations. A "point" remains undefined *as such*.[12] In fact, in the projective plane, the "points" and "lines" may be interchanged without changing the geometry. Similar notions apply to painting. The painter paints no leaves, but foliage-like texture (think of Fragonard or Corot, for instance). You "read" the texture as "leafiness," the total blob of paint as a treetop. The treetop depends upon the leafiness (a uniform green blob would hardly appear "tree-like"), and the leafiness depends on its being part of the treetop (a square filled with the same texture might not read as "leafiness" at all). The same remarks apply to drawing (figure 1.2). Notice how scribbles and blobs of ink "depict" in a large variety of different ways and how large parts (about one half of the "woman" at bottom left) remain undrawn but are hallucinated by the observer. Thus the mereology of iconic symbolic forms (presentations) is *circular*, indeed necessarily so because they have no independent parts. The internal part of perception remains largely unexplored territory (see Albertazzi, 2008), and formal descriptions are largely lacking.

Properties

In the external (i.e., by an observer of the perceiver) description, one attempts to correlate relations between qualities with physical structural relations. Such relations may be arbitrarily complicated and need make little sense from the *a priori* perspective of the physicist. A trivial example of the laboratory type is Kanizsa's triangle (see figure 1.3). It is often held that the triangle presents itself in the "absence of stimulation" ("amodally"), but this is nonsense. In order for the triangle to present itself the optical structure available to the observer has to be of a very special kind. The relevant physical structures that admit the presentation of Kanizsa's triangle are well understood. The confusion arises from the fact that the necessary structures are unexpected to the scientist with a narrow reductionist mind set.

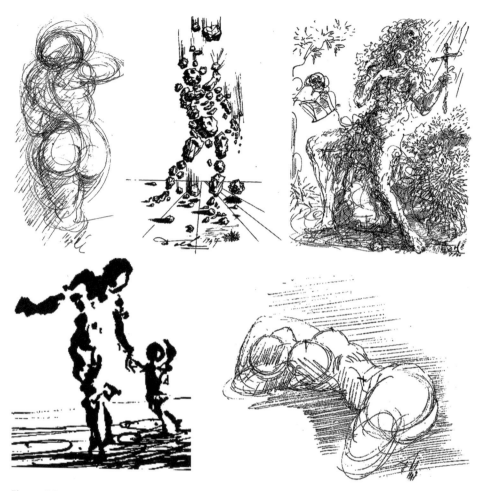

Figure 1.2
A small set of drawings by Dali (from the *50 secretos magicos para pintar*), all depicting human bodies. Notice the meaning of the various scribbles and blobs, also the function of the white spaces.

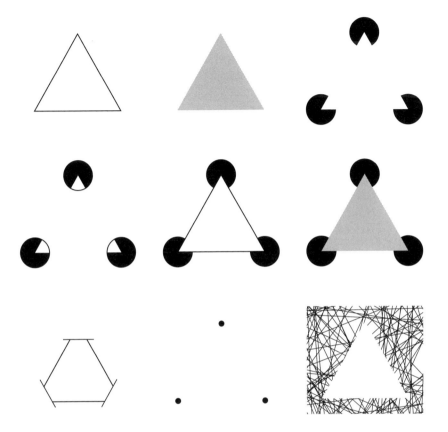

Figure 1.3
Some scenes that give rise to presentations containing a "triangle." Notice that the scenes are quite different as planar pigment distributions go. Top right is the Kanizsa triangle; it looks similar to the triangle at bottom right, lighter than the paper. Center left is also similar but largely occluded because seen through three holes. Top left has the color of the paper but looks less material than top center. The "materiality" improves a lot in the versions at center and center right. Bottom left is a triangle with tips inserted in slits in the paper and looks more "real" than bottom center. The latter is perhaps the least salient as a triangle, it appears more like an afterthought as it were. It would be easy to continue this series ad infinitum. What is the "adequate stimulus" for a phenomenal triangle?

"Properties" belong to "objects" as actual parts of the (physical) world. The objects of your presentations do not have "properties," they have "qualities." For instance, the Kanizsa triangle apparently has a lightness that exceeds that of the paper it is printed on. Because the Kanizsa triangle exists only in your presentation, this quality cannot be correlated with any "corresponding" property. It might seem different for the case of the paper. You see it as having a certain "lightness." Because a corresponding object exists in the world (a flattish sheet of wood pulp) that has a certain physical property known as "reflectance," classical psychophysics treats the lightness quality as causally related to the reflectance property. In folk psychology, one says that you "see the lightness of the paper" *in the world*. Because the paper is always taken as "given" it is sometimes said that the lightness (in the mind) is "attributed" to the paper (in the world). There is not a *little* confusion here.

To avoid unfortunate confusions, one needs to keep the level of physical description strictly separate from the level of presentations. Because presentations are prior to physics, it makes little sense to explain presentations on the basis of physics, yet this is the classical praxis. Hard-nosed scientists even believe that (eventually) perceptions will be "reduced" to physics. It makes more sense to look for correlations in the physical description with the qualities of presentations. Such correlations need not be obvious, as the example of the lightness of Kanizsa's triangle indicates.

Toward a New Psychophysics

The concept of "veridical vision" cannot be given any sense at all, contrary to the conventional assumptions in the vision sciences. What would it have to be, the quantum mechanical wave function of the universe perhaps? All vision is but the act of some agent. The building blocks of vision are threads of experience that are possible for that agent. What is possible for the agent again depends on the agent's evolutionary history and its life's experience as much as the structure of its biotope. Of course, these are closely knit together. *Euglena*'s optical world is exhausted by the local radiation density and the net radiation flux vector (or "light vector") (Gershun, 1936), the cat's optical world is rather more differentiated. This is why Bertrand Russell's (1912) notion of "sense data" as clean, value–free data, untinged by cognition, is utterly useless; there can be no such things.

The fact that the observer may blindly rely on the structure of its Umwelt (based on immensely long evolutionary time spans) means that the Holmes' type of information gathering is likely to be fast and effective (Riedl, 1975). Essentially *any* question serves to start the process. Almost any misdirected question will lead to a negated expectation at the first try. Almost any applicable expectation will grow to certainty after a few verifications. Because the Umwelt is highly and hierarchically structured, questions can be generated in an informationally (in Shannon's sense) optimal way, much like in the game of "20 questions."[13] This is generally not acknowledged in vision science because the important questions to ask are so obvious that the human observer handles them fully preconsciously. It is Brunswik's (1955) "ratiomorphic apparatus" that handles the bulk of perception without our even noticing. The research problems pursued in the study of vision implicitly take all of this for granted and only start where cognition kicks in. To begin to study the fundamental structure of perception, one needs an understanding of the human Umwelt. Here visual artists have reached a pragmatic understanding that far outstrips the scarce explicit scientific knowledge. Biology may yield the best handles on the problem because it allows one to study observers, which have Umwelts that are much reduced relative to the human one and have senses alien to the human, which much promotes an objective approach. A famous example is the tick whose recognition of a "mammal" is triggered by the coincidence of the scent of butyric acid and a 37°C temperature. This is rather (and surprisingly) different from my own definition (would *you* ever have thought of the tick's one?). If the tick and I are said to share the "same" world, then the concept "world" becomes almost irrelevant and has to be replaced with that of "interface," the "other side" of the interface being largely superfluous.

Ecological Optics

The "material properties" of science (physics and chemistry) do not structure the Umwelt as they do the physical world. For instance, the nature of a "material" depends on distance: A "distant forest" has a certain velvety character that is missing in "treetops at a distance," which often have a peculiar fluffy character, quite different from "foliage," which again appears very different from a leafy branch. As a painter, you will paint different materials, although the physical objects may be the same. Again, the basic dichotomy between dielectrics and metals (conductors) fails to structure the Umwelt as is evident from the "silvery" appearance of moonlight on a rippled lake. The notion of a "homogeneous substance" is likewise different and depends on size (or, better, the span of simultaneous attention). "Granite" is a homogeneous substance (e.g., has a color, etc.) in large chunks but a conglomerate of differently colored mineral grains in sufficiently small pieces. Similar observations apply to spatial and temporal properties (topological or metrical), numerosity, colors, and so forth. Thus "inverse optics" as usually understood is ill suited as a prolegomena to psychophysics (as it indeed is to "machine vision" [Forsyth and Ponce, 2002]) and has to be replaced with an "ecological optics" that has yet to be developed in *optima forma*, although various shreds exist. In summary, it is the observer's "interface" that has to be described (in terms of itself!), and whether the "world beyond the interface" can be described (by us who only know the world through the interface) at all is a moot question (Hoffman, 2009) (anyway, that is the proper task of physics, not of psychology). The common objections against such a view derive from the reification of the "physical world" as distinct and independent from any observer's experiences.

An "information theory" of visual perception will largely have to coincide with such an "ecological optics." It will naturally divide into multitudinous branches, at least as many as there are Umwelts. Here is the basis for a viable psychophysics.

Acknowledgments

I am grateful to Liliana Albertazzi, Andrea van Doorn, Joseph Lappin and Whitman Richards for their critical remarks on (earlier versions of) the chapter.

Notes

1. Shakespeare, W. *Hamlet*, Act III. Scene ii, 1602.

2. *Oxford American Dictionaries*, Version 1.0.1 (1.0.1). Copyright © 2005 Apple Computer, Inc. All rights reserved.

3. Ibid.

4. Ibid.

5. Ibid.

6. Ibid.

7. Ibid.

8. Plotinus ca. 205–270, *Ennead* I.6 [1], On Beauty, Translated by Stephen MacKenna, http://eawc .evansville.edu/anthology/beauty.htm.

9. On von Uexküll's "*Lebenskreisen*"; see his "*Umwelt und Innenwelt der Tiere.*" 1921. 2ed. Berlin: Springer.

10. Shakespeare, W. *Romeo and Juliet*, Act II, Scene ii, 1597.

11. See the catalog from the Bonnard retrospective held at the Museum of Modern Art in 1998.

12. David Hilbert in a letter to Frege writes: "If I take for my points any system of things, for example, the system love, law, chimney-sweep, . . . and I just assume all my axioms as relations between these things, my theorems—for example, the theorem of Pythagoras—also hold of these things," 29 December 1899.

13. On the game of "20 questions," see: http://barelybad.com/20questions.htm.

References

Adelson, E. H., and Bergen, J. R. 1991. "The Plenoptic Function and the Elements of Early Vision." In *Computational Models of Visual Processing*, edited by M. Landy and J. A. Movshon. Cambridge, Mass.: MIT Press, 3–20.

Albertazzi, L. 2006. "Das rein Figurale—The Shadowy Scheme of the Form." *Gestalt Theory* 28: 123–151.

Albertazzi, L. 2008. "The Ontology of Perception." In *TAO–Theory and Applications of Ontology, Vol. 1, The Philosophical Stance*, edited by R. Poli, J. Seibt and J. Symons. Berlin: Springer.

d'Arcy Thompson, W. 1917. *On Growth and Form*. Cambridge: Cambridge University Press.

Antonioni, M. (Director, writer), *Blow up* (movie), 1966. (Producer Carlo Ponti, Cinematographer Carlo di Palma)

Bachelard, Gaston. 1938. *La formation de l'esprit scientifique*. (The Formation of the Scientific Spirit) Paris: Vrin.

Baring–Gould, William S. 1967. *The Annotated Sherlock Holmes*. New York: Clarkson N. Potter, Inc. & London: John Murray Publishers.

Barlow, H. B. 1972. "A Speculative Attempt to Account for the Performance of Complex Perceptual Tasks on Terms of Known Properties of Nerve Cells." *Perception* 1: 371–394.

Bayes, T. 1763. "An Essay Towards solving a Problem in the Doctrine of Chances. By the late Rev. Mr. Bayes, F. R. S. communicated by Mr. Price, in a letter to John Canton, A. M. F. R. S." *Philosophical Transactions, Giving Some Account of the Present Undertakings, Studies and Labours of the Ingenious in Many Considerable Parts of the World* 53: 370–418.

Bell, J. L. 1998. *A Primer of Infinitesimal Analysis*. Cambridge: Cambridge University Press.

Berkeley, G. 1709. *An Essay Towards a New Theory of Vision*. Dublin: Printed by Aaron Rhames, at the Back of Dicks Coffee–House, for Jeremy Pepyat, Bookseller in Skinner-Row.

Block, N. 2003. "Mental Paint." In *Reflections and Replies, Essays on the Philosophy of Tyler Burge*, edited by M. Hahn and B. Ramberg. Cambridge Mass: MIT Press.

Blyth, R. H. 1996. *Zen and Zen Classics*, Vol. 4: Mumonkan. Japan: The Hokuseido Press.

Bradley, D. R., and Petry, H. M. 1977. "Organizational Determinants of Subjective Contour: The Subjective Necker Cube." *American Journal of Psychology* 90: 253–262.

Braitenberg, V. 1984. *Vehicles: Experiments in Synthetic Psychology*. Cambridge Mass: MIT Press.

Brentano, F. 1995. *Psychology from Empirical Standpoint*. London: Routledge (original 1874).

Bridgman, P. W. 1959. *The Way Things Are*. Cambridge Mass: Harvard University Press.

Brown, J. W. 2002. *Self–Embodying Mind: Process, Brain Dynamics and the Conscious Present*. Barytown NY: Barytown Ltd.

Brunswik, E. 1955. "Representative Design and Probabilistic Theory in a Functional Psychology." *Psychological Review* 62: 193–217.

Cassirer, E. 1923–1929. *Philosophy of Symbolic Forms*. Berlin: Bruno Cassirer.

Cortazar, J. 1959. *Las Armas Secretas* (Secret Weapons). Buenos Aires: Editorial Sudamericana.

Costall, A. 2006. "'Introspectionism' and the Mythical Origins of Scientific Psychology." *Consciousness and Cognition* 15: 634–654.

Denis, M. 1998. "Definition of Neo-Traditionalism." In *Art in Theory 1815–1900: An Anthology of Changing Ideas*, edited by Ch. Harrison, P. Wood and J. Gaiger. Oxford: Blackwell Publishing Ltd, 862–869.

Forsyth, D. A., and Ponce, J. 2002. *Computer Vision: A Modern Approach*. Upper Saddle River NJ: Prentice–Hall.

Gershun, A. 1939. (Moscow, 1936). "The Light Field." Translated by P. Moon and G. Timoshenko in *Journal of Mathematics and Physics*, Vol. XVIII: 51–151.

Gibson, J. J. 1950. *The Perception of the Visual World*. Boston: Houghton Mifflin.

Goethe, J. W. 1789/1790. "Versuch, die Metamorphose der Pflanzen zu erklären" (Attempt to Explain the Metamorphosis of Plants). "Versuch über die Gestalt der Tiere (1790)" (Essay on the Shape of Animals). "Erster Entwurf einer allgemeinen Einleitung in die vergleichende Anatomie, ausgehend von der Osteologie (1795)" (First Draft of a General Introduction to Comparative Anatomy, Based on the Osteology). See http://www.steinerschule.ch/goethe/werke.html.

Goethe, J. W. 1808–1810. *Zur Farbenlehre. Didaktischer Teil.* (The Theory of Colour. Didactic Part). Tübingen: J. G. Cotta.

Goethe, J. W. 1978. "Zahmen Xenien." (Tame Reminders). In *Goethes Werke*, Band I, 367, Hamburg: Christian Wegner Verlag.

Gombrich, E. 1960. *Art and Illusion: A Study in the Psychology of Pictorial Representation*. London: Phaidon.

Hadamard, J. 1902. "Sur les problèmes aux dérivées partielles et leur signification physique" (On the Problems with Partial Derivatives and their Physical Meaning). *Princeton University Bulletin*: 49–52.

Hartmann, N. 1942. "Neue Wege der Ontologie" (New Ways of Ontology). In *Systematische Philosophie*, edited by N. Hartmann. Stuttgart, Germany: Kohlhammer: Stuttgart-Berlin. 1–17.

Hebb, D. O. 1966. *Textbook of Psychology*. Philadelphia: Saunders.

Helmholtz, H. von. 1860. *Handbuch der Physiologischen Optik* (Handbook of Physiological Optics). Leipzig: Voss.

Hoffman, D. D. 2009. "The Interface Theory of Perception: Natural Selection Drives True Perception to Swift Extinction." In *Object Categorization: Computer and Human Vision Perspectives*, edited by S. Dickinson, M. Tarr, A. Leonardis, and B. Schiele. Cambridge UK: Cambridge University Press.

Hoyle, F. 1968. *October the First is Too Late*. Harmondsworth: Penguin Books.

Hubel, D. 1989. *Eye, Brain, and Vision*. New York: W. H. Freeman.

Kandinsky, W. 1926. *Punkt und Linie zu Fläche, Beitrag zur Analyse malerischen Elemente* (Point and Line to Plane, Contribution to the Analysis of Pictorial Elements). Bauhaus Bücher Bnd. 9. München: Verlag Albert Langen.

Kant, I. 1968. *Werke*. Gruyter Verlag. Akademie Textausgabe (Nachdruck 1968, 9 Bnde. Photo-mechanischer Abdruck des Textes der von der Preussischen Akademie der Wissenschaften 1902 begonnenen Ausgabe von Kants gesammelten Schriften. Band 3: Kritik der reinen Vernunft (Nachdruck der 2. Auflage 1787); Band 4: u.a.: Kritik der reinen Vernunft (Nachdruck der 1. Auflage 1781).

Kant, I. 1783. *Prolegomena zu einer jeden künftigen Metaphysik, die als Wissenschaft wird auftreten können* (Prolegomena to Any Future Metaphysics that will Occur as a Science). Riga: Johann Friedrich Hartknoch.

Kheirandish, E. 1998. *The Arabic Version of Euclid's Optics*. New York: Springer.

Knill, D. C., and Richards, W. 1996. *Perception as Bayesian Inference*. Cambridge, UK: Cambridge University Press.

Langer, S. 1942. *Philosophy in a New Key: A Study in the Symbolism of Reason, Rite, and Art*. Cambridge, Mass.: Harvard University Press.

Langer, S. 1953. *Feeling and Form: A Theory of Art*. New York: Scribner.

Leonardo da Vinci. 1796 (orig. ca. 1680). *A Treatise on Painting by Leonardo da Vinci*. London: I. and J. Taylor.

Leyton, M. 1992. *Symmetry, Causality, Mind*. Cambridge, Mass.: MIT Press.

Lorenz, K. 1973. *Die Rückseite des Spiegels: Versuch einer Naturgeschichte des menschlichen Erkennens* (The Backside of the Mirror: Essay of a Natural History of Human Understanding). München: Piper Verlag.

Lotze, H. 1876. *Mikrokosmos. Ideen zur Naturgeschichte und Geschichte der Menschheit. Versuch einer Anthropologie*. Leipzig: Hirzel.

MacKay, D. M. 1950. "Quantal Aspects of Scientific Information." *Philos. Mag.* 41: 293–311.

MacKay, D. M. 1969. *Information, Mechanism and Meaning*. Cambridge, Mass. and London: MIT Press.

Marr, D. 1982. *Vision*. San Francisco: W. H. Freeman.

McCarthy, J. 1959. "Programs with Common Sense." In *Mechanisation of Thought Processes, Proceedings of the Symposium of the National Physics Laboratory*. London, UK: Her Majesty's Stationery Office, 77–84.

Metzger, W. 1953. *Gesetze des Sehens* (Laws of Vision). Frankfurt am Main: Kramer Verlag.

Meyer–Eppler, W. 1969. *Grundlagen und Anwendungen der Informationstheorie* (Fundaments and Applications of Information Theory). Berlin: Springer.

Minsky, M. 1974. "A Framework for Representing Knowledge." *MIT–AI Lab Memo* 306.

Nagel, T. 1974. "What is it Like to be a Bat?" *Philosophical Review* 83: 435–450.

Neisser, U. 1967. *Cognitive Psychology*. New York: Appleton–Century–Crofts.

Nietzsche, F. 1901. *Der Wille zur Macht* (The Will to Power). Leipzig: hg. von E. Förster–Nietzsche und P. Gast.

Nietzsche, F. 1977. *Umwertung aller Werte, 2. Auflage* (Reappraisal of all Values). München: Deutscher Taschenbuch Verlag.

Palmer, S. E. 1999. *Vision Science: Photons to Phenomenology*. Cambridge, MA: MIT Press.

Pestilli, L. 1993. "Ut Pictura Non Poesis: Lord Shaftesbury's "Ridiculous Anticipation of Metamorphosis" and the Two Versions of "Diana and Actaeon" by Paolo de Matteis." *Artibus et Historiæ* 14, no. 27: 131–139.

Pierce, C. S. 1955. *Philosophical Writings of Pierce*, edited by J. Buchler. New York: Dover.

Poggio, T. 1984. "Low-level Vision as Inverse Optics." In *Proceedings of Symposium on Computational Models of Hearing and Vision*, edited by M. Rauk. Academy of Sciences of the Estonian S.S.R. 123–127.

Poli, R. 2001. "The Basic Problem of the Theory of Levels of Reality." *Axiomathes* 12: 261–283.

Proust, M. 1913–1927. *À la recherche du temps perdu* (In Search of Lost Time). Paris: Grasset and Gallimard.

Purves, D., Lotto, R. B., Williams, S. M., Nundy, S., and Yang, Z. 2001. "Why we See Things the Way we Do: Evidence for a Wholly Empirical Strategy of Vision." *Phil. Trans. Roy. Soc. London B–Bio Sci* 356: 285–297.

Riedl, R. 1975. *Die Ordnung des Lebendigen. Systembedingungen der Evolution* (The Order of the Living. System Conditions of Evolution). Hamburg: Paul Parey.

Rosenberg, A. 2000. *Philosophy of Science: A Contemporary Introduction*. London, UK: Routledge.

Ruskin, J. 1843–1860. "The Fullness and Mystery of Turner's Distances." In *Modern Painters*, Volume 1, Part II, Section II, Ch. V, §11. London: George Routledge & Sons.

Russell, B. 1912. *The Problems of Philosophy*. London: Hazell, Watson and Viney (Home University Library).

Schopenhauer, A. 1818/1819 (vol 2, 1844). *Die Welt als Wille und Vorstellung* (The World as Will and Presentation). Leipzig: Brockhhaus.

Schrödinger, E. 1944. *What is Life?* Cambridge, UK: Cambridge University Press.

Searle, J. 1983. *Intentionality: An Essay in the Philosophy of Mind*. Cambridge, UK: Cambridge University Press.

Shannon, C. E. 1948. "A Mathematical Theory of Communication, Part I." *Bell Systems Technical Journal* 27: 379–42.

Skinner, B. F. 1945. "The Operational Analysis of Psychological Terms." *Psychological Review* 52: 270–277, 290–294.

Tinbergen, N. 1951. *The Study of Instinct*. Oxford: Clarendon Press.

Tinbergen, N. 1975. *The Animal and its World*, Vol. 1. Cambridge, Mass.: Harvard University Press.

Tolhurst, D. J. 1972. "On the Possible Existence of Edge Detector Neurones in the Human Visual System." *Vision Research* 12: 797–804.

Uexküll, J. v. 1940/1982. "The Theory of Meaning." *Semiotica* 42, no. 1: 25–82.

VanCleave, J. 1997. *Janice VanCleave's Guide to the Best Science Fair Projects*. New York: John Wiley & Sons, Inc.

Vico, G. 2002. *The First New Science*, edited and translated by Leon Pompa. Cambridge, UK: Cambridge University Press. (Original, 1725.)

Watson, J. B. 1920. "Is Thinking Merely the Action of Learning Mechanisms?" *British Journal of Psychology* 11: 87–104.

Young, H. D., Freedman, R. A., Sandin, T. R., and Ford, L. A. 1999. *Sears and Zemansky's University Physics*. San Francisco: Addison Wesley.

I Time and Dynamics

2   Riddle of the Past, Puzzle for the Future

Ilona Kovács

The Riddle of the Dome[1]

In 1418, the *Opera del Duomo* (the office of works in charge) in Florence announced a competition to find a master builder who could erect the dome of Santa Maria del Fiore (figure 2.1). In fact, the construction of the cathedral started much earlier, in 1269. It was decided in 1376, that the dome would have to be built on a 52-meter-high drum, and the curvature of the dome should be calculated by the *quinto-acuto* or pointed-fifth measure (Gartner, 1998). The pointed-fifth implied that the radius of curvature had to be at a four-fifth diameter distance from the perimeter of the dome at the base, which results in a pointed arch that is taller than a circular arch and distributes the stresses along the arches into the ground, thereby greatly reducing hoop stresses (Director, 2003). The diameter of the octagon-shaped drum was 42 meters on the inside, and the planned height of the dome without the lantern was more than 80 meters (Gartner, 1998). All these parameters suggested that the cupola should be erected *senza armadura*—without internal scaffolding. Wooden or stone supporting structures of such enormous dimensions were considered either impossible or expensive. Calculations suggested that such *armadura* might even collapse under its weight. Among the competing masters, there was only one—Filippo Brunelleschi (figure 2.2)—who proposed to build the dome without scaffolding. After two years of bitter competition, Brunelleschi was assigned to build the cupola in 1420, and it was completed in 1436. Today, nearly 600 years later, Brunelleschi's cupola is still the largest masonry dome of the world.[2]

Unfortunately, there is little information on how this wonderful three-dimensional shape was constructed from bricks and mortar. The dome was built using approximately 4 million specially designed bricks weighing about 37,000 tons. Brunelleschi's brilliant masonry techniques[3] have been great contributions to architecture, and his work is probably the best example of Renaissance engineering (King, 2000). However, he was also secretive and never revealed his methods in detail. Although the dome is probably the most studied building on the planet, it is still uncertain how it was

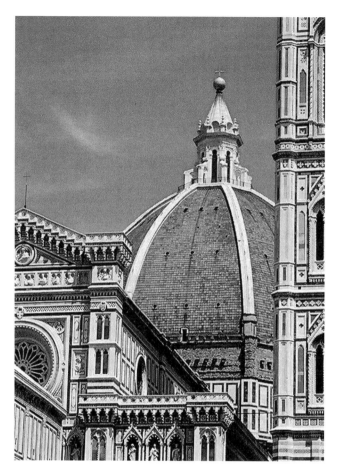

Figure 2.1
The dome of Santa Maria del Fiore, Florence (photo contributed by the author). The construction of the Florence Cathedral started in 1296, and the grand dome crowned it in 1436. Although Florentine pride at the time only wanted to surpass Pisa and Siena in the size and decoration of the cathedral, the cupola is still the largest masonry dome in the world.

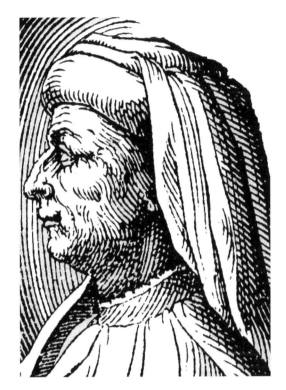

Figure 2.2
Filippo Brunelleschi (portrait by Giorgio Vasari, 1568). Filippo Brunelleschi (1377–1446), also known as "Pippo," was a Florentine goldsmith and architect. His most important architectural work is the dome of the Florence Cathedral. This Renaissance genius left us with exceptional architectural constructs and also with many questions. It is still not fully understood how he was able to erect the great dome of Florence without scaffolding.

built. It is not known exactly, for example, what instruction was given to the—assumedly—eight groups of bricklayers raising the cupola's eight sides. How were they to know the exact positioning of each brick? Walls are easy to raise vertically, although some quasi-global reference (e.g., a mason's level or a plumb line) is needed from time to time. However, when the wall is curved, there are three dimensions to control: (1) longitudinal curvature of the dome; (2) circumferential curvature; and (3) course by course, precise, and non-uniform change of the inward tilt of the bricks (figure 2.3). A simple plumb line, even if it is combined with a level, obviously cannot control these three dimensions.

Brunelleschi was a great geometer, and the plan of the dome was probably perfect. He even took care to design the shapes of the bricks for each new course himself.

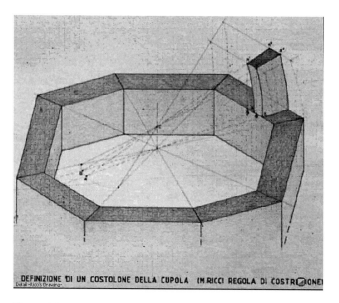

Figure 2.3

The three dimensions of the curved wall (with Massimo Ricci's kind permission). The *longitudinal curvature* of the dome of Santa Maria del Fiore is determined by the pointed-fifth measure: The radius of curvature in the intersecting arches is four fifths of the diameter. *Circumferential curvature* was approximately circular, with smaller and smaller circle diameters as height increased and with centers of curvature for each new course of bricks at the symmetry axis of the dome extending from the center of the drum to the lantern. Each new course of bricks had an increasing *inward angle*, reaching 60 degrees at the top. It is a true riddle how a bricklayer would be able to place *each individual brick* correctly according the requirements of these three dimensions.

However, even with the best planning and greatest care, bricklayers make slight errors, and if they only use local references (e.g., the previous course of bricks or the ribs of the dome), these small errors will add up. Even an error of a hundredth of a degree in any of the previously mentioned three dimensions would result in a catastrophe in the case of 4 million bricks. In fact, such a catastrophe was observed in Siena after a massive addition to the existing cathedral and dome was started in 1339. Although Sienese ambition was at least as high at that time as Florentine ambition, Brunelleschi's ingenuity only served Florence, and the great dome of Siena serves as a parking area in the back of the comparatively smaller cathedral today. Just how did Brunelleschi manage to control the global shape of the dome and achieve this unprecedented and still unequaled construction?

   With respect to the global shape of the dome, it may have seemed a good idea to use some central reference during the construction. However, wooden centering or scaffolding, which could have served to support as well as guide the overall arches, was not

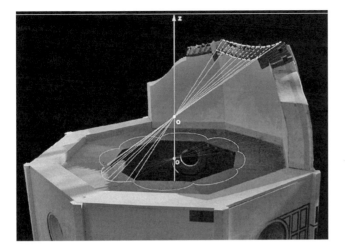

Figure 2.4
The flower theory (with Luciana Burdi's kind permission based on Massimo Ricci theory). The flower-shaped "skeleton" and many ropes between the flower and the wall serve to adjust the spatial position of the bricks according to the requirements of longitudinal, circumferential, and inward tilts. It is the symmetry axis of the shape that is employed as a global reference; however, the axis does not have to be there, it is determined with the help of ropes.

employed. How had the shape of the dome been preserved without any scaffolds to guide it? How does the complicated pattern of bricks fill the spaces between the corners of the dome? Imagine that eight bricklayer groups are working on the wall, and, other than along the circumference of the wall, they cannot compare notes. If there is no central pole of any kind (and there was none for sure because the dome is more than 80 meters high) to use as a reference and the masons cannot communicate with each other directly, how are the eight sides going to meet at the top? Perhaps there was some central reference, and communication through this reference after all, a reference which was removed after the dome was finished?

Massimo Ricci, a contemporary Italian architect, spent almost as much time trying to figure out the secret of the dome as did Brunelleschi building it. It took Ricci fifteen years of perplexity to come up with an idea that might be the practical solution of the dome riddle. According to him, the real secret of Santa Maria del Fiore is an extremely simple, although, in this context, surprising shape: the flower (figure 2.4). The eight petals of the flower grew out of a circle, centered within the octagonal base, with a diameter three-fifth of the octagon diameter (remember that the dome is based on a *quinto-acuto*, four-fifth measure). The flower was probably made of metal, and had long ropes attached to it, traversing the internal space of the dome. The shape of the petal controlled the circumferential curvature (dimension [2], as mentioned earlier), the length of the ropes attached to the petals controlled the longitudinal curvature (dimension [1]), and the tilt angle of the ropes controlled the inward tilt of the bricks (dimension [3]). Each rope, connecting a certain location of the wall to the petal across the base of the dome, was adjusted to cross the central axis of the cupola. This was achieved by centering ropes between the corners of the cupola and the vertices of the flower. When a bricklayer wanted to align a new brick, he would move his rope to the new position, and his apprentice would shift the other end of the rope along the petal until the rope crossed the central axis again in a straight line. Perhaps the procedure was not repeated for each individual brick, but whenever it was done, the brick adjusted this way must have fallen to its correct place according to the global reference point, and earlier local errors did not accumulate any further. This sounds like the solution indeed!

Even if historical evidence for the flower theory is missing, Ricci's scale model of the dome attests to the feasibility of it. The idea is simple: *When only local operators are given, use an axis-based global reference in order to achieve a global shape and avoid the accumulation of local errors.* According to Ricci, this is the only way to construct such a shape. Even if appearing ambitious, the usefulness of symmetry axes in avoiding the accumulation of local errors is clearly illustrated with this example, and that was our aim.

The Puzzle of "Closure"[4]

Among the many unsolved issues of vision, the issue of segmentation might be one of the toughest. Although it does not sound difficult to parse an image into different regions that correspond to objects and ground, machine or computer vision systems still cannot match the capabilities of the human visual system in this respect, not to talk about categorization and image comprehension that are strongly linked to segmentation. Human segmentation of visual images might indeed be dependent on acquired knowledge and proceed interactively with object recognition (e.g., Ullman, 2007). However, the explicit manner in which these higher level knowledge systems communicate with low-level feature extractors has not been clarified yet.

The problem is similar to Brunelleschi's riddle. On the one hand, there is obviously some higher order intentionality (paralleling the conceptualization of the three-dimensional structure of the dome) globally organized by the brain. On the other hand, there is the continuous sensing of the environment, the first steps of presenting potentially meaningful features of some sort (parallel laying of the individual bricks of the dome). Just how will these different levels of processing—global organization versus local analysis (or global analysis vs. local organization)—meet and interact to result in the visual world as we relate to it? How is the accumulation of local errors avoided in cortical processing?

According to the "standard" view of visual processing, visual information is first transmitted from the retina through several parallel pathways to the brain in a compressed version, emphasizing edge information at a number of spatial scales. A crucial second step is carried out by cortical area 17 (or primary visual cortex) that is assumed to extract a set of local features based on the retinal input. Although the "standard" view then proceeds to progressively more complex representations, let us now take a look at the second step and the cortical "mosaic" generated by the primary visual cortex. It has been known for more than 40 years that the receptive fields of the primary visual cortex are composed of elongated antagonistic zones (Hubel and Wiesel, 1959). The shape and layout of these receptive fields furnish the cells with selectivity for oriented line segments, and receptive field size determines the spatial scale of orientation information.

The primary visual cortex thus provides a neural description of oriented edge primitives and their locations at a number of spatial scales. This can be viewed as an enormous puzzle containing millions of pieces to be put together into figure and ground. A possible candidate for assembling local information already within the primary visual cortex is the plexus of long-range horizontal connections (e.g., Gilbert, 1992). These connections are suspected to establish connections between neighboring processing units and help the segmentation process. However, we find the same problem that the bricklayers had to face when constructing a curved wall: Tiny errors in the local interactions might add up, and the boundaries of a visual object will never meet (figure 2.5). Local interactions help a great deal, just as plumb lines and mason's levels; however, some global reference might be needed.

Earlier, we designed a psychophysical paradigm to challenge the local filters and local interactions model of the primary visual cortex, and to investigate the type of integration that might be carried out at this "early" cortical level (Kovács and Julesz, 1993). The stimulus used in this paradigm consisted of a closed chain of collinearly aligned Gabor signals (contour) and a background of randomly oriented and positioned Gabor signals (noise) (figure 2.6). Gabor signals roughly model the receptive field properties of orientation selective simple cells in the primary visual cortex. Therefore, they are appropriate stimuli for the examination of these small spatial filters and their interactions. Notice that the contours cannot be detected purely by local filters or by neurons with large receptive field sizes corresponding to the size of the contour. The long-range orientation correlations along the path of the contour can only be found by the integration of local orientation measurements. The noise forces the observer to rely on local measurements at the scale of the individual Gabor signals and on long-range interactions between local filters while connecting the signals as a whole.

Because the "contour in noise" stimulus was designed to isolate long-range interactions subserving spatial integration of orientation information in the primary visual cortex, all we expected was that human observers would be able to detect the contours

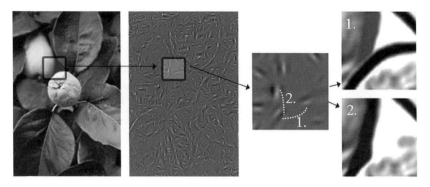

Figure 2.5
The cortical puzzle. The primary visual cortex provides a neural description of oriented edge primitives and their locations at a number of spatial scales. The natural image in the first panel will activate a large number cortical filters; however, those that receive input according to their selectivities will be more active. The second panel shows the most activated filters for each location within the image. Neural interactions within the primary visual cortex are assumed to connect the most active filters in an orientation-selective, facilitatory manner (e.g., similar-to-similar orientations). However, when viewed locally within the inset, it seems that these connections might be ambiguous. Should there be a strong facilitatory connection there according to 1 or 2? 1 is a good choice; the central object will be well segmented. However, 2 would be a very bad choice, connecting the boundaries of two independent objects. Is there some global reference guiding these local decisions (remember the bricklayer's problem in adjusting the position of each brick in 3D)?

even if noise density is greater than contour density (in other words, when noise elements are closer to each other than contour elements). This was indeed observed, but another surprising observation surfaced: Closed contours in these images were much easier to see than open ones (Kovács and Julesz, 1993). We called this a "closure superiority" effect: Closure superiority can be measured at perceptual thresholds. Threshold effects are difficult to illustrate. Figure 2.6 is an attempt to illustrate the results of the experiments in an example demonstration. According to the results, despite the locally equivalent parameters (same elements and same space spacing parameters), closed contours are perceived differently—they seem to get a kick during the segmentation process.

Here is the puzzle for the future: If local features are detected by local filters, and their interactions are also local (between neighbors), what makes the elements of a closed contour jump out and the same types of elements along an open one remain blend with noise? Closure is a global shape property (similarly to the shape of the dome). Local filters and local interactions—even if they form long chains—cannot deal with a global shape property. Local errors will accumulate along the chains of

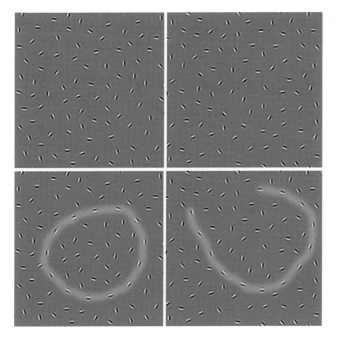

Figure 2.6
The closure effect. The top two panels both have a contour embedded in noise. The solutions are
presented in the bottom panels. Most observers find the closed contour in the upper left panel
easy to see, whereas it is difficult to trace the open contour even in the presence of the solution
(because of individual variability in noise tolerance, certain individuals might need different
noise levels for the closure effect to show up).

local interactions, and the result will be uncertain. Top-down instructions arriving
from higher levels of the cortical hierarchy may not be helpful either. The higher level
"hypotheses" about the shape will meet unsegmented local orientation signals (contour
+ noise), and, in such a dense field of elements, any global suggestion can take shape,
and the result will be uncertain again. Are there more than just local interactions during segmentation in the primary visual cortex? Is there some kind of global reference
serving segmentation the same way as the Brunelleschi–Ricci flower served the erecting
of the dome? If there is such a reference system, what are the strings (taking the analogy further) in the brain connecting the flower and the bricks?

The answer might be in computational models (e.g., Li, 2005) or the careful investigation of cortical microcircuits (e.g., Angelucci et al., 2002). However, one should not
forget the warning of a great Gestaltist: "If a line forms a closed, or almost closed, figure, we see no longer merely a line on a homogeneous background, but a surface figure
bounded by the line" (Koffka, 1935, p. 150). The riddle of the dome and the puzzle of

closure are, indeed, aptly related to the Brentanian idea of *Prägnanz*: The wonderful shape of the dome is not simply a collection of arches, it is a three-dimensional volume; the closed line is not simply a collection of line segments, it is a circular whole. Ricci's flower theory presents us with a good suggestion as to how the Gestalt of the dome can be assembled from millions of bricks using an ingeniously simple line of reference: the main symmetry axis of the dome. Do symmetry axes play a crucial role in vision as well? In a series of experiments, we asked this question with respect to the cortical representation of simple two-dimensional shapes. For example, how is a closed circle represented in the activity pattern of orientation tuned neurons possessing small receptive fields? Simultaneous activity of a large number of interacting neural elements can be revealed by tracking the activity of several units in search of their higher order correlations, such as in electrophysiological cross-correlation and multiunit studies. An alternative is to estimate how the activity of one unit is affected in the context of the activity of other units. We used the latter approach in a psychophysical reverse-mapping technique, where the activity of one unit is measured as a function of the gradually changing context. Psychophysically measured local contrast sensitivity reflects the local activity of neurons, and the context of the interaction pattern can be manipulated by changing the overall stimulus design. We employed closed contours (illustrated in figure 2.6) as context and single Gabor signals to obtain local contrast sensitivity of human observers (Kovács and Julesz, 1994). The position of the local signals varied within the closed contours, and by measuring sensitivity for many locations within these contours, a map of contrast sensitivity was obtained for each investigated shape (circle, ellipse, cardioid [i.e., heart shape], triangle) (described in detail in Kovács, Fehér, and Julesz, 1998; Kovács, 1996).

To be able to see whether any sensitivity change within these contours is related to the symmetry axes of the shape, we used a medial–axis-type transformation (see e.g., Blum, 1967; Leymarie and Kimia, 2008; Leyton, 1992). The medial-axis type or skeletal representation of shape was introduced to vision science by Blum (1967) and was derived by the so-called grassfire transformation. The grassfire transformation has several modern versions also known as the medial-axis transformation (MAT) (see e.g., Ogniewicz, 1993). The advantages of the MAT are that it is compact and captures important properties, such as symmetry and complexity, in a translation- and rotation-invariant manner. Following Blum's early studies, it has been shown in several excellent studies, ranging from computer science through psychophysics to neurophysiology, that a medial–axis-type representation might indeed have biological relevance and might be important in perceptual processing (see e.g., Burbeck and Pizer, 1996; Lee et al., 1998; Leymarie and Kimia, 2008; Leyton, 1992; Van Tonder, Lyons, and Ejima, 2002). Our procedure was intended to advance the MAT-type descriptions by increasing locality and compactness and easing the computational costs of a multiscale representation. The goal was to find the most informative points along the skeleton (medial axis) of a

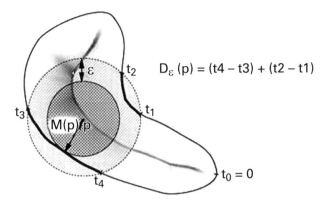

$$D_\varepsilon (p) = (t4 - t3) + (t2 - t1)$$

Figure 2.7
The D_ε function. D_ε is defined for each internal point by the percentage of the boundary points that are equidistant from the internal point within a tolerance of $_\varepsilon$.

shape. The D_ε function, as shown in figure 2.7, is based on an equidistance metric, where the D_ε value of each internal point represents the degree to which this point can be considered as the center of the local boundary segment around it. The transformation provides a non-uniform skeleton of the shape with one or more peak values. The peaks are important; they are equidistant from the longest segments of the boundary. In other words, these points are the most informative (Leyton, 1987), and long contour segments can be traded for them. We used the maxima of the D_ε function, which we called the medial-point representation, to predict potential sensitivity changes within the simple shapes mentioned earlier. If there is any symmetry axis-related change in local contrast sensitivity, it should be around these maxima.

To our great surprise, the D_ε function was a wonderful predictor of psychophysical performance. The prediction worked for the simple shapes shown in figure 2.8, for other ellipses, and for shapes with curved and branching symmetry axes as well (Kovács et al., 1998). The contrast sensitivity changes were extremely specific, not simply some inside-specific enhancements. The maxima of the sensitivity changes corresponded to the maxima of the D_ε function. Neural correlates of these results have also been found in the modulation profiles of single-cell activity in the primary visual cortex (Lee, 2003; Lee et al., 1998), although further confirmation of these correlates would be useful. The psychophysical and neurophysiological data at least indicate that the primary visual cortex, in addition to processing global shape properties such as closure and figure-ground relationships, is capable of processing specific shape properties and hosting a medial–point-type representation. The most provocative possibility is that this early cortical area provides a sparse skeletal, symmetry-based code of shape (also see Leyton, 1992).

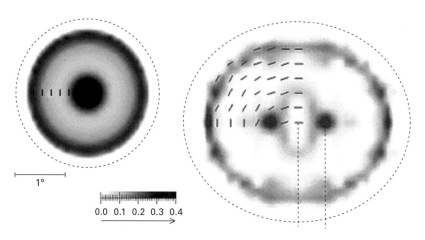

Figure 2.8
Sensitivity maps. Sensitivity maps for a perfect circle and an ellipse of 1.2 aspect ratio. The dotted lines show the contours within which contrast sensitivity was measured for local probes. The vertical lines within the circle and the tilted lines within the upper left quadrant of the ellipse show the relative locations of the test probes within the shapes. Measurements carried out at those test-probe locations were used to plot the map of sensitivity changes. Light shading represents an increase in contrast sensitivity, and scale is in log units (replotted from Kovács and Julesz, 1994).

Conclusion

However, the puzzle for the future remains: Are the closure superiority effect and the related contrast sensitivity maps merely epiphenomena or are they the pulse of purposeful contribution by the primary visual cortex toward the process of vision? If the latter, how is it implemented precisely in the cortex? Perhaps some non-oscillatory but synchronous firing of orientation-tuned neurons mediates the compression and provides "hot-spots" in the neural representation of the segmented visual input. In what neural form would these "hot-spots" then be transmitted to more abstract levels of processing to meet with linguistic representations and semantic memory? How would the enriched information then proceed through the feedback pathways to enhance segmentation? In trying to answer these questions, it is useful to remember Brentano's message: Higher levels of organization might not be understood purely by accounting for the elements—organizational rules between these elements need to be discovered.

Acknowledgments

I.K. was supported by TAMOP-4.2.2-08/1/KMR-2008-0007.

Notes

1. This is also the title of a BBC Open University video (1999, ISBN: 9780749233358), which takes the viewers into the secrets of the Florence Cathedral. The video reveals the ideas of a contemporary architect, Massimo Ricci, who claims to have solved the riddle.

2. The other great masonry dome of Saint Peter's Cathedral in Rome (finished in 1590) reaches higher from the ground; however, the cupola of Santa Maria del Fiore, as measured from the top of the drum, is taller. Michelangelo planned the dome in Rome to be a hemispheric one. Later, Giacomo della Porta modified the plans, and the cupola has an elliptic curve between the hemispheric and *quinto-acuto* measures (Norwich, 1975). Both domes were based on a 42-meter-wide drum. Therefore, the Florentine dome, with its gothic pointed fifth, is, in fact, taller.

3. Two important techniques helped to provide the static balance of the dome during the process of building. The tool of *corda banda* (a loose rope or hanging chain between the ribs of the dome; in modern geometry, the catenary line) ensured that the wall was self-supporting during the course of its development because of equal physical tension at each point (Director, 2003). A special *herringbone* pattern in laying the bricks helped to keep them from falling inside at the increasing inward angle of the wall.

4. "Closure" is an old Gestaltist term used, for example, by Kurt Koffka in his 1935 book, *Principles of Gestalt Psychology*. The term refers to the superiority of closed contours over open ones.

References

Angelucci, A., Levitt, J. B., Walton, E. J. S., Hupé, J.-M., Bullier, J., and Lund, J. S. 2002. "Circuits for Local and Global Signal Integration in Primary Visual Cortex." *The Journal of Neuroscience* 22 (19): 8633–8646.

Blum, H. J. 1967. "A New Model of Global Brain Function." *Perspectives in Biology and Medicine* 10: 381–407.

Burbeck, C. A., and Pizer, S. M. 1996. "Object Representation by Cores: Identifying and Representing Primitive Spatial Regions." *Vision Research* 35 (13): 1917–1930.

Director, B. 2003. "The Long Life of the Catenary: From Brunelleschi to La Rouche." *Fidelio* XII (1): 100–111.

Gartner, P. J. 1998. *Filippo Brunelleschi 1377–1446*. Koln: Konemann.

Gilbert, C. D. 1992. "Horizontal Integration and Cortical Dynamics." *Neuron* 9 (1): 1–13.

Hubel, D. H., and Wiesel, T. N. 1959. "Receptive Fields of Single Neurons in the Cat's Visual Cortex." *Journal of Phisiology* (London) 148: 574–591.

King, R. 2000. *Brunelleschi's Dome: How a Renaissance Genius Reinvented Architecture*. New York: Penguin Books.

Koffka, K. 1935. *Principles of Gestalt Psychology*. New York: Harcourt, Brace.

Kovács, I. 1996. "Gestalten of Today: Early Processing of Visual Contours and Surfaces." *Behavioral Brain Research* 82 (1): 1–11.

Kovács, I., Fehér, A., and Julesz, B. 1998. "Medial-Point Description of Shape: A Representation for Action Coding and Its Psychophysical Correlates." *Vision Research* 38 (15–16): 2323–2333.

Kovács, I., and Julesz, B. 1993. "A Closed Curve Is Much More Than an Incomplete One: Effect of Closure in Figure-Ground Segmentation." *Proceedings of the National Academy of Sciences USA* 90 (16): 7495–7497.

Kovács, I., and Julesz, B. 1994. "Perceptual Sensitivity Maps Within Globally Defined Visual Shapes." *Nature* 370 (6491): 644–646.

Lee, T. S. 2003. "Computations in the Early Visual Cortex." *Journal of Physiology* 97 (2–3): 121–139.

Lee, T. S., Mumford, D., Romero, R., and Lammme, V. 1998. "The Role of Primary Visual Cortex in Object Representation." *Vision Research* 38 (15–16): 2429–2454.

Leymarie, F. F., and Kimia, B. B. 2008. "From the Infinitely Large to the Infinitely Small." In *Medial Representations Mathematics, Algorithms and Applications*, edited by K. Siddiqi and S. M. Pizer. New York: Springer. 369–406.

Leyton, M. 1987. "Symmetry-Curvature Duality." *Comp. Vis. Graph. Image Proc.* 38: 327–341.

Leyton, M. 1992. *Symmetry, Causality, Mind*. Cambridge, MA: MIT Press.

Li, Z. 2005. "The Primary Visual Cortex Creates a Bottom-up Saliency Map." In *Neurobiology of Attention*, edited by L. Itti, G. Rees, and J. K. Tsotsos. Burlington, VT: Academic Press. 570–575.

Norwich, J. J. 1975. *Great Architecture of the World*. New York: Random House.

Ogniewicz, R. L. 1993. *Discrete Voronoi Skeletons*. Konstanz: Hartung-Gorre Verlag.

Ullman, S. 2007. "Object Recognition and Segmentation by a Fragment-Based Hierarchy." *Trends in Cognitive Science* 11 (2): 58–64.

Van Tonder, G. J., Lyons, M. J., and Ejima, Y. 2002. "Perception Psychology: Visual Structure of a Japanese Zen Garden." *Nature* 419: 359–360.

3 Extending *Prägnanz*: Dynamic Aspects of Mental Representation and Gestalt Principles

Timothy L. Hubbard

Although examples of Gestalt principles of perceptual grouping (e.g., principles of proximity, similarity, good continuation, etc.) found in many textbooks involve static figures, these principles actually reflect dynamic processes (Kohler, 1938, 1940, 1969). Indeed, Gestalt theory more broadly suggests that the perceptual act involves a dynamic unfolding of the structure of phenomenal space (Albertazzi, 2002a, 2002b, 2006). Research with visual (Palmer, 2002) or auditory (Deutsch, 1999) stimuli reveals that Gestalt principles influence spatial organization, and research on perceived rhythms in auditory streaming reveals that Gestalt principles influence temporal organization (Bregman, 1990). Thus, Gestalt principles involve spatiotemporal information and result in spatiotemporal biases. More recently, other spatiotemporal biases that also appear to involve a dynamic unfolding of phenomenal space have been documented. One such spatiotemporal bias, representational momentum, is considered in detail, and it is shown that representational momentum exhibits properties and consequences similar to properties and consequences of Gestalt principles of perceptual grouping. These similarities suggest that Gestalt principles of perceptual grouping and spatiotemporal biases such as representational momentum might be assimilated into a broader anticipatory framework based, in part, on dynamic information within mental representation.

The concept of "information" within cognitive and psychological sciences traditionally involved static abstract or symbolic content manipulated by various processes within a given level of representation or mapped between representations at different levels of processing (e.g., Kolers and Smythe, 1979; Pylyshyn, 1984; Shanon, 2008). However, the concept of "information" can be applied equally well to dynamic concrete spatiotemporal content. Viewed in this light, the unfolding of phenomenal space involves the presence of dynamic information in perception. The ideas of information and dynamic representation and of an incorporation of dynamic information within mental representation are considered, and it is suggested that an expanded view of *Prägnanz* and isomorphism can account for traditional Gestalt principles of perceptual grouping and for spatiotemporal biases such as representational momentum. The first section ("Information and Dynamics") reviews ideas of *Prägnanz*, information, and dynamics. The second section ("Dynamic Information within Mental Representation") reviews examples of dynamic influences within mental representation and introduces a distinction between intrinsic dynamics (involving shape and structure of a stimulus) and extrinsic dynamics (involving physical principles and the context within which a stimulus is embedded). The third section ("Gestalt Principles and Representational Momentum") examines similarities of the properties and consequences of Gestalt principles of perceptual grouping with the properties and consequences of representational momentum. The final section provides a brief summary and conclusions.

Information and Dynamics

Gestalt principles of perceptual grouping are based on a general notion of *"Prägnanz"* (van Tuijl, 1980), which is a bias to interpret a stimulus to be as regular, simple, and symmetrical as possible (Koffka, 1935). Stimuli that are high in regularity, simplicity, and symmetry are said to be high in "figural goodness." In this section, traditional ideas relating information and *Prägnanz* in Gestalt theory and a more contemporary idea of dynamic mental representation are considered.

Information and *Prägnanz*

Figure 3.1 shows the relationship between the amount of information required to describe a stimulus and the figural goodness of that stimulus. There are three panels, each of which contains a stimulus consisting of a black figure on a white background. Given that the stimulus in each panel is created by coloring each of the cells within an 8×8 grid black or white, it might initially be suspected that each stimulus requires the same amount of information to specify (alternatively, that each stimulus contains the same amount of information). However, that is not correct. To specify (encode, reproduce) the stimulus in panel A, it is necessary to encode whether each cell of the 8×8 grid is black or white (64 bits of information). To specify the stimulus in panel B, it is necessary to encode only the information in the left half of the stimulus. The information in the left side could then be reflected across the vertical axis to re-create the entire stimulus (32 bits of information plus notation of vertical symmetry). To specify the stimulus in panel C, it is necessary to encode only the information in the upper left quadrant of the stimulus. The information in that quadrant could be reflected across the horizontal axis and the resultant pattern reflected across the vertical axis to re-create the entire stimulus (16 bits of information plus notation of vertical and horizontal symmetry).

The rating of figural goodness for each of the stimuli in figure 3.1 increases from left to right, but the amount of information required to specify each of the stimuli in figure 3.1 decreases from left to right. Thus, there is an inverse relationship between the fig-

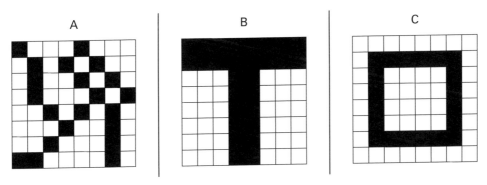

Figure 3.1
An example of the relationship between figural goodness and the information required to specify
a figure. Figural goodness is lowest and the amount of information required to specify the figure
are highest in panel A. Figural goodness and the amount of information needed to specify a figure
are intermediate in panel B. Figural goodness is highest and the amount of information required
to specify the figure are lowest in panel C. As figural goodness increases, the amount of information necessary to specify that figure decreases. Adapted from Coren, Ward, and Enns (2004).

ural goodness of a stimulus and the amount of information required to specify that
stimulus (see also Attneave, 1955; Hochberg and McAlister, 1953; Hochberg and
Brooks, 1960). As a consequence, there is less information in a stimulus high in figural
goodness than there is in a stimulus low in figural goodness. This pattern is consistent
with findings that more regular and more symmetrical figures are more easily recognized (Pomerantz, Sager, and Stoever, 1977), imaged (Finke, Johnson, and Shyi, 1988),
and remembered (Howe and Brandau, 1983; Howe and Jung, 1986) than are less regular
or less symmetrical figures. The decreased information in good figures might be related
to the bias to interpret figures as more regular: Simpler representations require fewer
cognitive resources (Hatfield and Epstein, 1985), and given the 7 ± 2 limits of working
memory, it would be adaptive to minimize the amount of information processing required to specify a stimulus. Therefore, a bias in favor of interpreting figures to be as
simple, regular, and symmetrical as possible (i.e., a bias for *Prägnanz*) developed.

One of the most striking examples of how *Prägnanz* and a preference for minimizing
information processing can influence perception is the existence of illusory (subjective) contours,[1] and an example of this based on Kanizsa (1979) can be seen in figure
3.2. The stimulus in panel A is composed solely of three circles with missing wedges
and three angle shapes. Most observers perceive a solid white triangle on top of a black
outline triangle and three circles. Observers typically perceive boundaries at the points
marked by the arrows in panel B, but no such boundaries actually exist in the physical
stimulus. Rather, those boundaries are interpolated by observers, and this phenomenon
occurs because the existence of such boundaries makes the stimulus a more regular,

A

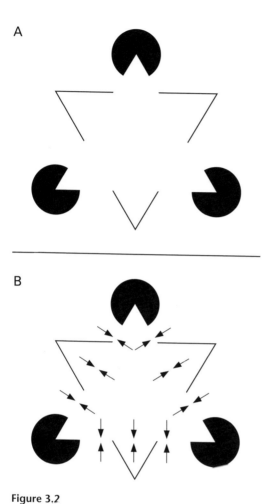

B

Figure 3.2
An example of illusory contours. Panel A illustrates the basic stimulus display. With continued inspection, a white triangle appears even though such a triangle is not actually physically present in the display. The boundaries of the perceived white triangle are indicated by the arrows in panel B. Adapted from Kanizsa (1979).

simple, and symmetrical form. In the absence of such interpolation, observers would have to accept the existence of several irregular shapes and multiple coincidental alignments of apparently unrelated elements. Such multiple coincidences would be highly unlikely, and so the visual system "invents" a white triangle that it inserts into the percept to regularize and simplify (the interpretation of) the stimulus. Although invention of the white triangle adds content to the percept, such an addition actually decreases the total amount of information necessary to specify or encode that content.[2]

Dynamic Information

Gestalt theory (e.g., especially the writings of Brentano and of Wertheimer) suggests the perceptual act is dynamic, and that this dynamic quality is characterized by an unfolding of phenomenal space or structure that is governed by an intrinsic coherence and meaning (see Albertazzi, 2005, 2006). The characterization of the perceptual act, and of mental representations underlying the perceptual act, as exhibiting intrinsic coherence and meaning is consistent with suggestions that information does not exist without an associated meaning and without a purpose.[3] In the case of a dynamic unfolding of phenomenal space exemplified by Gestalt principles, information regarding the surrounding environment (and objects in that environment) is represented by the observer; the meaning and purpose of that information might be to increase adaptation and survival of an observer by decreasing information-processing demands and increasing cognitive efficiency. Several authors have previously considered dynamics of cognition within the context of complex, self-organizing, or nonlinear systems (Kelso, 1995; Port and van Gelder, 1995; Spivey, 2007; Thelen and Smith, 1994), but the focus here is on a simpler and more basic issue: dynamics as information reflecting and reflected by spatiotemporal properties of mental representation and the meaning encoded by such dynamics.

One view of dynamic mental representation relevant to the current concern is that of Freyd (1987), who suggests that mental representation is dynamic (or incorporates dynamic information) if temporal information is intrinsic to and a necessary part of the representation (indeed, traditional views of mental representation have been criticized for ignoring temporal information, e.g., see Shanon, 2008). To be intrinsic to the representation, temporal information must be represented by a dimension or feature that has the same inherent temporal structure as the represented object. There are two criteria of such intrinsic representation. The first criterion involves direction—time is asymmetrical, and the dynamic unfolding of a mental representation is similarly asymmetrical (i.e., time flows one way). Evidence for an asymmetrical influence of time on mental representation is found in studies of mental imagery: If experimental participants image actions or processes (e.g., flowing water [Schwartz and Black, 1999], actions of pulley and gear systems [Hegarty, 1992]), it is easier to imagine such actions or processes in the direction of natural motion and casual progression than in the direction opposite to natural motion and causal progression. To the extent that actions or processes unfold in time, Freyd's emphasis on intrinsic inclusion of temporal information is consistent with Gestalt theory, as Wertheimer (1922/2002; cited in Albertazzi, 2006) referred to "whole processes possessed of specific inner intrinsic laws."

The second criterion of intrinsic representation is continuity. Time, at least at the experiential level, seems continuous (i.e., between any two points in time, there is a third point). Evidence for continuity in mental representation is found in studies of mental imagery: Studies of mental rotation (Shepard and Cooper, 1982) and image scanning (Kosslyn, 1980) suggest that intermediate orientations or locations are functionally represented within a mental image. If experimental participants viewed two stimuli and judged whether the stimuli were identical except for a difference in orientation or whether the stimuli were different, then the further the first object had to rotate to match the orientation of the second object, the longer were the participants' response times (Shepard and Metzler, 1971). If experimental participants imaged a stimulus rotating to a specified orientation, and if during this process a probe was presented, then judgment comparing the probe to the image was facilitated if the orientation of the probe matched the (presumed) orientation of the imaged object (Cooper, 1976). If experimental participants scanned from one location on an image to a second location, then the farther the second location was from the first location, the longer were the participants' response times (Kosslyn, Ball, and Reiser, 1978). In general, such findings suggest that intermediate orientations or locations were represented, and this pattern is consistent with the continuity criterion.

Having temporal information be intrinsic to the representation is one of two major properties of dynamic mental representation. The other major property of dynamic mental representation is that temporal information is necessarily included within the representation. If temporal information is necessarily included within mental representation, then that information (or any temporal property) does not emerge as a function of processes applied to that representation but instead emerges as part of the representation's functional architecture (see also Jones, 1976). An interpretation of findings of studies on mental rotation that is based on nondynamic mental representation suggests that the linear function relating response time to angular distance arises from a transformation (rotation) applied to a spatial and static representation. However, an interpretation of those same results that is based on dynamic mental representation suggests that the linear function arises from the representation's structure (i.e., the representation would have a temporal component) rather than from a transformation or process applied to an otherwise static structure (Freyd, 1987). In the latter case, removal of temporal information would render the representation no longer useful. Along these lines, it has been persuasively argued that a lack of temporal information in the traditional (nondynamic) view of representation revealed that view was incorrect (e.g., see Shanon, 2008).

Dynamic Information within Mental Representation

The existence of dynamic information in mental representation is consistent with the notion in Gestalt theory that a perceptual act involves a dynamic unfolding of phenomenal space. In this section, two different types of dynamic information in mental representation are distinguished: One type of dynamic involves intrinsic forces that arise from the shape and structure of a stimulus, and a second type of dynamic involves extrinsic forces or other stimuli that act on the stimulus as a function of stimulus behavior or the context within which the stimulus is embedded.

Intrinsic Dynamics—Shape and Structure

Arnheim (1966, 1974, 1988, 1996) addressed dynamics arising from the structure and shape of objects. Many of these dynamics are based on the structural skeleton (i.e., principle axes) of the object, and some examples are shown in figure 3.3. Just as

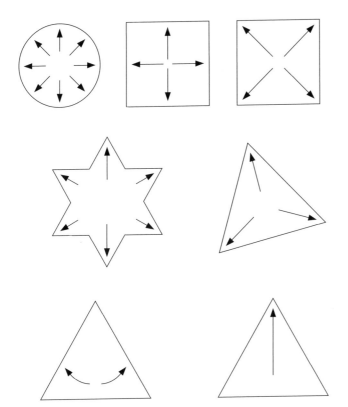

Figure 3.3
Examples of structural dynamics based on shape and structure; arrows indicate the direction of the perceived dynamics. Adapted from Arnheim (1974).

Prägnanz can give rise to illusory contours, some intrinsic dynamics can also give rise to illusions. For example, the outward dynamic along a radius of a circle is consistent with gamma motion, an illusion in which a circle that suddenly appears is perceived to unfold from the center outward, and conversely, when a circle suddenly disappears, it is perceived to vanish from the periphery inward (e.g., Bartley and Wilkinson, 1953; Harrower, 1929; Winters, 1964). Similarly, a triangle often appears to "point" in a particular direction (e.g., Attneave, 1968; Palmer, 1980; Palmer and Bucher, 1981, 1982), and the direction of pointing can influence the direction of subsequent apparent motion of that triangle (McBeath and Morikawa, 1997; McBeath, Morikawa, and Kaiser, 1992) and subsequent memory for the location of that triangle (Freyd and Pantzer, 1995; Nagai and Yagi, 2001). Also, the perceived pointing of a triangle along a given axis is enhanced with motion of the triangle along that axis (Bucher and Palmer, 1985). Thus, dynamics arising from shape or structure can combine and influence an observer's mental representation of the size, shape, and location of a stimulus.

If the shape or structure of an object incorporates or specifies information regarding forces (dynamics) that previously acted on that object, then observers might perceive that dynamic information (cf. Freyd, 1992, 1993), and observers' mental representations might reflect that dynamic information. For example, figure 3.4 shows the winding and twisting growth of trees in a windy area, and the shapes of the trees preserve unambiguous information regarding the direction of the prevailing winds. Similarly, traces of waves on a beach and sculpting of sand dunes by the wind preserve information regarding the forces that shaped those structures. Dynamic information can be found in human artifacts; for example, shapes and connecting lines in calligraphy or in handwriting preserve information regarding the creation and ordering of strokes in those shapes (Babcock and Freyd, 1988; Tse and Cavanagh, 2000). Arnheim suggested

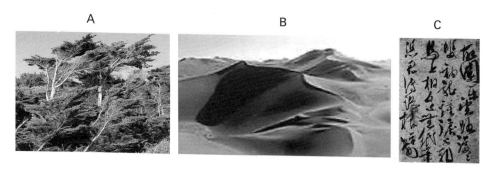

Figure 3.4

Examples of stimuli that embody intrinsic dynamics that reflect the forces that shaped those objects. In panel A, the prevailing winds shaped the growth of trees. In panel B, the shapes of sand dunes were sculpted by wind. In panel C, the ordering of strokes in a sample of calligraphy is evident.

that such dynamic information is perceived and, furthermore, that modulation of such dynamic information is a major contributor to artistic expression (Arnheim, 1966). Along these lines, Leyton convincingly argued that when we perceive an object, we perceive not just that object but also the history of the forces that acted on that object (e.g., when we perceive a dent in an otherwise smooth surface, we also represent the force that produced that dent) (Leyton, 1989, 1992).

Extrinsic Dynamics—Physical Principles

Observers are also sensitive to forces currently acting on an object. Although forces currently acting on a stimulus can result in changes in the shape or configuration of a stimulus similar to changes related to intrinsic dynamics (e.g., leaves and small branches blown by the wind), sensitivity to forces currently acting on a stimulus can also be seen in the absence of changes in shape or configuration. Perhaps the most well-known example of the latter involves the influence of implied momentum on memory for location. More specifically, memory for the final location of a moving target is displaced slightly farther along the anticipated trajectory of that target. This has been referred to as *representational momentum* (Freyd and Finke, 1984; for review, see Hubbard, 2005) and was initially attributed to an analogue of physical momentum within the mental representation of motion. Much as a physical object could not be immediately stopped because of the momentum of that object, so too the mental representation of motion could not be immediately stopped because of an analogue of momentum within the representation of motion (Finke, Freyd, and Shyi, 1986).[4] However, subsequent research revealed variables other than implied momentum could modulate forward displacement (Hubbard, 2005). Representational momentum typically increases in magnitude during the first few hundred milliseconds after a target has vanished (e.g., Freyd and Johnson, 1987), and this demonstrates a dynamic unfolding of phenomenal space.

Physical principles other than momentum can also influence mental representation. For example, in addition to the larger forward displacement previously noted, memory for the location of a horizontally moving target is also displaced slightly downward. Forward displacement in memory for the location of a descending target is larger than forward displacement in memory for the location of an ascending target (Hubbard, 1990; Hubbard and Bharucha, 1988). Also, memory for the location of a stationary target is displaced downward (Freyd, Pantzer, and Cheng, 1988; Hubbard and Ruppel, 2000). These patterns are consistent with the direction of implied gravitational attraction, and this phenomenon has been referred to as *representational gravity* (Hubbard, 1995b, 1997). Forward displacement in memory for the location of a horizontally (Hubbard, 1995a) or vertically (Hubbard, 1998) moving target is largest when the target does not contact a surface, is decreased when the target slides along one surface, and is decreased even more when the target slides between two surfaces; this has been referred to as *representational friction*. Memory for the location of a target moving along a circular orbit is displaced inward, and this has been referred to as *representational centripetal force* (Hubbard, 1996a). Although there is disagreement regarding the mechanisms of displacements that appear related to physical principles (cf. Hubbard, 2006b; Kerzel, 2006; for review, see Hubbard, 2010), the existence of such displacements is consistent with a sensitivity to dynamic information.

Extrinsic Dynamics—Context
Representational momentum, representational friction, and representational centripetal force can be viewed as involving forces attributable (at least in part) to behavior of the target. In a sense, such forces would be internal (and specific) to the target. In contrast, representational gravity can be viewed as a more external extrinsic dynamic because such a force would be external (and not specific) to the target. Other spatiotemporal biases provide evidence of additional external extrinsic dynamics based on the presence of other stimuli. One example of a dynamic unfolding of phenomenal space regarding a target based on the presence of an additional stimulus is illusory line motion (e.g., Christie and Klein, 2005; Downing and Treisman, 1997; Hikosaka, Miyauchi, and Shimojo, 1993). In illusory line motion, a cue directing attention to a specific location appears, and then a stationary line appears (all at once) near the cued location. The line is perceived to "unfold" or "expand" from the end closest to the cue to the end farthest from the cue. Illusory line motion has been attributed to a variety of mechanisms (for a brief discussion, see Fuller and Carrasco 2009). Regardless of the mechanism, the dynamic unfolding of phenomenal space in illusory line motion occurs at a rate slow enough that observers perceive the actual dynamic unfolding as motion (growth) of (what is actually) a stationary line.

Another example of a dynamic in mental representation related to context is boundary extension (for review, see Hubbard, Hutchison, and Courtney, 2010; Intraub, 2002). If observers view a photograph or drawing of a scene, memory for that scene incorporates information not actually present within the scene, but that would likely have been present just beyond the boundaries of that scene. If observers judge whether the viewpoint within a subsequent probe photograph or probe drawing is the same as the viewpoint within the original photograph or drawing, they are more likely to respond *same* to probes with a slightly wider-angle view (i.e., probes in which the boundaries have been extended outward). If observers produce from memory a drawing of the remembered view, they are likely to incorporate within their drawings information (e.g., objects) that was not visible within the original photograph or drawing but that probably would have been visible just beyond the boundaries of the original photograph or drawing. Boundary extension is dependent on context and does not occur for objects not in a scene (Gottesman and Intraub, 2002). Also, boundary extension typically occurs rapidly after a target has vanished (within 42 milliseconds) and might aid in integration of successive views (Dickinson and Intraub, 2008), and this demonstrates a dynamic unfolding of phenomenal space.

Extending *Prägnanz:* Dynamics as Simplicity

Mental representation preserves or includes dynamic spatiotemporal information. Adding or incorporating dynamic information might initially make a representation more complex, and so it might appear that adding or incorporating dynamic information would be opposed to *Prägnanz*. However, and as discussed in greater detail in the third section, additional information provided by dynamic aspects of mental representation can actually simplify processing of a stimulus and decrease the amount of information processing required. If mental representation is dynamic, then temporal information is an intrinsic and necessary part of the representation. By including temporal information as part of the representation, the need to store temporal information separately and for additional processes to apply temporal manipulations or processing to an otherwise static representation is eliminated. If dynamic information is part of the structure (functional architecture) of mental representation, then that information can be recovered by activating the representation without retrieving or adding additional information or processes.[5] Thus, although incorporation of dynamic information might make the structure of the representation initially appear more complex, the presence of dynamic information can actually decrease overall processing demands. The net result of adding dynamic information is an increase in simplicity, and such a result is consistent with *Prägnanz*.

Gestalt Principles and Representational Momentum

If dynamic information within mental representation reflects *Prägnanz*, then properties and consequences of a dynamic spatiotemporal bias such as representational momentum should be similar to properties and consequences of Gestalt principles of perceptual grouping. In this section, similarities of Gestalt principles of perceptual grouping and representational momentum are considered. Numerous similarities are discussed, and these involve (1) displacement in remembered location, (2) reflection of environmental regularities, (3) decreases in the amount of information that must be processed, (4) a possible basis in second-order isomorphism, (5) a possible contribution to aesthetics and artistic expression, (6) effects of configuration and context, (7) interpretation as laboratory-based illusions or as adaptive strategies, and (8) automaticity in application.

Displacement in Remembered Location

As noted earlier, representational momentum results in displacement of the represented location of an object in the direction of motion. Application of Gestalt

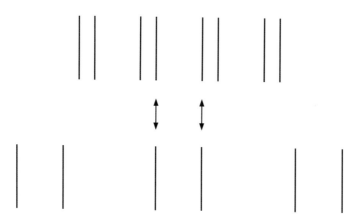

Figure 3.5
An example of a Gestalt illusion based on the principle of proximity. The two lines indicated by
the arrows in the top row are the same horizontal distance apart as the two lines indicated by the
arrows in the bottom row. However, the lines in the top row are grouped into different pairs and
the lines in the bottom row are grouped into the same pair. The distance between lines in different pairs (i.e., not grouped together) is usually remembered as slightly larger than is the distance
between lines in the same pair (i.e., grouped together). Adapted from Coren and Girgus (1980).

principles also results in displacement in remembered location; such displacement has
been referred to as a *Gestalt illusion* (Coren and Girgus, 1980), and one example is
shown in figure 3.5. In the top row are eight lines, and the principle of proximity results in these lines being grouped into four pairs. In the bottom row are six lines, and
the principle of proximity results in these lines being grouped into three pairs. Consider the lines indicated by arrows. The lines indicated in the top row are separated by
the same distance as the lines indicated in the bottom row; however, in the top row
these lines are not grouped into the same pair, whereas in the bottom row these lines
are grouped into the same pair. Participants reproduced the distance between these
lines, and when the lines were not grouped into the same pair (as in the top row), the
reproduced distance was slightly larger than when the lines were grouped into the
same pair (as in the bottom row). Similar examples involving other Gestalt principles
have been reported; in each case, the reproduced distance between elements was larger
when elements were not grouped together than when elements were grouped together
(Coren and Girgus, 1980; Enns and Girgus, 1985).

Reflecting Environmental Regularities
The existence of Gestalt principles suggests that observers perceive objects according to
rules that reflect regularities or invariants in the environment (e.g., Goldstein, 1999;
Lowe, 1985; Palmer, 1983). Regularities exploited by Gestalt principles involve proper-

ties of objects and forms and reflect the broader notion of *Prägnanz*, and so Gestalt principles aid object and form recognition and identification. For example, in everyday experience, parts of the same object tend to be closer to other parts of the same object than to other objects, and this gives rise to the principle of proximity. Objects tend to be fairly homogenous in lightness and texture, with changes in lightness or texture associated with boundaries between objects or parts of an object, and this gives rise to the principle of similarity. Objects tend to follow along smooth or continuous paths rather than abruptly changing direction, and this gives rise to the principle of good continuation. Portions of stimuli can be occluded or in shadow, but such stimuli continue behind the occluder or through the shadow, and this gives rise to the principle of closure. Multiple elements that move in the same direction are typically part of the same object, and this gives rise to the principle of common fate.

The existence of representational momentum suggests that observers perceive objects according to rules that reflect regularities or invariants in the environment (e.g., Hubbard, 1999, 2005, 2006a). Regularities exploited by representational momentum involve (subjective aspects of) dynamics involved in object motion and reflect the broader notion of environmentally invariant physical principles, and so representational momentum aids spatial localization. Consider the situation depicted in figure 3.6. As shown in panel A, when an observer initially senses a moving target, that target is at position P1. This initiates a cascade of sensory, perceptual, cognitive, and perhaps motor processes that are very rapid but nonetheless require some minimal amount of time. If the observer is going to respond to the target (e.g., by hitting, blocking, or catching the target), then that response should be calibrated to where the target will be when the response reaches the target and not where the target was when it was initially sensed. However, a target will not typically pause at the position where it was initially sensed and wait for the observer to finish processing before continuing further; rather, as shown in panel B, the target will continue to move. The observer needs a way to bridge the gap between the position where the target was sensed (P1) and where the target would be when a response from the observer would reach that target (P2); representational momentum aids this bridging.

Decreasing Information

As noted earlier, stimuli high in figural goodness require less information to specify. Does representational momentum similarly decrease the amount of information necessary to specify a stimulus? Consider a target moving from left to right. In the absence of sensitivity to the effects of momentum, the search space for the subsequent location of such a target would be a large area centered on the target's previous location, and the target would be perceived as equally likely to subsequently appear to the right of, left of, above, or below the previous location. There would be no reason to consistently search a particular region prior to searching any other region, and so observers might

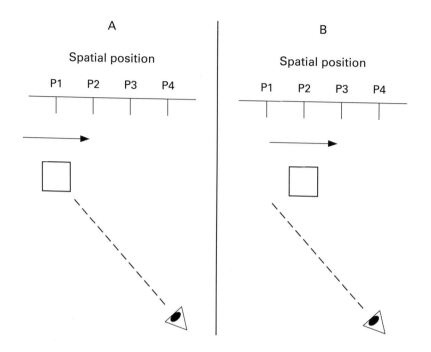

A

Spatial position

P1   P2   P3   P4

B

Spatial position

P1   P2   P3   P4

Observer initially senses moving target and initiates perceptual/ cognitive/motor processing Target located at P1.

Observer ready to respond to moving target. Perceptual/cognitive/ motor processing complete. Target located at P2.

Figure 3.6
An illustration of how displacement aids spatial localization. In panel A, a moving target is initially sensed, and perceptual and cognitive processing begins. During this processing, the target continues to move. In panel B, the initial perceptual and cognitive processing is complete, but the target is no longer at the position where it was initially sensed. For a response to the target such as catching, blocking, hitting, or intercepting to be maximally effective, an observer must compensate for the movement of the target during the time between when perceptual processing was initiated and when that processing is completed and a motor response initiated. Representational momentum might aid in this compensation. Adapted from Hubbard (2005).

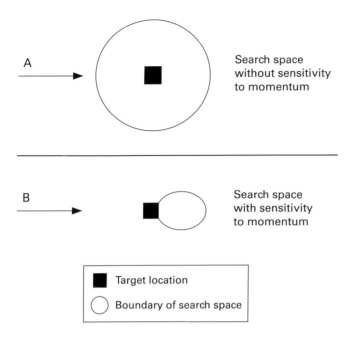

Figure 3.7

An example of how sensitivity to momentum decreases the amount of information needed to specify a target. Panel A illustrates the search space for the subsequent location of a target moving from left to right in the absence of a sensitivity to momentum. The search space is centered on the current location of the target, and the search for the subsequent location is equally likely to be to the right, left, above, or below the current location. Panel B illustrates the search space for the subsequent location of a target moving from left to right in the presence of a sensitivity to momentum. The search space is focused in the area immediately in front of the current location. The search space is much smaller in panel B than in panel A, and observers would on average detect the subsequent location of the target much faster given the situation in panel B than given the situation in panel A.

be equally likely to initially search to the right of, left of, above, or below the previous location for the subsequent location. This is illustrated in panel A of figure 3.7. However, if observers are sensitive to the effects of momentum, this decreases the size of the search space. Instead of searching a relatively large area centered on the previous location of the target, observers search a relatively small area in the direction specified by that momentum (i.e., along the anticipated trajectory). This is illustrated in panel B of figure 3.7. The target will probably be in that area, and so observers do not waste time or resources first searching other locations.[6] Thus, sensitivity to dynamics acting on a stimulus decreases the amount of information that must be processed to detect and specify the stimulus.

A Basis in (Second-Order) Isomorphism

Gestalt theorists speculated on the correspondence between structures in the nervous system and structures of perceived objects (e.g., Kohler, 1938, 1969), and they referred to such a correspondence as an *isomorphism*. Despite some theorists' suggestions (e.g., Gregory, 1974), the Gestalt view of isomorphism does not involve a "picture in the head," in which brain structure literally mirrors the stimulus (e.g., an image of a green elephant is not literally green and shaped like an elephant) but instead involves a more functional preservation of information (for a discussion, see Henle, 1984). Indeed, the "picture in the head" was explicitly rejected by Gestalt theorists (e.g., Kohler, 1938) and others (e.g., Shepard, 1968). The "picture in the head" is untenable in neural terms, but consideration of intrinsic dynamics and extrinsic dynamics that were discussed in the previous section suggests the possibility of functional correspondences between dynamics that acted or are acting on the stimulus and dynamics of the representation (i.e., the represented shape and location of an object preserves information regarding forces that acted or are acting on that object). Such a consideration is consistent with a dynamic unfolding of phenomenal space and suggests the correspondence between a stimulus and the representation of that stimulus involves functional isomorphism rather than structural isomorphism.

The Gestalt notion of isomorphism is consistent with the notion of second-order isomorphism within the literature on mental imagery. Shepard referred to preservation of functional information in imagery as *second-order isomorphism* (preservation of structural information would be *first-order isomorphism*), and he suggested that such isomorphism reflected internalization of geometry and kinematics (Shepard, 1975, 1984, 1994). As shown in figure 3.8, a physical object that rotates from orientation A to orientation C must pass through intermediate orientation B, and this reflects constraints on physical transformation. Similarly, mental representation of an object that rotates from orientation A* to orientation C* must pass through intermediate orientation B*, and this reflects constraints on mental transformation. Hubbard (2006a) suggested the notion of second-order isomorphism be broadened to include dynamics and forces, as well as geometry and kinematics. In this broadening, representational momentum reflects second-order isomorphism between forces that influence a physical object and a mental representation of that object. A physical object that rotates from orientation A to orientation C must possess momentum, and this reflects a constraint on physical transformation. The mental representation of an object that rotates from orientation A* to orientation C* would thus exhibit a functional analogue of momentum (i.e., representational momentum).

Aesthetics and Artistic Expression

The notion of intrinsic dynamics discussed in the previous section suggests traces of forces that acted on a stimulus could be perceived in the shape and structure of that

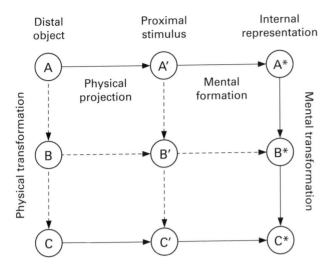

Figure 3.8
Shepard's illustration of the correspondence between mental and physical transformations. A distal physical object at orientation A must pass through intermediate orientation B before reaching orientation C. Similarly, a mental representation of an object in orientation A* must pass through orientation B* before reaching orientation C*. The mental representation of the physical transformation is a functional analogue of the physical transformation (i.e., mental rotation is second-order isomorphic to physical rotation). Similarly, a distal physical object rotating from orientation A to orientation C must exhibit momentum, and so mental representation of a physical object rotating from orientation A* to orientation C* must exhibit a functional analogue of momentum (i.e., representational momentum). Adapted from Shepard and Cooper (1982).

stimulus. Arnheim (1966, 1974) sketched a Gestalt theory of artistic expression in which such traces of dynamics play a central role, and he suggested that artistic expression is "the psychological counterpart of the dynamic processes that result in the organization of the perceptual stimuli" (Arnheim, 1966, p. 62). Methods used in studies of representational momentum can be adapted to examine intrinsic structural dynamics (e.g., Hubbard and Blessum, 2001) as well as aesthetics and artistic expression (e.g., Hubbard and Courtney, 2006). One such methodology involves use of a frozen-action photograph drawn from a longer motion sequence (e.g., Futterweit and Beilin, 1994; Thornton and Hayes, 2004). As shown in figure 3.9, in such a methodology, observers view a frozen-action photograph and then view a probe photograph that is from slightly earlier in the motion sequence, the same as the original photograph, or from slightly later in the motion sequence. Observers judge whether the probe photograph is the same as the original photograph, and they are typically more likely to respond *same* to probes from slightly later in the motion sequence than to probes from slightly earlier in the motion sequence. The distribution of *same* responses as a

Possible probes

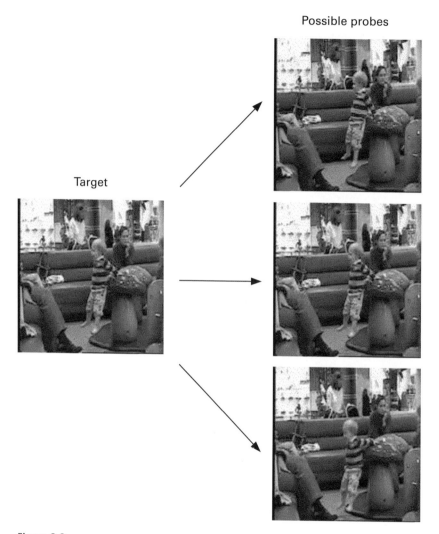

Target

Figure 3.9
Examples of frozen action stimuli. On the left is a target photograph. On the right are three possible probe photographs, with the top probe from slightly earlier in the motion sequence, the middle probe the same as the target, and the bottom probe from slightly later in the motion sequence. When observers judge whether a probe is the same as the original target, they are more likely to respond *same* to a probe from slightly later in the motion sequence than to a probe from slightly earlier in the motion sequence.

A   B   C

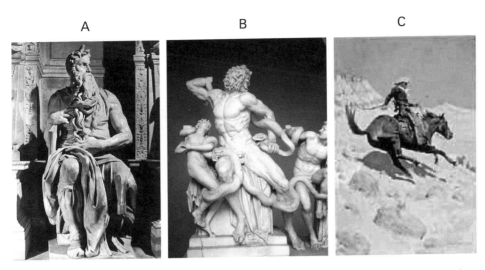

Figure 3.10

Examples of aesthetic artwork that look like frozen action stimuli. Panel A is a Renaissance sculpture of a seated Moses who appears to be turning toward his left (created by Michelangelo and located in the church of San Pietro in Vincoli in Rome). Panel B is the ancient Greek sculpture of Laocoon and his sons battling a sea serpent (created by Athanadoros, Hagesandros, and Polydoros of Rhodes and located in the Vatican Museum in Rome). Panel C is a nineteenth-century painting of a cowboy riding a horse along a steeply sloping hill (created by Frederic Remington and located in the Amon Carter Museum in Fort Worth, TX). Adapted from Hubbard and Courtney (2006).

function of probe position can then be used to quantify direction and magnitude of displacement in memory for the content of the original photograph.[7]

An aesthetic work of art often appears as if it were a single frame drawn from a larger motion sequence, that is, an aesthetic work of art often looks like a frozen-action photograph. For example, the works of art shown in figure 3.10 are considered highly aesthetic, and each captures a single moment of time out of a larger motion sequence. In the statues of Moses and of Laocoon, and in the painting of the cowboy on the horse, the strain and force of the muscles of each of the depicted figures can be clearly perceived, and the direction of motion if the muscle action continued is obvious. This latter point is consistent with the notion that (sensitivity to) dynamic information might engage an observer's own motor programs. Indeed, the idea that perception involves activation of an observer's own motor programs has been discussed for stimuli in several domains (e.g., Knoblich and Sebanz, 2006; Liberman and Mattingly, 1985; Wilson and Knoblich, 2005). What is especially relevant for the current concern is that a stimulus containing more dynamic information might be more effective at activating an observer's motor programs, and so stimuli containing more dynamic information

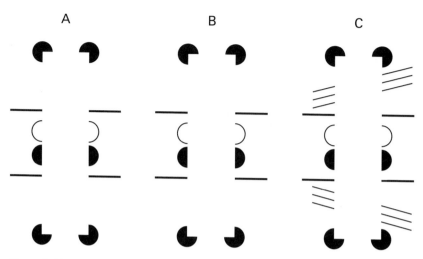

Figure 3.11

An example of the importance of context on the strength of illusory contours. The number of cues suggesting the presence of an overlapping white rectangle, and the strength of the illusory contours, are lowest in panel A and highest in panel C. This indicates that the more cues that suggest the presence of an overlaying figure, the stronger the perception of illusory contours. Adapted from Schiffman (2001).

would be more efficiently perceived or processed than would stimuli containing less dynamic information. Thus, the presence of dynamic information would lead to more efficient processing.

Configuration and Context

It is a truism in Gestalt theory that the context within which a stimulus is embedded influences perception of that stimulus. For example, the strength of illusory contours is greater when there are more cues (i.e., there is more context) suggesting existence of an overlapping figure (e.g., Kennedy, 1988; Lesher and Mingolla, 1993). Figure 3.11 shows three versions of a Kanizsa-type stimulus. In panel A, there are several cues suggesting the existence of a white rectangle. In panel B, more cues are added, and in panel C, even more cues are added. The strength of illusory contours increases as more cues suggesting the existence of an overlapping white rectangle are added. In figure 3.12, the context within which stimuli are embedded influences the structural dynamics of those stimuli. The orientations of the analogous lines of each of the six individual equilateral triangles in panel A are the same, but the triangles on the left are usually perceived as pointing toward the left, whereas the triangles on the right are usually perceived as pointing toward the upper right. Similarly, in panel B, the triangles on the left are usually perceived as pointing toward the right, and the triangles on

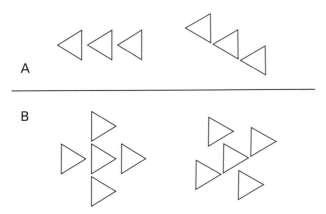

A

B

Figure 3.12
Examples of the effects of orientation and shape of surrounding elements on the direction of
perceived pointing. In panel A, the stimuli on the left are more likely to be perceived as pointing
toward the left, and the stimuli on the right are more likely to be perceived as pointing toward the
upper right. In panel B, the effects of alignment with a configural line are shown; the stimuli on
the left are more likely to be perceived as pointing toward the right, and the stimuli on the right
are more likely to be perceived as pointing toward the upper left. Adapted from Palmer (1980) and
Palmer and Bucher (1981, 1982).

the right are usually perceived as pointing toward the upper left. In figures 3.11 and
3.12, the direction an equilateral triangle is perceived to point is influenced by the surrounding context; more broadly, the whole (i.e., the configuration) influenced perception of the parts and relationships between the parts.

Although representational momentum can be observed for a single target on a blank
background, displacement in memory for a target is strongly influenced by the context
within which that target is embedded. If target motion is embedded in a larger sequence in which that motion oscillates, displacement at the moment of an anticipated
reversal of target motion is in the direction of the expected reversal and opposite to the
direction of actual target motion (e.g., Hubbard and Bharucha, 1988; Johnston and
Jones, 2006; Verfaillie and d'Ydewalle, 1991). Motion of a surrounding context in the
form of an enclosing window or frame increases forward displacement of a target when
that context moves in the direction of target motion and decreases forward displacement of a target when that context moves in the direction opposite to target motion
(Hubbard, 1993; Whitney and Cavanagh, 2002). Forward displacement is increased
when a target moves toward a stationary landmark and decreased when a target moves
away from a stationary landmark (Hubbard and Ruppel, 1999). Cognitive context in
the form of conceptual knowledge regarding target identity (Nagai and Yagi, 2001;
Reed and Vinson, 1996; Vinson and Reed, 2002), verbal cues regarding subsequent

target behavior provided prior to target appearance (Hubbard, 1994), and whether the source of target motion is autonomous or attributed to another object (Hubbard, Blessum, and Ruppel, 2001; Hubbard and Favretto, 2003; Hubbard and Ruppel, 2002) also influence displacement in memory for the target.

Laboratory-Based Illusions or Adaptive Strategies

Just as *Prägnanz* can lead to illusions of form and shape (e.g., illusory contours), representational momentum can lead to illusions of location. Indeed, representational momentum has been characterized as a "memory illusion" (Roediger, 1996), and as noted earlier, displacement of location resulting from an application of Gestalt grouping principles has been referred to as a "Gestalt illusion." In studies of Kanizsa-type stimuli or representational momentum, laboratory stimuli are usually atypical of "real-world" stimuli (e.g., numerous unexplained alignments are unlikely, visible targets do not suddenly vanish, etc.). Such laboratory stimuli allow better experimental control, and, more intriguingly, the existence of illusory effects with such laboratory stimuli also demonstrates the robustness of these properties of mental representation (e.g., computer-animated targets do not possess mass and so do not experience the effects of physical momentum or physical gravity, but mental representations involving such targets nonetheless exhibit representational momentum and representational gravity). However, although Gestalt principles and representational momentum might be considered to result in illusions if the information content of the representation is compared to the information content of the stimulus, such influences on representation could alternatively be viewed as adaptive strategies for subsequent object recognition and localization. Indeed, providing such adaptive strategies could be the purpose or meaning of dynamic information in mental representation.

Automaticity in Application

In studies on representational momentum in which participants were given feedback about their performance (Finke and Freyd, 1985; Ruppel, Fleming, and Hubbard, 2009), instructed about representational momentum prior to experimental trials and asked to compensate for its effects (Courtney and Hubbard, 2008), or explicitly cued where a target vanished or would vanish (Hubbard, Kumar, and Carp, 2009), such information did not eliminate representational momentum. Also, representational momentum is increased under conditions of divided attention (i.e., increased when less attention was allocated to the target; Hayes and Freyd, 2002). The failure of explicit feedback and of instruction to eliminate representational momentum, coupled with increases in representational momentum with decreases in the amount of attention allocated to the target, suggests that representational momentum reflects automatic processes rather than conscious or controlled processes,[8] and that attention is necessary to halt the forward displacement (Finke and Freyd, 1989; Finke, Freyd, and Shyi, 1986). Similarly, the common observation of the robust emergence of illusory contours even when observers know the nature of the stimuli and that those contours are not present in the stimulus suggests consequences of Gestalt principles reflect automatic processes rather than conscious or controlled processes.

Summary and Conclusions

There are numerous similarities of properties and consequences of Gestalt principles of perceptual grouping with properties and consequences of representational momentum. Both Gestalt principles of perceptual grouping and representational momentum (1) lead to displacement in remembered location, (2) reflect environmental regularities, (3) decrease the amount of information needed to specify a stimulus, (4) have a potential basis in second-order isomorphism, (5) are potentially related to aesthetics and artistic expression, (6) are influenced by configuration and context, (7) can be interpreted as laboratory-based illusions or as adaptive strategies, and (8) involve automaticity in application. The existence of such similarities is consistent with an expanded view of *Prägnanz*, in which previously unconsidered types of dynamic information (e.g., representational momentum) are also viewed as increasing the simplicity or regularity of a stimulus (thus decreasing processing demands and increasing cognitive efficiency).[9] Indeed, given numerous similarities in properties and consequences of Gestalt principles of perceptual grouping and of representational momentum, and given a basis for representational momentum in *Prägnanz*, representational momentum could be considered a new Gestalt principle and an exemplar of a new class of Gestalt principle involving localization rather than identification.

Several of the similarities of properties and consequences of Gestalt principles of perceptual grouping with properties and consequences of representational momentum involve a dynamic unfolding of phenomenal space within mental representation. This process of unfolding is based on expectations grounded in experience of environmental regularities. In the case of Gestalt principles of perceptual grouping, the unfolding of phenomenal space reflects rapid parsing and identification of stimuli (which often adds new information to perception; e.g., illusory contours, amodal perception). In the case of representational momentum, the unfolding of phenomenal space reflects rapid extrapolation of an anticipated state (which often results in displacement in remembered qualities or quantities from the actual value to an expected value). Dynamics in the physical environment unfold in time, and so the idea of information within a mental representation that unfolds in time is consistent with Freyd's view, in which a dynamic mental representation intrinsically and necessarily includes temporal information. Interestingly, many examples of the inclusion of dynamic information in mental representation came from the literature on mental imagery, and this suggests a possibility of deeper connections among Gestalt notions, mental imagery, and dynamics (e.g., such as a second-order isomorphism that reflects dynamics and forces, as well as kinematics and geometry).[10]

The similarities of properties and consequences of Gestalt principles of perceptual grouping with properties and consequences of representational momentum suggest that the notion of *Prägnanz* could be extended to include recent findings on dynamic aspects of mental representation. Recent work on dynamics in cognitive systems has focused primarily on dynamics within the operation of those cognitive systems and has not focused on how dynamics in mental representation are related to dynamics in the physical world. However, it is this latter focus (i.e., the correspondence between dynamics in mental representation and dynamics in the physical world) that motivated Gestalt theorizing on isomorphism. Although Gestalt principles and the underlying idea of *Prägnanz* were originally discussed as involving dynamic processes, much of the recent research on dynamic processes in cognition has not connected with this earlier work. The large number of similarities of properties and consequences of Gestalt principles with properties and consequences of representational momentum suggests it might be possible to incorporate historical Gestalt theory and contemporary theories and findings regarding dynamic aspects of mental representation into a single larger and more comprehensive theoretical framework involving anticipatory structures.

Notes

1. An illusion reflects a mismatch or miscalibration between the information content in the stimulus and the information content in the percept. However, as discussed in the introduction to this volume, such mismatches or miscalibrations are relevant only in inferential or other models in which the information content of the precept is required to be identical with (or is not otherwise distinguished from) the information content of the stimulus. To the extent that the perceptual act is not solely based on or computed from information in the stimulus, then illusions per se do not exist in phenomenal perception. Nonetheless, several phenomena discussed in this chapter have traditionally or historically been referred to as "illusory" or "illusions" (e.g., illusory contours, gamma motion, Gestalt illusions), and so this nomenclature is retained.

2. The length of a description of the stimulus offers an initial approximation of the degree of information and figural goodness: Stimuli higher in figural goodness require fewer words (i.e., less information) to describe than do stimuli lower in figural goodness. Compare a description when illusory contours are present (e.g., a white triangle above a black outline triangle and partially overlapping three black circles) with a more objective description of the stimulus in which illusory contours are not present (e.g., three black circles with equal-sized wedges missing from them and which are aligned so that the edges of the wedge in each circle align with edges of the wedges in the other circles, and three open angle stimuli that are aligned so that each line in an angle aligns with lines in the other two angles and the terminator of each line would be along a line connecting the wedges missing from the two nearest circle shapes, etc.).

3. For an additional discussion regarding meaningfulness in information, see Roederer (2003). On a related point, and as discussed in the introduction to this volume, perceptual information involves qualitative and semantic (i.e., meaningful) elements in addition to any purely quantitative elements, but current theories of the perceptual act do not include qualitative or semantic information (an analogous discussion that theories of mental imagery do not include semantic information was developed in Hubbard, 1996b). The importance of qualitative elements in perception is also demonstrated in the existence of metathetic continua in psychophysics.

4. Many researchers do not accept, and there has subsequently been evidence reported that does not support, the hypothesis that an analogue of momentum might be incorporated or internalized into mental representation (for an overview of theories of representational momentum, see Hubbard, 2010). However, the conclusions drawn in this chapter do not depend on a literal incorporation of momentum into mental representation and should be compatible with whatever mechanisms are suggested by a more developed or final theory of representational momentum.

5. Such a claim is consistent with notions that (1) dynamic information is not computed separately from other elements of the perceptual act, and (2) the perceptual act reflects a larger unitary experience based on the embedding of the perceiver and the perceived within the physical world.

6. There are two strands of evidence consistent with the idea that representational momentum leads an observer to attend more to locations along the anticipated trajectory. One strand involves judgments of locations primed by representational momentum. Kerzel, Jordan, and Müsseler (2001) presented horizontally moving targets and a subsequent probe. The probe was a circle with a gap at the top or bottom, and observers judged whether the gap was at the top or bottom of the probe. Observers were faster and more accurate when the probe was slightly in front of the actual final position of the target than when the probe was slightly behind the actual final position of the target. A second strand involves inhibition of return, in which processing of stimuli in locations previously attended to is less efficient than processing of stimuli in novel locations (Klein, 2000; Posner and Cohen, 1984). If the normal trajectory of a target is considered, locations behind the target would have been previously attended (as the target moved through those positions), and so observers should be less likely to subsequently attend those locations. If observers are less likely to attend locations behind a target, they presumably are more likely to attend locations in front of that target.

7. Evidence consistent with a perception of dynamics that previously acted on a stimulus can also be found in data already in the literature but not previously interpreted as reflecting such dynamics. For example, findings regarding effects of cardioidal strain on perception of youthfulness (e.g., Pittenger, Shaw, and Mark, 1979) suggest a sensitivity to the duration of exposure of a stimulus to gravity. Moreover, such an interpretation would be consistent with Leyton's (1989, 1992) view that perception involves the history of the forces that operated on an object.

8. In an alternative view, Kerzel (2003) argued that attention is necessary to generate or maintain forward displacement. However, in the experiments on which his argument is based, Kerzel presented a distractor after the target vanished, whereas Hayes and Freyd (2002) used a divided attention methodology in which participants attended to the target and to a secondary task concurrent with target presentation. It could be argued that a divided attention task offers a purer measure of

the effects of attention to the target than does presentation of a distractor after the target already vanished. There were also other methodological differences between Kerzel's task and Hayes and Freyd's task (for further discussion, see Hubbard, 2005; Hubbard et al., 2009).

9. Although comparison of spatiotemporal biases with Gestalt principles of perceptual grouping used representational momentum as the example of a spatiotemporal bias, other spatiotemporal biases exhibit similar properties and consequences. For example, boundary extension (1) results in displacement in remembered location (of the edges of the scene outward), (2) reflects environmental regularities of spatial continuity (when viewing a picture, observers know the scene continues beyond the edges of the picture, and when viewing a scene though a window, observers know the scene continues beyond the edges of the window; Intraub, 2002), (3) decreases the amount of information to be processed by priming objects and elements of a scene likely to be encountered in the next moment of time or with the next fixation, (4) could reflect a second-order isomorphism to the extent that represented space exhibits continuity similar to that of physical space, (5) is sensitive to context (a target object must be within a scene, that is, there must be a meaningful context surrounding the object, (6) has been classified as a memory illusion by Roediger (1996), and (7) occurs automatically even in observers who are informed about the phenomenon prior to viewing pictures and asked to guard against boundary extension in their responding (Intraub and Bodamer, 1993).

10. In one suggestive study, Munger, Solberg, and Horrocks (1999) found a positive correlation between the velocity of mental rotation and the magnitude of representational momentum. This pattern is consistent with the possibility that a common form of representation or representational structure might underlie both mental imagery and representational momentum.

References

Albertazzi, L. 2002a. "Continua." In *Unfolding Perceptual Continua*, edited by L. Albertazzi. Amsterdam: Benjamins Publishing Company. 1–28.

Albertazzi, L. 2002b "Towards a Neo-Aristotelian Theory of Continua: Elements of an Empirical Geometry." In *Unfolding Perceptual Continua*, edited by L. Albertazzi. Amsterdam: Benjamins Publishing Company. 29–79.

Albertazzi, L. 2005. *Immanent Realism*. New York: Springer.

Albertazzi, L. 2006. "Das rein figurale—The Shadowy Scheme of the Form." *Gestalt Theory* 28: 123–151.

Arnheim, R. 1966. *Toward a Psychology of Art*. Berkeley, CA: University of California Press.

Arnheim, R. 1974. *Art and Visual Perception: A Psychology of the Creative Eye*. Berkeley, CA: University of California Press.

Arnheim, R. 1988. *The Power of the Center: A Study of Composition in the Visual Arts*. Berkeley, CA: University of California Press.

Arnheim, R. 1996. *The Split and the Structure*. Berkeley, CA: University of California Press.

Attneave, F. 1955. "Symmetry, Information and Memory for Patterns." *American Journal of Psychology* 68: 209–222.

Attneave, F. 1968. "Triangles as Ambiguous Figures." *American Journal of Psychology* 81: 447–453.

Babcock, M. K., and Freyd, J. J. 1988. "Perception of Dynamic Information in Static Handwritten Forms." *American Journal of Psychology* 101: 111–130.

Bartley, S. H., and Wilkinson, F. R. 1953. "Some Factors in the Production of Gamma Movement." *Journal of Psychology* 36: 201–206.

Bregman, A. S. 1990. *Auditory Scene Analysis: The Perceptual Organization of Sound*. Cambridge, MA: MIT Press.

Bucher, N. M., and Palmer, S. E. 1985. "Effects of Motion on Perceived Pointing of Ambiguous Triangles." *Perception & Psychophysics* 38: 227–236.

Christie, J., and Klein, R. M. 2005. "Does Attention Cause Illusory Line Motion?" *Perception & Psychophysics* 67: 1032–1043.

Cooper, L. A. 1976. "Demonstration of a Mental Analog of an External Rotation." *Perception & Psychophysics* 19: 296–302.

Coren, S., and Girgus, J. S. 1980. "Principles of Perceptual Organization: The Gestalt Illusions." *Journal of Experimental Psychology: Human Perception and Performance* 6: 404–412.

Coren, S., Ward, L. M., and Enns, J. T. 2004. *Sensation and Perception*. 6th ed. New York: Wiley.

Courtney, J. R., and Hubbard, T. L. 2008. "Spatial Memory and Explicit Knowledge: An Effect of Instruction on Representational Momentum." *Quarterly Journal of Experimental Psychology* 61: 1778–1784.

Deutsch, D. 1999. "Grouping Mechanisms in Music." In *The Psychology of Music*, edited by D. Deutsch. 2nd ed. New York: Academic Press. 299–348.

Dickinson, C. A., and Intraub, H. 2008. "Transsaccadic Representation of Layout: What Is the Time Course of Boundary Extension?" *Journal of Experimental Psychology: Human Perception and Performance* 34: 543–555.

Downing, P. E., and Treisman, A. M. 1997. "The Line-Motion Illusion: Attention or Impletion?" *Journal of Experimental Psychology: Human Perception and Performance* 23: 768–779.

Enns, J. T., and Girgus, J. S. 1985. "Perceptual Grouping and Spatial Distortion: A Developmental Study." *Developmental Psychology* 21: 241–246.

Finke, R. A., and Freyd, J. J. 1985. "Transformation of Visual Memory Induced by Implied Motion of Pattern Elements." *Journal of Experimental Psychology: Learning, Memory, and Cognition* 11: 780–794.

Finke, R. A., and Freyd, J. J. 1989. "Mental Extrapolation and Cognitive Penetrability: Reply to Ranney and Proposals for Evaluative Criteria." *Journal of Experimental Psychology: General* 118: 403–408.

Finke, R. A., Freyd, J. J., and Shyi, G. C. W. 1986. "Implied velocity and acceleration induce transformations of visual memory." *Journal of Experimental Psychology: General* 115: 175–188.

Finke, R. A., Johnson, M. K., and Shyi, G. C. W. 1988. "Memory Confusions for Real and Imaged Completions of Symmetrical Visual Patterns." *Memory & Cognition* 16: 133–137.

Freyd, J. J. 1987. "Dynamic Mental Representations." *Psychological Review* 94: 427–438.

Freyd, J. J. 1992. "Dynamic Representations Guiding Adaptive Behavior." In *Time, Action, and Cognition: Towards Bridging the Gap*, edited by F. Macar, V. Pouthas, and W. J. Friedman. Dordrecht: Kluwer. 309–323.

Freyd, J. J. 1993. "Five Hunches about Perceptual Process and Dynamic Representations." In *Attention and Performance XIV: Synergies in Experimental Psychology, Artificial Intelligence, and Cognitive Neuroscience*, edited by D. Meyer and S. Kornblum. Cambridge, MA: MIT Press. 99–119.

Freyd, J. J., and Finke, R. A. 1984. "Representational Momentum." *Journal of Experimental Psychology: Learning, Memory, and Cognition* 10: 126–132.

Freyd, J. J., and Johnson, J. Q. 1987. "Probing the Time Course of Representational Momentum." *Journal of Experimental Psychology: Learning, Memory, and Cognition* 13: 259–269.

Freyd, J. J., and Pantzer, T. M. 1995. "Static Patterns Moving in the Mind." In *The Creative Cognition Approach*, edited by S. M. Smith, T. B. Ward, and R. A. Finke. Cambridge, MA: MIT Press. 181–204.

Freyd, J. J., Pantzer, T. M., and Cheng, J. L. 1988. "Representing Statics as Forces in Equilibrium." *Journal of Experimental Psychology: General* 117: 395–407.

Fuller, S., and Carrasco, M. 2009. "Perceptual Consequences of Visual Performance Field: The Case of the Line Motion Illusion." *Journal of Vision* 9: 1–17.

Futterweit, L. R., and Beilin, H. 1994. "Recognition Memory for Movement in Photographs: A Developmental Study." *Journal of Experimental Child Psychology* 57: 163–179.

Goldstein, E. B. 1999. *Sensation & Perception*. 5th ed. Pacific Grove, CA: Brooks/Cole.

Gottesman, C. V., and Intraub, H. 2002. "Surface Construal and the Mental Representation of Scenes." *Journal of Experimental Psychology: Human Perception and Performance* 28: 589–599.

Gregory, R. L. 1974. "Choosing a Paradigm for Perception." In *Handbook of Perception. Vol. 1. Historical and Philosophical Roots of Perception*, edited by E. C. Carterette and M. P. Friedman. New York: Academic Press. 255–283.

Harrower, M. R. 1929. "Some Experiments on the Nature of Gamma Movement." *Psychologische Forschung* 13: 55–63.

Hatfield, G., and Epstein, W. 1985. "The Status of the Minimum Principle in the Theoretical Analysis of Visual Perception." *Psychological Bulletin 97*: 155–186.

Hayes, A. E., and Freyd, J. J. 2002. "Representational Momentum When Attention Is Divided." *Visual Cognition* 9: 8–27.

Hegarty, M. 1992. "Mental Animation: Inferring Motion From Static Displays of Mechanical Systems." *Journal of Experimental Psychology: Learning, Memory, and Cognition* 18: 1084–1102.

Henle, M. 1984. "Isomorphism: Setting the Record Straight." *Psychological Research/Psychologische Forschung* 46: 317–327.

Hikosaka, O., Miyauchi, S., and Shimojo, S. 1993. "Focal Visual Attention Produces Illusory Temporal Order and Motion Sensation." *Vision Research* 33: 1219–1240.

Hochberg, J. E., and Brooks, V. 1960. "The Psychophysics of Form: Reversible-Perspective Drawings of Spatial Objects." *American Journal of Psychology* 73: 337–354.

Hochberg, J. E., and McAlister, E. 1953. "A Quantitative Approach to Figural Goodness." *Journal of Experimental Psychology* 46: 361–364.

Howe, E. S., and Brandau, C. J. 1983. "The Temporal Course of Visual Pattern Encoding: Effects of Pattern Goodness." *Quarterly Journal of Experimental Psychology* 35A: 607–633.

Howe, E. S., and Jung, K. 1986. "Immediate Memory Span for Two-Dimensional Spatial Arrays: Effects of Pattern Symmetry and Goodness." *Acta Psychologica* 61: 37–51.

Hubbard, T. L. 1990. "Cognitive Representation of Linear Motion: Possible Direction and Gravity Effects in Judged Displacement." *Memory & Cognition* 18: 299–309.

Hubbard, T. L. 1993. "The Effects of Context on Visual Representational Momentum." *Memory & Cognition* 21: 103–114.

Hubbard, T. L. 1994. "Judged Displacement: A Modular Process?" *American Journal of Psychology* 107: 359–373.

Hubbard, T. L. 1995a. "Cognitive Representation of Motion: Evidence for Friction and Gravity Analogues." *Journal of Experimental Psychology: Learning, Memory, and Cognition* 21: 241–254.

Hubbard, T. L. 1995b. "Environmental Invariants in the Representation of Motion: Implied Dynamics and Representational Momentum, Gravity, Friction, and Centripetal Force." *Psychonomic Bulletin & Review* 2: 322–338.

Hubbard, T. L. 1996a. "Representational Momentum, Centripetal Force, and Curvilinear Impetus." *Journal of Experimental Psychology: Learning, Memory, and Cognition* 22: 1049–1060.

Hubbard, T. L. 1996b. "The Importance of a Consideration of Qualia to Imagery and Cognition." *Consciousness and Cognition* 5: 327–358.

Hubbard, T. L. 1997. "Target Size and Displacement Along the Axis of Implied Gravitational Attraction: Effects of Implied Weight and Evidence of Representational Gravity." *Journal of Experimental Psychology: Learning, Memory, and Cognition* 23: 1484–1493.

Hubbard, T. L. 1998. "Some Effects of Representational Friction, Target Size, and Memory Averaging on Memory for Vertically Moving Targets." *Canadian Journal of Experimental Psychology* 52: 44–49.

Hubbard, T. L. 1999. "How Consequences of Physical Principles Influence Mental Representation: The Environmental Invariants Hypothesis." In *Fechner Day 99: The End of 20th Century Psychophysics. Proceedings of the 15th Annual Meeting of the International Society for Psychophysics*, edited by P. R. Killeen and W. R. Uttal. Tempe, AZ: The International Society for Psychophysics. 274–279.

Hubbard, T. L. 2005. "Representational Momentum and Related Displacements in Spatial Memory: A Review of the Findings." *Psychonomic Bulletin & Review* 12: 822–851.

Hubbard, T. L. 2006a. "Bridging the Gap: Possible Roles and Contributions of Representational Momentum." *Psicologica* 27: 1–34.

Hubbard, T. L. 2006b. "Computational Theory and Cognition in Representational Momentum and Related Types of Displacement: A Reply to Kerzel." *Psychonomic Bulletin & Review* 13: 174–177.

Hubbard, T. L. 2010. "Approaches to Representational Momentum: Theories and Models." In *Space and Time in Perception and Action*, edited by R. Nijhawan and B. Khurana. Cambridge, UK: Cambridge University Press. 338–365.

Hubbard, T. L., and Blessum, J. A. 2001. "A Structural Dynamic of Form: Displacements in Memory for the Size of an Angle." *Visual Cognition* 8: 725–749.

Hubbard, T. L., Blessum, J. A., and Ruppel, S. E. 2001. "Representational Momentum and Michotte's (1946/1963) 'Launching Effect' Paradigm." *Journal of Experimental Psychology: Learning, Memory, and Cognition* 27: 294–301.

Hubbard, T. L., and Bharucha, J. J. 1988. "Judged Displacement in Apparent Vertical and Horizontal Motion." *Perception & Psychophysics* 44: 211–221.

Hubbard, T. L., and Courtney, J. R. 2006. "Evidence Suggestive of Separate Visual Dynamics in Perception and in Memory." In *Visual thought*, edited by L. Albertazzi. Amsterdam: Benjamins. 71–97.

Hubbard, T. L., and Favretto, A. 2003. "Naive Impetus and Michotte's 'Tool Effect:' Evidence From Representational Momentum." *Psychological Research/Psychologische Forschung* 67: 134–152.

Hubbard, T. L., Hutchison, J. L., and Courtney, J. R. 2010. "Boundary Extension: Findings and Theories." *Quarterly Journal of Experimental Psychology* 63: 1467–1494.

Hubbard, T. L., Kumar, A. M., and Carp, C. L. 2009. "Effects of Spatial Cueing on Representational Momentum." *Journal of Experimental Psychology: Learning, Memory, and Cognition* 35: 666–677.

Hubbard, T. L., and Ruppel, S. E. 1999. "Representational Momentum and Landmark Attraction Effects." *Canadian Journal of Experimental Psychology* 53: 242–256.

Hubbard, T. L., and Ruppel, S. E. 2000. "Spatial Memory Averaging, the Landmark Attraction Effect, and Representational Gravity." *Psychological Research/Psychologische Forschung* 64: 41–55.

Hubbard, T. L., and Ruppel, S. E. 2002. "A Possible Role of Naive Impetus in Michotte's 'Launching Effect:' Evidence From Representational Momentum." *Visual Cognition* 9: 153–176.

Intraub, H. 2002. "Anticipatory Spatial Representation of Natural Scenes: Momentum Without Movement?" *Visual Cognition* 9: 93–119.

Intraub, H., and Bodamer, J. L. 1993. "Boundary Extension: Fundamental Aspect of Pictorial Representation or Encoding Artifact?" *Journal of Experimental Psychology: Learning, Memory, and Cognition* 19: 1387–1397.

Johnston, H. M., and Jones, M. R. 2006. "Higher Order Pattern Structure Influences Auditory Representational Momentum." *Journal of Experimental Psychology: Human Perception and Performance* 32: 2–17.

Jones, M. R. 1976. "Time, Our Lost Dimension: Toward a New Theory of Perception, Attention, and Memory." *Psychological Review* 83: 323–355.

Kanizsa, G. 1979. *Organization in Vision: Essays on Gestalt Psychology*. New York: Praeger.

Kelso, J. A. S. 1995. *Dynamic Patterns: The Self-Organization of Brain and Behavior*. Cambridge, MA: MIT Press.

Kennedy, J. M. 1988. "Line Endings and Subjective Contours." *Spatial Vision* 3: 151–158.

Kerzel, D. 2003. "Attention Maintains Mental Extrapolation of Target Position: Irrelevant Distractors Eliminate Forward Displacement After Implied Motion." *Cognition* 88: 109–131.

Kerzel, D. 2006. "Why Eye Movements and Perceptual Factors Have to Be Controlled in Studies on 'Representational Momentum.'" *Psychological Bulletin & Review* 13: 166–173.

Kerzel, D., Jordan, J. S., and Müsseler, J. 2001. "The Role of Perception in the Mislocalization of the Final Position of a Moving Target." *Journal of Experimental Psychology: Human Perception and Performance* 27: 829–840.

Klein, R. M. 2000. "Inhibition of Return." *Trends in Cognitive Sciences* 4: 138–147.

Knoblich, G., and Sebanz, N. 2006. "The Social Nature of Perception and Action." *Current Directions in Psychological Science* 15: 99–104.

Koffka, K. 1935. *Principles of Gestalt Psychology*. New York: Harcourt Brace.

Kohler, W. 1938. *The Place of Value in a World of Facts*. New York: Liveright.

Kohler, W. 1940. *Dynamics in Psychology*. New York: Liveright

Kohler, W. 1969. *The Task of Gestalt Psychology*. Princeton, NJ: Princeton University Press.

Kolers, P. A., and Smythe, W. E. 1979. "Images, Symbols, and Skills." *Canadian Journal of Psychology* 33: 158–184.

Kosslyn, S. M. 1980. *Image and Mind*. Cambridge, MA: Harvard University Press.

Kosslyn, S. M., Ball, T. M., and Reiser, B. J. 1978. "Visual Images Preserve Metric Information: Evidence From Studies of Image Scanning." *Journal of Experimental Psychology: Human Perception and Performance* 4: 47–60.

Lesher, G. W., and Mingolla, E. 1993. "The Role of Edges and Line-Ends in Illusory Contour Formation." *Vision Research* 33: 2253–2270.

Leyton, M. 1989. "Inferring Causal History From Shape." *Cognitive Science* 13: 357–387.

Leyton, M. 1992. *Symmetry, Causality, Mind*. Cambridge, MA: MIT Press.

Liberman, A. M., and Mattingly, I. G. 1985. "The Motor Theory of Speech Perception Revised." *Cognition* 21: 1–36.

Lowe, D. 1985. *Perceptual Organization and Visual Recognition*. Dordrecht: Kluwer Academic.

McBeath, M. K., and Morikawa, K. 1997. "Forward-Facing Motion Biases for Rigid and Nonrigid Biologically Likely Transformations." *Perceptual and Motor Skills* 85: 1187–1193.

McBeath, M. K., Morikawa, K., and Kaiser, M. K. 1992. "Perceptual Bias for Forward-Facing Motion. *Psychological Science* 3: 362–367.

Munger, M. P., Solberg, J. L., and Horrocks, K. K. 1999. "The Relationship Between Mental Rotation and Representational Momentum." *Journal of Experimental Psychology: Learning, Memory, and Cognition* 25: 1557–1568.

Nagai, M., and Yagi, A. 2001. "The Pointedness Effect on Representational Momentum." *Memory & Cognition* 29: 91–99.

Palmer, S. E. 1980. "What Makes Triangles Point: Local and Global Effects in Configurations of Ambiguous Triangles." *Cognitive Psychology* 12: 285–305.

Palmer, S. E. 1983. "The Psychology of Perceptual Organization: A Transformational Approach." In *Human and Machine Vision*, edited by J. Beck, B. Hope, and A. Rosenfeld. New York: Academic Press. 269–339.

Palmer, S. E. 2002. "Perceptual Organization in Vision." In *Stevens Handbook of Experimental Psychology. Vol. 1. Sensation and Perception*, edited by H. Pashler and S. Yantis. 3rd ed. New York: Wiley. 177–234.

Palmer, S. E., and Bucher, N. M. 1981. "Configural Effects in Perceived Pointing of Ambiguous Triangles." *Journal of Experimental Psychology: Human Perception and Performance* 7: 88–114.

Palmer, S. E., and Bucher, N. M. 1982. "Textural Effects in Perceived Pointing of Ambiguous Triangles." *Journal of Experimental Psychology: Human Perception and Performance* 8: 693–708.

Pittenger, J. B., Shaw, R. E., and Mark, L. S. 1979. "Perceptual Information for the Age Level of Faces as a Higher Order Invariant of Growth." *Journal of Experimental Psychology: Human Perception and Performance* 5: 478–493.

Pomerantz, J. R., Sager, L. C., and Stoever, R. J. 1977. "Perception of Wholes and of Their Component Parts: Some configural superiority effects." *Journal of Experimental Psychology: Human Perception and Performance* 3: 422–435.

Port, R. F., and van Gelder, T. (Eds.). 1995. *Mind as Motion: Explorations in the Dynamics of Cognition*. Cambridge, MA: MIT Press.

Posner, M. I., and Cohen, Y. 1984. "Components of Visual Orienting." In *Attention and Performance X: Control of Language Processes*, edited by H. Bouma and D. Bouwhuis. London: Erlbaum. 531–556.

Pylyshyn, Z. W. 1984. *Computation and Cognition*. Cambridge, MA: MIT Press.

Reed, C. L., and Vinson, N. G. 1996. "Conceptual Effects on Representational Momentum." *Journal of Experimental Psychology: Human Perception and Performance* 22: 839–850.

Roederer, J. G. 2003. "On the Concept of Information and Its Role in Nature." *Entropy* 5: 3–33.

Roediger, H. L. 1996. "Memory Illusions." *Journal of Memory and Language* 35: 76–100.

Ruppel, S. E., Fleming, C. N., and Hubbard, T. L. 2009. "Representational Momentum Is Not (Totally) Impervious to Error Feedback." *Canadian Journal of Experimental Psychology* 63: 49–58.

Schiffman, H. R. 2001. *Sensation and Perception: An Integrated Approach*. 5th ed. New York: Wiley.

Schwartz, D. L., and Black, T. 1999. "Inferences Through Imagined Actions: Knowing by Simulated Doing." *Journal of Experimental Psychology: Learning, Memory, and Cognition* 25: 116–136.

Shanon, B. 2008. *The Representational and the Presentational*. 2nd ed. Charlottesville, VA: Imprint-Academic.

Shepard, R. N. 1968. "Review of Cognitive Psychology by U. Neisser." *American Journal of Psychology* 81: 285–289.

Shepard, R. N. 1975. "Form, Formation, and Transformation of Internal Representations." In *Information Processing and Cognition: The Loyola Symposium*, edited by R. L. Solso. Hillsdale, NJ: Erlbaum. 87–122.

Shepard, R. N. 1984. "Ecological Constraints on Internal Representation: Resonant Kinematics of Perceiving, Imagining, Thinking, and Dreaming." *Psychological Review* 91: 417–447.

Shepard, R. N. 1994. "Perceptual-Cognitive Universals as Reflections of the World." *Psychonomic Bulletin & Review* 1: 2–28.

Shepard, R. N., and Cooper, L. A. (Eds.). 1982. *Mental Images and Their Transformations*. Cambridge, MA: MIT Press.

Shepard, R. N., and Metzler, J. 1971. "Mental Rotation of Three-Dimensional Objects." *Science* 171: 701–703.

Spivey, M. 2007. *The Continuity of Mind*. New York: Oxford University Press.

Thelen, E., and Smith, L. B. 1994. *A Dynamic Systems Approach to the Development of Cognition and Action*. Cambridge, MA: MIT Press.

Thornton, I. M., and Hayes, A. E. 2004. "Anticipating Action in Complex Scenes." *Visual Cognition* 11: 341–370.

Tse, P. U., and Cavanagh, P. 2000. "Chinese and Americans See Opposite Apparent Motions in a Chinese Character." *Cognition* 74: B27–B32.

Van Tuijl, H. 1980. "Perceptual Interpretation of Complex Line Patterns." *Journal of Experimental Psychology: Human Perception and Performance* 6: 197–221.

Verfaillie, K., and d'Ydewalle, G. 1991. "Representational Momentum and Event Course Anticipation in the Perception of Implied Periodical Motions." *Journal of Experimental Psychology: Learning, Memory, and Cognition* 17: 302–313.

Vinson, N. G., and Reed, C. L. 2002. "Sources of Object-Specific Effects in Representational Momentum." *Visual Cognition* 9: 41–65.

Wertheimer, M. 2002. "The General Theoretical Situation." In *A Source Book of Gestalt Psychology*, edited by W. Ellis. London: Routledge. 12–16. (Original work published 1922)

Whitney, D., and Cavanagh, P. 2002. "Surrounding Motion Affects the Perceived Locations of Moving Stimuli." *Visual Cognition* 9: 139–152.

Wilson, M., and Knoblich, G. 2005. "The Case for Motor Involvement in Perceiving Conspecifics." *Psychological Bulletin* 131: 460–473.

Winters, J. J. 1964. "Gamma Movement: Apparent Movement in Figural Aftereffects Experiments." *Perceptual and Motor Skills* 19: 819–822.

4 Informing through an Imperfect Retina

Gert J. van Tonder

The visual constancies we associate with perception—at the level of ecological surfaces and objects, such as the pine tree, the shaded velvety moss on its bark, the patches of sky seen through its branches, dipping in the breeze—are accepted as the outcome of a system of brain mechanisms that, much like a weavery, has its spindles whizzing busily, the waft separating as programmed by a prior design. On the other end of all this activity emerges a finely woven cloth: silky, shiny, the intricately colored florals and beasts of its design all dancing in unison. This is perception. None of its visual richness is apparent in the formless bales of unspun fibers that eventually become the woven cloth. One might be tempted to consider the retina in these terms: Like the gaping difference between preprocessed silk and a decorated cloth, information at the retinal level seems so raw that, ironically, the eye could be considered practically blind compared with the perceptual richness attributed to the cerebral cortex.

Even phrases such as "the seeing eye" or "psychology of the eye" are now frowned upon, the consensus being that the brain, not the eye, is the seat of vision. The true creation of information is considered not a sensory but a cortical feat. In this chapter, I hypothesize that proto-categories of the visual divisions externally observed within the lower level visual cortex already arise in the eye; in fact, at the first level where light meets a neural structure—the retinal cones—leaving serious questions about the actual role of the cortex in visual perception.

Because we are specifically interested in "information," let me clarify my position on the terminology. I still remember the first university lecture on the standard information theory (Weaver and Shannon, 1963). My whole being tingled with the feeling that common sense was being flogged alive. How was it possible that what appears most informative to me could be labeled as a redundancy? True, one needs a maximal number of memory bits to accurately transmit a screen of white noise between a sender and a receiver, but why on earth call that a maximal *information* load when all those noise dots appear so meaningless? Why not call it a maximal *decorrelation* load? The more meaningless something is, the more tedious the task of transmitting it. This use of terminology reminds me of the trend in the financial world to call high-risk investments "securities" in a bid to attract investors. In contrast, even if a large number of points on a closed circle—a highly redundant (noninformative) structure in standard information theory but quite meaningful to me as a perceiving human—were corrupted between sender and receiver, its circularity could still be effortlessly confirmed.

The stance in this chapter is opposite to the standard information theory. In terms of perceptual information, I could actually rearticulate it as the standard decorrelation theory: The more decorrelated a structure, the greater the channel capacity needed to accurately transmit it between a sender and a receiver. Highly decorrelated structures, such as screens of white noise, are accordingly more redundant because individual structural elements are less likely to contribute robustly to the context of the structure while also clogging the transmission channel.

Intuitively, information implies meaning. In a true theory of information, the most meaningful structures should have the highest informational content. Instead of the concept of redundancy, one could rather use *consistency* as a measure of how well a structure retains information (i.e., remains meaningful when it becomes corrupted, deformed, or fragmented). Thus, a shiny metal teapot remains roughly equally meaningful regardless of the intricate patterns reflected from its surface, whether the reflections are of a kitchen interior or the scenery around a park bench. The standard information theory is concerned with transmitting each of the miniscule variations in the reflection on the teapot surface accurately while perceptually to me they do not mean much: The object and its material properties remain more or less the same.

Indeed, meaning, and thus information, implies subjective experience; it can therefore not be externally measured or analyzed by looking at the structure and activity of either the eye or the brain. At best—as far as external measurement is concerned—one can compare internally experienced percepts with physical measurements to find *possible correlations* between measurements and what is subjectively experienced. This will be the stance from which I view all model simulations in this chapter. What is shown in the following sections is not the information (or meaning) created by the visual system but mere computational structures open for comparison with one's own perceptual content in an attempt to elucidate some of their mutual underpinnings. I do not intend to equate the content of perception with the output of a computational algorithm.

The stance on a theory of information is important for interpreting the role of the eye in vision. In the standard information theory, the eye is on the wrong side of a vast bottleneck. Not only does the retina fail to correctly encode "information" (decorrelations) due to shortcomings such as spatial blurring, temporal smearing together of structures that occur at different intervals, and sampling the incoming light at suboptimal resolutions; at a signal compression rate of at least 140:1 across the optic nerve, the retinal signals reaching the brain are thought at best to retain only a corrupted facsimile of the exact "information" needed to accurately reconstruct the so-called veridical physical reality. Hence, a vast complex of cortical divisions (Livingstone and Hubel, 1988; DeYoe and van Essen, 1988) streaming into dedicated pathways for object and spatial vision (Ungerleider and Mishkin, 1982) or perception and action (Goodale and Milner, 2004)—thought to house prior assumptions about the external reality—is necessary for inferring what was lost through the imperfect sampling and transmission by the retina. Deblurring, reconstructing, and interpolating are part of the solution (Rogers-Ramachandran and Ramachandran, 1998); sifting between the infinity of possible scenarios that could have given rise to the image of the natural scene constitutes the other main part of the problem. Even if the brain received a perfect image of the world, reverse engineering of that image back into the original physical layout is considered a vastly underconstrained or ill-posed problem to computationally solve. Hence, the formidable *problem of vision* (Marr, 1982).

My eyes tell me that vision does not have a problem, and that the bark of the ill-defined nature of the supposed problem is far worse than its bite. First, the postretinal bottleneck is probably overstated because it is not yet clear what exactly the retina functionally achieves. Looking at the sufficiency of most evolved systems around us, our scientific intuition should actually be that the eye is so efficient in performing its function that a thin bundle of nerves suffices as its connection to the brain while thus also facilitating easy movement of the eyes. Science should be seriously concerned with finding out more about what exactly that efficient retina achieves.

The fact that we can see convincing visual worlds even when the shading, perspective, and other visual structure deviate wildly (e.g., in pictures) from that of physical reality implies that visual perception does not hinge on veridicality but comfortably proceeds with open-ended visual information that differs from the punctual structural arrays deemed necessary for computational models of vision.

In addition, the eye does not take snapshots of the world as if it were a serious of frozen visual frames (Schnapf et al., 1990), and the eye certainly does not sit still—it is like a curious child in a toy store. The correspondence problem and the consequently ill-posed problem of vision are always posed from a stationary frame in which any part within the visual scene is accessed at equal levels of optical focus, hence vastly different from the problem solved by the eye.

In what follows, I want to show that by looking externally at the response of a *dynamic* eye, one finds the correlate of a rich set of potential cues for cortical vision. I also show how the dynamic nature of the eye—specifically, the spatiotemporal response at the retinal level—may contribute toward steering clear of some of the problems identified in conventional computer vision. Whatever the philosophical heritage of the readership, I hope that this chapter offers an original interpretation of low-level vision that will instill a new awareness of the creative impact of the retina on visual perception.

The Problem of Transitory Contrast

Let me start with a practical perceptual demonstration. Numerous perceptual effects spontaneously occur when viewing figure 4.1A: Faint-colored rainbows may appear to shift between the black and white lines, the whole figure may appear as an undulating three-dimensional wave, but the appearance of vivid transitory ribbons of high contrast—especially when the figure is jigged around—is perhaps the most salient effect observed. In fact, the effect was first described by Purkinje (1823); later by Helmholtz (1856), who incorrectly ascribed it to temporary astigmatism of the lens; and consequently by various investigators (Wade, 1978), each of whom gave different examples and explanations of the effect (see Gosselin and Lamontagne [1997] for an overview of the history of the scientific investigation). The explanations mainly attribute transitory contrast effects to either the eye or the brain.

The retina, thought unable to cope with the constant bombardment of light, confuses the incoming "image" with the previous image it just registered (Cobbold, 1881), and the averaged image (Gosselin and Lamontagne, 1997) results in transitory contrast patterns as seen in figure 4.1A. It also may result from the retina confusing the presently incoming light with an afterimage of the previous image (MacKay, 1958; Gregory, 1998), resulting in a Moiré pattern of successive images (Oster and Nishijima, 1963). Claims that motion detectors drive the perceived transitory contrast (Zanker, 2004) remain to be supported by experimental evidence. Alternatively, transitory contrast patterns are ascribed to cortical mechanisms (Zeki, 1994), although these hypotheses remain uncertain and without experimental evidence (as pointed out by Fermuller, Pless, and Aloimonos, 1997; Gregory, 1995).

Recent progress (Van Tonder and Ohtani, 2007) suggests that retinal cones are the source of transitory contrast effects. Take figure 4.1A and move it quickly up and down; you should see horizontal bands of transitory contrast. Next, rotate the figure, around its center, clockwise and anti-clockwise in quick succession while fixating the center; a different set of transitory loci appear. Finally, move the figure closer and farther away (scaling) in quick succession while fixating the center; this time a vertically snaking locus of contrast should appear. The observed contrast effect is not a random fluctuation but depends strictly on the relative displacement between observer and stimulus. For each type of movement, a fixed but unique set of transitory contrast loci appear.

Consider the contrast pattern for scaling. The blue loci in figure 4.2B (plate 2) closely matches the spatial structure of the transitory contrast pattern that you saw. This pseudocolor picture was computed by using a rough second-order feedback approximation of a detailed model of the temporal dynamics of a macaque retinal cone (Schnapf et al., 1990). This model is theoretically blind: It simply computes a model response at each pixel in each frame of a movie sequence taken of figure 4.1 moving closer toward the camera as it would when you are scaling it and perceiving a snake-like transitory

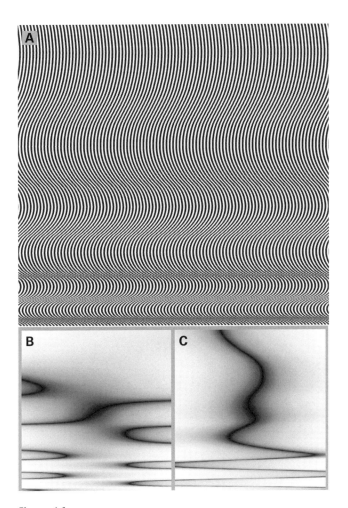

Figure 4.1
(A) A facsimile of *Fall*, a representative Op art work by Bridget Riley (1963) , now in the permanent collection of the Tate Gallery, London. Here, the author created an Adobe Photoshop image of stripes in which all the wavy black and white stripes are identical. In her original hand-painted work, small deviations in line width makes for a much more arresting aesthetic experience (Van Tonder, 2010). Effective duration of fluctuations between black and white stripes at each pixel, as figure 4.1A is (B) rotated and (C) scaled. Dark loci indicate locations where the duration is longer (i.e., stimulus regions that change less relative to a given location on the retina).

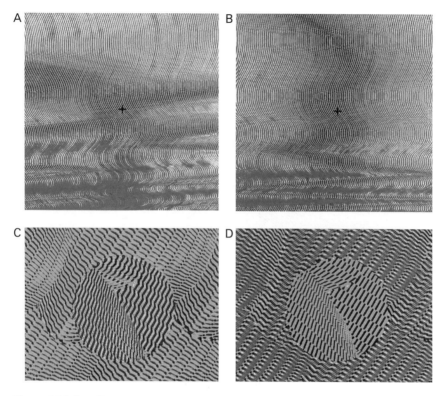

Figure 4.2 (plate 2)
Pseudocolor presentation of cone model simulations for (A) rotation and (B) scaling of figure 4.1.
Blue indicates high-contrast regions, red denotes lowest luminance contrast. Figure-ground segmentation in the Ouchi illusions (figure 4.5) is enhanced when moving the figure slightly. For
example, during (C) vertical and (D) oblique linear motion, different degrees of blur in the figure
and ground may play a role in the perceived relative motion between figure and ground. Visual
transduction in cones seems a proper candidate, albeit at a low level of vision for this selective
blur.

contrast locus in the middle of the figure. The model, a second-order feedback PID
controller that can be designed following standard control systems theory (Abramovici
and Chapksy, 2005), is set up to simulate a cone response to an incoming signal. The
response peaks 50 ms after onset of a change in incoming light, and the output signal
oscillation, at 5 Hz, stabilizes after 150 ms. With this blind dynamic model, a resemblance of the transitory contrast pattern can be computed. One would normally expect
a motion-detecting system to operate behind this; after all, transitory contrast appears
very *dynamic*, so why does a cone model work so well?

Cones respond slowly, rendering them unable to deal with fast changes between dark and light. Wherever a pattern of black and white stripes moves in a direction orthogonal to the orientation of the stripes, the fluctuation from black to white (e.g., at a point in the center of the pattern) occurs at a rate proportionally equivalent to the velocity of the motion of the grating. The faster this pattern moves, the quicker the succession between black and white; hence, a cone at the center of the pattern will have increasing difficulty in responding to either white or black. Its temporal dynamics produces an average of the two extremes: grey. Wherever this pattern of black and white stripes moves in a direction aligned with the orientation of the stripes, no fluctuation from black to white (e.g., at a point in the center of the pattern) occurs, and a cone would have sufficient time to respond appropriately to either black or white; where it moves at an angle of β relative to the orientation of the stripes, the fluctuation rate between black and white will be proportional to the product of velocity and the sine of β, and hence a cone will produce an increasingly weak (more grey) response for greater angles, β.

In other words, the duration for which either a white or dark stripe remains in front of a given cone will determine the strength of its response. This duration, computed as a function of stripe width, relative displacement velocity, and sin β (Van Tonder and Ohtani, forthcoming), is shown in figure 4.1B and 4.1C for rotation and scaling of figure 4.1A. This computation, unlike the cone model, is not blind, but a theoretical model, involving more abstract properties of the stimulus, such as line width, local orientation of stripes, and velocity vectors of displacements. The retina almost certainly does not explicitly rely on this theoretical computation, although implicitly its temporal dynamics has a conceptually related effect on its output signals. The theoretical model serves as evidence that the conclusion—that slow cone dynamics drives transitory contrast loci to appear in its output—is unlikely to be incorrect.[1] It further shows that transitory contrast loci appear along regions of the stimulus pattern that, for all practical purposes, remains stationary relative to the retina if one considers short *intervals* (about 200–500 ms). This conclusion is at first counterintuitive; transitory contrast appears so dynamic that one would not guess that it is the part of *least* flux in the stimulus.

Perception here noticeably agrees with and differs from the computational results in specific ways. First, it agrees in the sense that the spatial configuration—the geometrical structure—of perceived dynamic contrast loci bears a striking resemblance to the stationary geometrical structure seen in the computational result. This suggests that perception of the amount of light is deeply dependent on the retinal response to the extent where I cannot shut out the transitory contrast. I vividly perceive it as if it is—to borrow from naïve realism—a physical property of the surface material out of which the black and white stripes are made. Even if I know that it is veridically incorrect to see fluctuating contrast where there is only pure white and pure black, the effect persists.

Second, perception differs from the retinal response in that the transitory contrast structure appears so vividly *moving*. Here, the computational seriously facilitates insight into perception: It is as if vision frames the contrast structure within the knowledge that something is moving. This information seems to act as the reference, but the structure does not simply move: Transitory contrast appears as a moving element embedded in the black and white stripes; it takes on the meaning of an object with material properties—shimmering, metallic, flash-like, writhing, bending, and so on.

The retina captures stationary structure in clear detail while it temporally blurs changing structure. This effect, more widely known as *motion blur*, actually invites a whole new avenue of thinking about the role of retinal cones in vision.

The Informing Potential of Retinal Cones

Motion blur can be computed using the so-called signal averaging method (Burr, 1980; Gosselin and Lamontagne, 1997). It simply takes the average of a given number of successive image frames as a coarse approximation of retinal function. It differs in a significant way from the cone model (figure 4.3). Cones capture local asymmetries in the sharpness of leading and lagging edges of luminance gradients, analogous to the difference in slope of the water surface in front of, compared to the surface trailing behind,

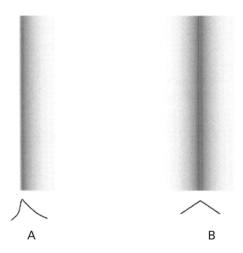

A   B

Figure 4.3
Motion smear during leftward motion of a vertical boundary contour as simulated with a model of visual transduction in retinal cones (A) and signal averaging (B). Note that (A) more closely resembles a traveling wave front (see insets at bottom of figure).

a breaking wave on the ocean (figure 4.3A). The effect is one of smearing rather than simply blurring and thus impresses cues of directionality into the existing visual structure (in the case of figure 4.3, the veridical structure would be a vertical luminance contour, moving toward the left). Note that wherever I mention "motion blur" from hereon in the chapter, I intend it to refer to directional smearing as obtained with a cone model.

The wave-like gradient of motion blur has many implications for what the eye conveys as information. As the retina sweeps around during every eye movement, the entire visual field is smeared. The generation of such false gradients is typically considered a problem that is somehow dealt with in later levels of visual processing or avoided altogether by suppression of retinal signals to the brain for the duration of the saccade (Burr, Morrone, and Ross, 1996). But not all visual channels—especially not the ones associated purely with cone-driven signals—are silenced during eye movements. How could this directional smearing that amounts to addition of false luminance gradients enrich the information created in the retina?

Motion Blur as Oriented Filtering

On a luminance contour of even width, deflection points and curvature maxima aligned with the direction of motion result in distinct smear markings of higher luminance contrast than over the rest of the contour (figure 4.4). This is evident from the fact that local contour segments around these points are parallel to the direction of motion and hence cover receptors at any of these points marginally longer than at any other location along the contour, exposing those receptors to the contour luminance values for a longer duration. Just as with developing photographs from film negatives, longer exposure means greater luminance intensities in regions exposed to light. At any other points along the contour, local contour segments move obliquely to the direction of motion and hence shift rapidly across receptors (i.e., exposing that given receptor to the least amount of contour structure).

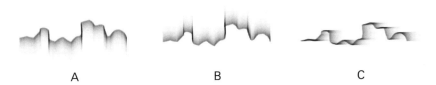

A   B   C

Figure 4.4
Smear lines simulated during upward (A), downward (B), and leftward (C) motion. The cone model generates stronger responses to deflection points and to regions around curvature maxima that locally align with the direction of motion. These high-contrast contour sections potentially convey cues of shape contour orientation and of motion orientation and direction.

Thus, smear lines around deflection points and curvature maxima explicitly mark locations on luminance contours. Whereas oriented filtering per se, such as one could expect for a V1 simple cell, would encode the orientation of every section along a contour such as shown in figure 4.4, smear lines significantly enhance some orientations and contour segments over others. Recall the transitory contrast loci perceived in figure 4.1A. Clearly, this is a form of proto-oriented filtering because some orientations are conveyed at much greater luminance contrast than others. Although retinal cones could hardly be regarded as detectors of orientation and direction, a model of their slow responsiveness thus clearly shows that an orientation bias for moving visual structure is introduced as if performing a narrow band of oriented filtering on input visual structures, suggesting that cortical orientation selectivity is not simply a response to natural image statistics but is also likely to be shaped by oculo-motor actions of the observer.

In the current scientific approach, receptive fields of retinal ganglia are regarded as isotropic, precluding the retina as the source of more sophisticated visual information (i.e., oriented filtering, marking locations on contours, recording oculo-motor action as a luminance contrast structure, etc.).

Motion Blur as an Object Motion Vector

Motion detectors in the visual system do not capture the direction of motion as reliably as one might expect given the range for which motion perception seems accurate and effortless. Geisler (1999) has shown that simulated simple and complex V1 cells accurately compute the direction of motion in complex natural scenes if the model input is not just a raw movie sequence of image frames but contains motion smears as one could expect from slow photoreceptors (e.g., retinal cones), contrary to various accepted neural models of motion detection that fail to compute direction of motion accurately in natural scenes.

Psychophysics supports this hypothesis. Geisler (1999) found that human subjects estimate motion direction far less accurately when the effect of motion smear is cancelled through appropriate masking during presentation of experimental stimuli.

For example, because the curvature-related smears shown in figure 4.4 are parallel to the direction of motion, these lines represent motion vectors: Their length gives a relative measure of velocity, their orientation indicates the orientation of motion, and their relative placement on either side of the contour indicates the direction of motion with respect to the contour.

Motion blur is therefore not simply a matter of corrupted or redundant visual data but signifies a source, independent of actual motion detection, for obtaining clues regarding motion over a wide range of motion velocities and, surprisingly, often more accurate than (hypothesized) direct motion detection.

Motion Blur as a Vector Field of Relative Displacement

Object and observer motion cause relative displacements between visual structures as registered by the retina, generating patterns of motion blur that constitute a potentially useful vector field description of the changing scenery facing the observer. For example, simple eye movements constitute linear displacement vector fields and induce straight smear lines. When an observer changes gait, shifts his weight, turns or walks while looking at something, slight rotations, foreshortening shears, and scaling displacements increase the complexity of the otherwise linear displacement regime, and consequently more complex smear lines result. Add to that movement of objects surrounding the observer, and the smear lines become even more complex. In fact, these smears explicitly resemble relative displacement vectors and should in that sense also be of utility to the visual system, especially in understanding the "shape" of the displacement field, its implications for optical flow immersing the observer, and for informing about stable structures within that flow.

The vector field of relative displacement is potentially highly informative for an observer acting in the environment. Unchanging visual structure in the changing vector field of relative displacement is significant because it reveals visual structure that is potentially synergetic to the observer's actions. For example, hand rails on a staircase constitute a comparatively stationary pattern in the retina while an observer is going down the stairs because the rails are roughly aligned with the radial vector field (scaling) of optical flow immersing the observer, whereas the stairs, roughly orthogonal to this field, are maximally blurred. The rails will thus implicitly be selected as an unchanging visual structure for the action of going down the stairs (and the same action—sliding or placing your hand on the rail—can be repeated again and again while going down the stairs to provide some stable interaction in that environment). The constancy of these structures may also be part of the reason that humans design such spaces. In any event, stable visual structures may be helpful when running down stairs while you try to catch a train in Tokyo station.

Segmenting Moving from Stationary Objects

Hypothetically, motion detectors segment natural scenes by negating stationary visual structure, thus differentiating moving from nonmoving parts. Motion detectors further segment among moving parts that move at different relative velocities (Fried, Münch, and Werblin, 2002). Motion based segmentation has been demonstrated in the retina (Ölveczky et al., 2003), although the actual mechanism involved, for example, a motion detector neural circuit, remains unclear).

Cones provide a base for the segmentation of stationary from moving objects, not through negation of moving structure but through motion blur. The faster a visual structure moves, the more blurred and transparent its registration becomes. The more blurred, the stronger the bias in the orientations constituting the visual data of that structure—another basis for segmentation of visual figure from the background.

Where relative visual motion is induced, such as when a walking observer looks at a house through a picket fence, the slow response of retinal cones would be useful in successfully segmenting the house from the picket fence because the structure of the moving planks of the picket fence will become smeared and thinned out to a far greater extent than that of the more stationary (and thus less blurred) house appearing in the background behind the picket fence.

Segmentation due to motion parallax is another inevitable consequence of motion blur. When the observer moves, distant objects move less across the retina than proximal objects. Hence, the latter will have stronger motion blur gradients, and these will be overlaid—as semitransparent smears—onto the less blurred features of objects in the background.

In fact, our vision may be so accustomed to interpret layers of structures that are blurred to different degrees as different moving structures that blur, if triggered appropriately, can set strong impressions of relative movement between objects, where in fact there is none.

The Ouchi illusion (figure 4.5) is an example where motion blur may cast new light on perception of texture, depth, and apparent relative motion. The figure shown here was adapted by Jacques Ninio from the original Ouchi illusion (Ninio, 2001) and presents a slightly more complex set of textural patterns that induces a strong illusion of

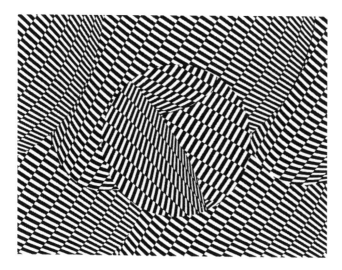

Figure 4.5
The Ouchi illusion adapted by Jacques Ninio (2001) into a more complex set of texture segments that still vividly evoke the impression of relative motion between figure and ground.

relative motion between the region included in the disc and the surrounding texture patches.

At least two interesting perceptual effects can be observed when shifting your gaze around this figure. One is the illusion of relative motion between figure and background, and another is the appearance of shimmering or bright high contrast patches that shift across the image, in both the figure and background textures. The latter is likely due to a combination of transitory contrast, as mentioned before, and spatial frequency-dependent contrast sensitivity (Campbell and Robson, 1968).

Simulated motion blur with the cone model (figure 4.2C and 4.3D) reveals that linear displacements—as eye movements typically induce—differentially smear textural patches either inside or outside the disk depending on the direction of the linear displacement. Thus, either figure or ground, but not both, appear in high contrast and relatively little blur.

Different degrees of smear or blur affect the degree of localization accuracy of textural features and may also serve as a low-level cue that either ground or figure is moving (Pinna and Spillmann, 2005). Motion blur thus (falsely) introduces visual data of relative motion and depth, useful in segmenting figure from ground, but constituting a surprisingly early possible neural origin for the generation of segmentation data that may underlie the Ouchi illusion.

Note that blur gradients further give an indication of direction of motion. The difference in the cone response to figure and ground results from the difference in the average orientation of their respective textural elements. In the stimulus image created by Ninio, the spatial frequency of textural elements seems to have been carefully chosen to locally mask global orientation gradients. This is perhaps an aesthetic choice because the illusion of motion seems all the more surprising when local textural gradients are not aligned with the direction of perceived relative motion in any obvious manner.

Enhancing Texture Gradients through Blur

Textures in natural scenes are typically distinguishable due to distinct signatures of density, intensity, orientation, and spatial frequency of textural elements. Because the properties of smear markings are directly dependent on these attributes, one could expect that retinal cones would enhance this differentiation in textures.

Using the model for visual transduction in cones, smear markings after linear displacement of an artificial line texture (figure 4.6, top) result in enhanced differences between textural regions (figure 4.6, bottom). In the computational results, higher textural densities appear relatively darker, whereas lower densities appear lighter according to the cone model. Spatial frequency is modulated in terms of image contrast: The lower spatial frequency textures appear at relatively higher image contrast. Orientation gradients appear at different luminance intensities and contrast after

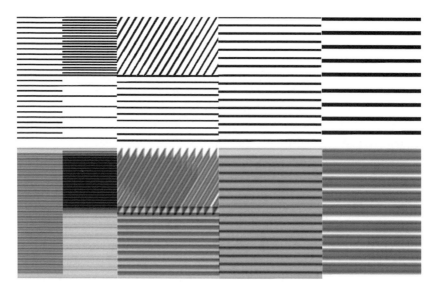

Figure 4.6
Differences between various texture patches (top) are enhanced as gradients in average luminance and contrast during simulated visual transduction (bottom). Note that this follows perceived differences in texture brightness. Also note how small irregularities in texture elements, such as the slightly thicker line segments in the oblique texture patch, become enhanced as a slightly darker blotch in the simulated result.

transduction modeling (figure 4.6, bottom third from left). Hence, motion blur provides important visual data for texture segmentation.

Selection of Irregularities
Motion blur further enhances small irregularities in texture element size and spacing that may go unnoticed during stationary viewing, especially if viewed at suboptimal spatial resolution. For example, slight differences in line width in the obliquely oriented texture patch show up as distinct light and dark regions in the simulated smear pattern, whereas slight variations in spacing between lines in the right-most texture patch show up as salient white bands in the simulated smear pattern. These artifacts become salient during motion or active exploration (involving eye movements) of the figure, and hence motion blur is a candidate source for enhancing both texture regions as wholes and outliers among texture elements.

Motion Blur as Spatial Filtering
What the above demonstrates is that a retinal cone not only operates as oriented filter, motion and optical flow recorder, or texture segmenter. It effectively functions as a multiscale spatial filter as long as it engages actively in the visual field.

Here, spatial filtering is proportionally dependent on motion. The faster any point moves, the lower the spatial frequency at which the cone structures it. Compare, for example, the appearance of a pattern of black and white stripes painted by hand (see Van Tonder, 2010, figure 1), with a facsimile of the same pattern where every black and white stripe is exactly identical (figure 4.1A). When viewed statically, such figures may not seem too different, although active visual exploration should quickly reveal significant differences in appearance.

The primary difference lies in the fact that the hand-painted stripes are irregular, constituting a multiscale structure. When moving the image slowly, the fast fluctuations between black and white of the highest spatial frequency structure cancels itself out as it moves in front of cones (except where transitory contrast loci occur). For increasingly faster movement, increasingly lower spatial frequency components cancel themselves in this way, so that with higher velocity, an increasingly low spatial frequency component of the image becomes the salient structure in the cone response.

Low-pass filtering of the two images confirms this difference (Van Tonder, 2010). Thus, especially when actively viewing the two images, the facsimile will appear increasingly hard and flat because it does not translate into a multiscale structure.

Although the facsimile contains just a slight modulation of structure along one dimension—and thus no multiscale structural reference that might be useful in stabilizing visual fixation—the original is teeming with structural articulations in all orientations and constitutes a figure and ground arrangement that would serve as a clear global reference of relative spatial arrangement between larger and finer spatial details. Fractal analysis shows that this structure, at least over the lower range of spatial scales, is also self-similar, whereas the facsimile is not (figure 4.7B and D). The increasingly finer cusps within the global scaffold of structure imbedded in the hand-painted composition are certain to improve gaze stability.

Most natural scenes exhibit multiscale structure characterized by many irregularities (Mandelbrot, 1977). The visual system should therefore be adapted to fixating with visual cues from various levels of spatial detail when an observer views natural scenes (Taylor, in press). Purely periodic line patterns, lacking in multiscale detail and irregularities, constitute visual environments deprived of nested spatial references for effortless visual orienting. Various lines of evidence suggest that periodic line patterns induce semi-psychotic eye movements. The rate and amplitude of saccades become affected, peak overshoot and oscillation amplitude around fixation locations are adversely affected, and the visual apparatus (and, consequently, perceptual apparatus as well) suffers a considerable amount of visual stress to maintain normal visual function (Zanker, Doyle, and Walker, 2003).

The slow transduction of cones therefore hints at another possibly significant function of the retina: spatial filtering. This function potentially reveals underlying visual structural frameworks for reducing visual confusion, especially when the observer experiences shifts in the visual field. It is an elegant approach to a difficult problem; the

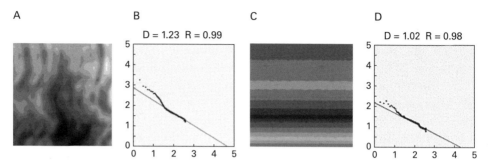

Figure 4.7
Lower spatial frequencies of a hand-painted composition (A) (discussed in Van Tonder, 2010), and its mechanistic computer facsimile (C), where all lines are identical (see figure 4.1A). The fractal dimension, D, and fractal strictness, R, computed via comparative Fourier power spectrum dropoff rate indicates that the hand-painted composition is more strictly self-similar (B) than the computer facsimile and has a higher fractal dimension than the computer generated image. The computer facsimile (C) has a dimension close to one (D) and, not surprisingly, looks rather flat.

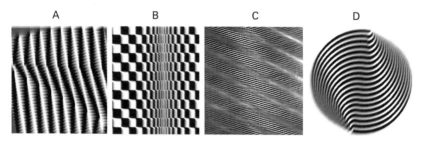

Figure 4.8
Simulated visual transduction in *Shift* (vertical motion, A), *Movement in Squares* (oblique upward motion, B), *Cataract 3* (rotation, C), paintings by Bridget Riley, and *Dynamique Circulaire* (oblique upward motion, D) by Maria Apollonio.

faster the movement—and the greater the potential confusion—the lower the spatial frequency of the structure captured by the cone response. Hence, the resulting information naturally becomes increasingly global, much like a shorthand description of a conversation, for larger changes in the visual field, and this facilitates visual perception in keeping track of what happens where.

Depth from Blur
Simulation of visual transduction in cones on four different works of Op art (figure 4.8) shows how smear lines serve as pseudoluminance contrast gradients that, at least intuitively, agree with some depth effects observed in these paintings. In *Shift* (figure

4.8A), smear lines enhance the luminance contrast between the central white spines and black grooves by leaving only a narrow central white band. The smearing resembles illumination flows and shadows (see e.g., Breton and Zucker, 1996), from which the visual system might normally reconstruct three-dimensional surface and depth data. Compared with the original painting (not shown here), motion smear induces false depth cues that cause the composition to appear as a dark, three-dimensional stair case spiraling around sets of white cantilevered axial spines.

In *Movement in Squares* (figure 4.8B), the luminance contrast generated due to smear is much lower around the center of the composition than elsewhere. Assuming that distant objects in natural scenes are typically seen at lower luminance contrast than proximal objects, smearing here induces at least one monocular depth cue. Otherwise, it introduces a pseudospecular quality suggestive of material reflectance.

Because smearing gradients bias spatial localization structure for edges of the central blocks more than for the larger blocks in the surround, the visual system may be falsely informed of a stable surround and of a central visual structure that cannot be as accurately located. Visual smear may thus give rise to the false impression that the central band moves relative to the entire pattern, as if in motion parallax, especially vivid when an observer makes eye movements.

Pseudosurfaces

The last two examples here (figure 4.8C and D) further demonstrate how visual smear literally highlights some parts in a line pattern while dimming others, thus inducing depth cues. In my subjective perception, the smeared images resemble objects in realistic scenes more closely than the images prior to motion blur. In stimuli rich in oriented edges, the transduction model strongly enhances some contour segments, and therefore some orientations, more than others. Such enhanced contrast regions may bias complex functions, such as contour and surface reconstruction, and even attention and further saccades, to start at these enhanced visual structures instead of any other location. Similar to Attneave (1954) points for shape perception from contour data, these may serve as key "Attneave loci" for shape perception from surface data.

Similarly, in a fragment from an etching by Dürer (figure 4.9A), different displacements of the image induce different smearing configurations (figure 4.9B, C, and D). Each instance enhances different qualities in the textures depicted. Where linear motion aligns with the texture contours of the cushions, the shimmering silkiness of their fabric covers become enhanced, whereas a different motion configuration enhances the granularity of the surface material in the window sill. Note that even if these induced motion smears do not constitute veridical cues of the depicted surfaces, smearing increases the impression of rich shading and texture flows. The fact that the resultant texture structures are slightly different during each displacement indicates that the effects of slow transduction in retinal cones could potentially enrich the range

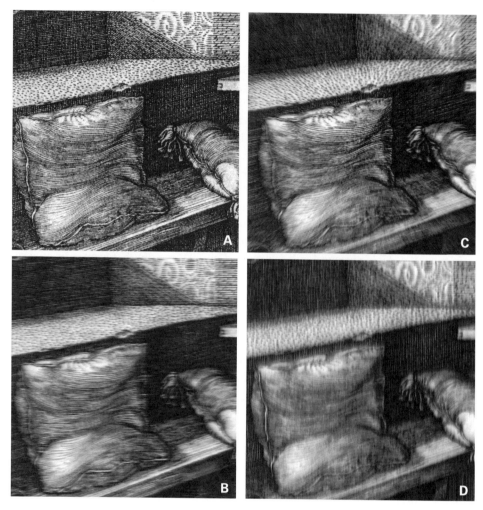

Figure 4.9
Simulated visual transduction in a section from an engraving of St. Jerome (A), by Albrecht Dürer, for the following displacement configurations: scaling around the center of the image (B), rightward motion (C), and downward motion (D).

of structures that the visual system has for segmenting and distinguishing different textural regions and surfaces even if the segmentation structures created are only pseudoversions of true shading and texture flows. The retina therefore generates textural structure in agreement with what I subjectively experience as visual textural "qualities."

In fact, Dürer's masterful technique in using etch lines at least suggests that he may have been sensitive to the dynamism that is added through the appropriate surface markings when the picture is actively explored (Van Tonder, 2005). The flowing lines of the cushion may well have been chosen because Dürer observed that these produce a striking shimmering effect as one would see on a real silken cushion or short-oriented lines to suggest the pitted appearance of an old oaken window sill, and that it is while one actively views this image that the surface markings most come to life—a case of a drawing for viewing by slow retinal cones.

Boundary Contour Completion

In theoretical modeling of so-called illusory figures, such as the Kanizsa triangle (see chapter 1, this volume), boundary contour reconstruction is often applied to a stationary stimulus figure (e.g., Grossberg and Mingolla, 1985; von der Heydt, R. 2003). When I look at these illusory figures, I am constantly making eye movements to fixate different regions of the figure as if my vision is continually confirming and testing the validity of the illusory contours perceived. Fixations between saccades would, of course, provide the opportunity for stationary contour reconstruction, but motion smear during saccades could also generate useful cues for boundary contour completion.

Illusory contours change significantly during motion. In my subjective experience, the Ehrenstein illusion and Kanizsa triangle, for example, both appear different when seen in motion. Depending on the direction of motion, the central bright region of the Ehrenstein illusion appears either like a rectangular strip, a rectangle with rounded corners, or a circular disc, and the bright triangle of the Kanizsa figure resembles an arrowhead—exactly what one would expect given the smear lines induced during linear motion of each stimulus. In this case, smear lines constitute concrete-oriented contour information that agrees with dynamically perceived shape. It concretizes the shapes that are generally considered *illusory* in the vision research literature.

Scintillating phase contours even more strongly demonstrate the possible role of an active retina in contour completion. Consider a figure delineated by a texture phase shift (figure 4.10A). Whereas stationary boundary completion models (e.g., Heitger et al., 1992) compute line inducers, or end points, and then reconstruct contour segments between these end points according to a predefined bipolar interpolation rule, the motion smear induced by the model of retinal transduction in cones provides a completely different means of arriving at a similar phase contour. It clearly enhances luminance contrast of phase texture contours relative to the surround (figure 4.10B and C). This does not depend on a unique displacement type for which the phase

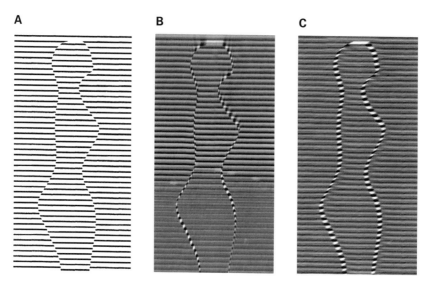

Figure 4.10

Texture phase contours are perceived as vivid, bright borders in this figure by Ehrenstein (A). Motion smear in simulated visual transduction during displacements generates high-contrast ridges that clearly delineate the phase contour, shown here for a transition from scaling to rotation (B) and oblique upward (C) motion. Note that perceptually phase contours appear to scintillate, and these simulation results suggest why: For the slightest relative displacement, the transitory contrast generated in this images fluctuate dramatically. Note that this segmentation occurs at the earliest level of visual processing—the retinal cone.

contour is accidentally emphasized but occurs to various degrees for almost any type of displacement of the original image. Note that the distortion of the image in this case, again, is one of biasing orientation cues, as if the retinal cones were creating visual structure tailored for orientation selective V1 simple cells.

The simulation result goes beyond suggesting the possible role of slow retinal transduction in the process of contour recovery or completion. It makes a novel suggestion as to the shimmering appearance of these phase contours—its qualitative appearance—a tricky issue to explain simply in terms of boundary contour completion models. When looking at the original figure (figure 4.10A), the phase contour is noticeably brighter than the rest of the textural regions—a percept that is especially clear while shifting one's gaze from one position to another. What I experience qualitatively appears as a flat transparent figurine placed on a striped background. When I look around, I see the optical deformations of the line pattern around the edges of the glass figurine. The effect has a strong quality of optical distortion through a transparent medium, although at the same time I can see it is not realistically rendered. For my eyes, there is no mys-

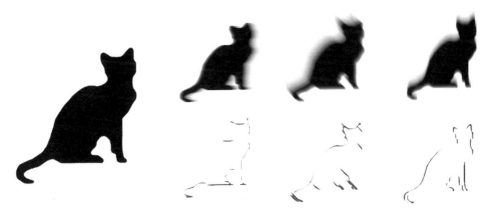

Figure 4.11
The enhancement of deflection points and curvature maxima, shown here for leftward, oblique downward, and downward motion of a black cat (top row) isolates potential sets of Attneave points—segments of boundary contour that are crucial for efficient shape recognition—separated in time and orientation.

tery involved. There is no illusory contour, just the obvious, even if it looks a bit off the mark.

Selection of "Attneave Points"

Smear lines indicate deflection points and curvature extrema in relation to the direction of displacement. It thus seems plausible that smear lines constitute a motion-defined set of so-called Attneave points (Attneave, 1954) (i.e., locations along the boundary contour that constitute characteristic cues for shape recognition of a contour figure). Smearing the silhouette of a cat, for example, in horizontal, oblique, and vertical directions (figure 4.11, left) generate smear profiles (figure 4.11, top) that, if filtered with isotropic edge filters (figure 4.11, bottom), leave edge segments that not only closely resemble the output of classical-oriented filters (although obviously no oriented filtering has been implemented here) but indicate subsets of points that may play a role in shape perception (Wagemans, De Winter, and Panis, 2002). Displacements such as eye movements therefore induce a process of precortical oriented filtering, resulting in an enhanced subset of object shape data that could potentially guide subsequent fixations and serve as starting points for cortical boundary contour processing.

Selection of Relations between Internal Parts of Objects

The selection of subsets of visual structure includes biases toward some internal configurations of object parts. Different linear displacements of an object image, such as a face, will enhance different sets of oriented visual structures, constituting a simple

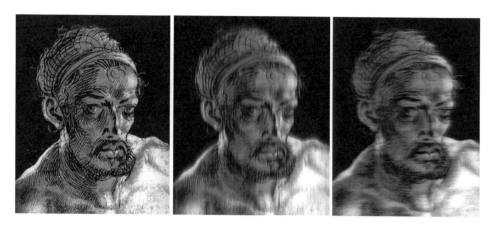

Figure 4.12
Self-portrait by Albrecht Dürer (left). Simulated transduction for vertical (middle) and horizontal (middle) linear motions. Different spatial relationships between facial features are enhanced for different displacements. Note the difference in appearance of facial expression and mood.

selection of that orientation during a given displacement (i.e., each eye movement selects structures of one given orientation over all others). This could bias the perception of the relationship between the constituent parts of a structural whole. Because complex visual percepts, such as understanding of facial expression, depend directly on the perceived relative relationship between local structures (Bruce and Young, 2000), motion smear from one saccade to the next may enhance subtly different expressions of the same face (figure 4.12, center and right; note again how different the qualities of textures, highlights, shadows, perceived motion, and other features of the face and accessories appear in each case), providing a richer set of visual cues and a potential source of perceived dynamism in a face at the earliest level of visual processing. This may hold true in general for perception of natural scenes.

Conclusion

The consensus that retinal ganglia, not to mention photoreceptors, operate as isotropic filters is probably not correct. Here I have argued that every mere retinal cone responds nonisotropically to luminance; acts as an oriented filter, a multiscale spatial filter, a motion detector, a velocity computer, and an optical flow recorder; senses texture gradients and irregularities; and provides potentially significant spatial depth structure, clues to the materials of textures and distinction between different surfaces, the shapes of objects and the relationships between their internal parts, and various other aspects of vision that are not associated with the retina. Just imagine what we may find in the retina if not just the cones but the entire repertoire of retinal cells were thoroughly considered. The critical condition needed for the retina to function at this level is that of *active vision*. Saccades, seen from this point of view, are the natural outcome of a system that functions at maximal meaningful complexity, not the compromise of a system bogged down by its little foveal keyhole to the world.

The fact that all these information categories are represented in cone responses raises the question of what function the visual cortex actually performs. Simple cells cannot simply be tuned to natural image statistics if retinal signals are already ripe with orientation bias. What does one find when the orientation-directional biases of cones are subtracted from the visual structures generated by simple cells, let us say in response to moving contrast gratings? If the cortex were constantly scanning retinal signals for such biases, instead of just passively filtering a map of retinal "pixels," one might come a step closer to decipher the seemingly spontaneous waves of cortical orientation selectivity that wash over the cortex in the absence of classical line stimuli (Kenet et al., 2003)—a startling observation that suggests we actually do not yet understand what simple cells are doing. I would suggest that simple cells must be doing more, perhaps relating knowledge about how the retina internally structures events with changes in our perceptions. The visual cortex may be specialized to *present*—in the Brentanian sense (Albertazzi, 2006)—the rich visual structuring that begins in the retina.

For visual arts, this chapter is relevant for various reasons. First, it underlines why modes of depicting smears and related deformations are so powerful in suggesting a sense of dynamism: Explicitly presenting the effects of retinal transduction elevates the visual traces of our own actions to a level above the subliminal threshold, as if that responsiveness is a physical structure for interaction with the observer. In this sense, various schools of visual art have literally reproduced the world as seen through the distortions of retinal cones. Second, it partially suggests that dynamism of some static artistic compositions originate from deformations introduced at the earliest levels of vision (and hence perhaps, the [ridiculed] notion held by various artists that they experience visual effects in their eyes, and not their brains) during active visual exploration; it reflects the dynamism of the observer, and the extent to which this dynamism can be controlled mirrors the extent to which the observer's actions can be voluntarily brought under control.

Nevertheless, when I see, I do not perceive a sea of motion blur (although it is perceptible if I really pay close attention). This might be the necessary outcome of having to interact with structures that are limited by the laws of physical interactions, not the laws of drawing pictures: One cannot interact with smear lines as if it were physical objects. It seems as if aware visual perception is limited to surfaces that potentially allow interaction with the observer.

This chapter is about how the structure of incident light becomes transformed into cone responses, as can be observed externally: structured visual smears; structures that will again be transformed into other structures in the cortex and so on, thus the external observations unfortunately do not transcend into the realm of consciousness no matter how tightly *action* and *perception* hold hands. At least, the ideas here lean slightly toward the inner realm of the mind insofar as the motion blur structures described here are quite unexpected if the eye were designed to optimally encode—in a physicalist sense—optical projections. Quite to the contrary, the retina *discards* the optical projection if the simulation results shown in this chapter and elsewhere are to be taken literally. Retinal responses (and visual perception, for that matter) do not merely substitute synergies between optical projection and bodily action. Instead, the responses all apparently encapsulate spatiotemporal structures. These relate more to what already has meaning in an embodied sense than to the properties of an optical projection. For example, if blur gradients were physical things and vision actually were like a hand that could reach out to touch them, they could be smooth or rough, solid or feathery, thick or tenuous. In this sense, the retina structures light into a repertoire of action-perception synergies: It is completely internal and accessible to qualitative experience. The retina seems to act like a child with crayons at a drawing board, drawing, smearing, and mixing. The brain's task is likely to know when, where, and how to appreciate the structures received from the retina.

Where along this path does consciously experienced subjectivity slip into the equation? It is certainly not by casting mantras such as "action-perception synergy!" The subjectivity of experience seems to lurk within even before I open my eyes. The answer to this question remains squarely evasive. But I can feel my nose pushing against the glass door of the explanatory gap!

Acknowledgments

This work was supported by the Japanese Society for the Promotion of Science and the Mitteleuropa foundation. Many thanks also to Dhanraj Vishwanavath for valuable commentary on the manuscript.

Notes

1. One other relatively successful model of transitory contrast exists: signal averaging. It simply averages a given number of image frames as a rough approximation of slow responsiveness in low-level vision. Their account failed to reach the level of insight gained through a theoretical model, such as presented here, but, more important, the results of a signal averaging model deviate from perception. Although the deviations are not huge, they are significant. For example, signal averaging results in bilaterally symmetric transitory contrast patterns for some test patterns, whereas subjects perceive bilateral asymmetry in these patterns. The cone model agrees with perception (Van Tonder and Ohtani, 2007), a result I ascribe to the fact that it responds to the temporal order in which light fluctuates, whereas signal averaging is blind to this temporal order; it simply averages light over a given interval. This shows that perception is sensitive to the

difference between incoming light as it is and a temporal averaged version of that light, contrary to the hypothesis by Burr (1980).

2. This is obviously a system of infinite feedback, a visual bootstrap of meaning. In robotics, the behavior of a robotic agent has been shown to stabilize comparatively fast if actions and pattern analysis units are behaviorally linked, such that self-motion of the agent preselects visual structures on which pattern analysis is based (Verschure et al., 2003). It is an enormous feat to achieve in an artificial system, yet it still seems framed within the Gibsonian concept of action-perception cycles (see Introduction, this volume).

References

Abramovici, A., and Chapksy, J. 2005. *Feedback Control Systems: A Fast-Track Guide for Scientists and Engineers*. Hingham, MA: Kluwer Academic Publishers.

Albertazzi, L. 2006. *Immanent Realism: An Introduction to Brentano*. Dordrecht, the Netherlands: Springer.

Attneave, F. 1954. "Some Informational Aspects of Visual Perception." *Psychological Review* 61: 183–193.

Breton, P., and Zucker, S. W. 1996, June 18–20. "Shadows and Shading Flow Fields." Proceedings of the 1996 Conference on Computer Vision and Pattern Recognition (CVPR '96), San Francisco, CA. 782.

Bruce, V., and Young, A. 2000. *In the Eye of the Beholder: The Science of Face Perception*. Oxford, UK: Oxford University Press.

Burr, D. C. 1980. "Motion Smear." *Nature* 284: 64–165.

Burr, D. C., Morrone, M., and Ross, J. 1996. "Selective Suppression of the Magnocellular Visual Pathway During Saccades." *Behavioral Brain Research* 80: 1–8.

Campbell, F. W., and Robson, J. G. 1968. "Application of Fourier Analysis to the Visibility of Gratings." *Journal of Physiology* 197: 551–566.

Cobbold, C. S. W. 1881. "Observations on Certain Optical Effects of Motion." *Brain* 4: 75–81.

DeYoe, E. A., and van Essen, D. C. 1988. "Concurrent Processing Streams in Monkey Visual Cortex." *Trends in Neurosciences* 11(5): 219–226.

Fermüller, C., Pless, R., and Aloimonos, Y. 1997. "Families of Stationary Patterns Producing Illusory Movement: Insights Into the Visual System." *Proc. R. Soc. Lond. B* 264: 795–806.

Fried, S. I., Münch, T. A., and Werblin, F. S. 2002. "Mechanisms and Circuitry Underlying Directional Selectivity in the Retina." *Nature* 420: 411–414.

Geisler, W. S. 1999. "Motion Streaks Provide a Spatial Code for Motion Direction." *Nature* 400: 65–69.

Goodale, M., and Milner, D. 2004. *Sight Unseen*. Oxford, UK: Oxford University Press.

Gosselin, F., and Lamontagne, C. 1997. "Motion-Blur Illusions." *Perception* 26: 847–855.

Gregory, R. L. 1995. "Brain-Created Visual Motion: An Illusion?" *Proc. R. Soc. Lond. B* 260: 167–168.

Gregory, R. L. 1998. *Eye and Brain*. 5th ed. Oxford, UK: Oxford University Press.

Grossberg, S., and Mingolla, E. 1985. "Neural Dynamics of Form Perception: Boundary Completion, Illusory Figures, and Neon Color Spreading." *Psychological Review* 92(2): 173–211.

Heitger, F., Rosenthaler, L., von der Heydt, R., Peterhans, E., and Kübler, O. 1992. "Simulation of Neuronal Contour Mechanisms: From Simple to Endstopped Cells." *Vision Research* 32: 963–981.

Helmholtz, H. von. 1856. *Handbuch der Physiologischen Optik* (Helmholtz's Treatise on Physiological Optics). Leipzig: Voss.

Kenet, T., Bibitchkov, D., Tsodyks, M., Grinvald, A., and Arieli, A. 2003. "Spontaneously Emerging Cortical Representations of Visual Attributes." *Nature* 425: 954–956.

Livingstone, M., and Hubel, D. H. 1988. "Segregation of Form, Movement, Color and Depth: Anatomy, Physiology, and Perception." *Science* 240(4853): 740–749.

MacKay, D. M. 1958. "Moving Visual Images Produced by Regular Stationary Patterns." *Nature* 181: 362–363.

Mandelbrot, B. B. 1977. *The Fractal Geometry of Nature*. New York: W. H. Freeman.

Marr, D. 1982. *Vision*. New York: W. H. Freeman.

Ninio, J. 2001. *The Science of Illusions*. London: Cornell University Press.

Ölveczky, B. P., Baccus, S. A., and Meister, M. 2003. "Segregation of Object and Background Motion in the Retina." *Nature* 423: 401–408.

Oster, G., and Nishijima, Y. 1963. "Moiré Patterns." *Scientific American* 208: 54–63.

Pinna, B., and Spillmann, L. 2005. "New Illusions of Sliding Motion in Depth." *Perception* 34(12): 1441–1458.

Purkinje, J. 1823. *Beobachtungen und Versuche zur Physiologie der Sinne. Beiträge zur Kenntniss des Sehens in subjectiver Hinsicht*. (Observation and Experiments on the Physiology of the Senses. Consideration on the Knowledge of Seeing from a Subjective Viewpoint). Prague: Calve.

Rogers-Ramachandran, D. C., and Ramachandran, V. S. 1998. "Psychopysical Evidence for Boundary and Surface Systems in Human Vision." *Vision Research* 38(1): 71–77.

Schnapf, J. L., Nunn, B. J., Meister, M., and Baylor, D. A. 1990. "Visual transduction in cones of the monkey *Macaca fascicularis*." *Journal of Physiology* 427: 681–713.

Taylor, R. P. in press. "Reduction of Physiological Stress Using Fractal Art and Architecture." In *Leonardo*. Cambridge, MA: MIT Press.

Ungerleider, L. G., and Mishkin, M. 1982. "Two Cortical Visual Systems." In *Analysis of Visual Behavior*, edited by D. J. Ingle, M. A. Goodale, and R. J. W. Mansfield. Cambridge, MA: MIT Press. 549–586.

Van Tonder, G. J. 2005. "Dürer's Choice: Representing Surface Attitude in Engravings." *Perception* 34: 89.

Van Tonder, G. J. 2010. "Perceptual Disruption and Composure in *Fall*." In *Leonardo* 43:3. Cambridge, MA: MIT Press.

Van Tonder, G. J., and Ohtani, Y. forthcoming. "Effective Velocity and Transitory Contrast Loci."

Van Tonder, G. J., and Ohtani, Y. 2007, October 20–23. "A Second Order Feedback Model of Visual Transduction in Cones of the Monkey *Macaca fascicularis*." Proceedings of the 23rd meeting of the International Society of Psychophysics, Tokyo, Japan.

Verschure, P. F. M. J., Voegtlin, T., and Douglas, D. J. 2003. "Environmentally Mediated Synergy Between Perception and Behaviour in Mobile Robots." *Nature* 425: 620–624.

von der Heydt, R. 2003. *Image Parsing Mechanisms of the Visual Cortex*. In *The Visual Neurosciences*, edited by J. S. Werner and L. M. Chalupa. Cambridge, MA: MIT Press. 1139–1150.

Wade, N. J. 1978. "Op Art and Visual Perception." *Perception* 7: 21–46.

Wagemans, J., De Winter, J., and Panis, S. 2002. "The Awakening of Attneave's Sleeping Cat: Identification of Everyday Objects on the Basis of Straight-Line Versions." Proceedings of the annual meeting of the Vision Science Society, Abstract No. 679.

Weaver, W., and Shannon, C. E. 1963. *The Mathematical Theory of Communication*. Champaign-Urbana, IL: University of Illinois Press.

Zanker, M. J. 2004. "Looking at Op Art From a Computational Viewpoint." *Spatial Vision* 17(1–2): 75–94.

Zanker, M. J., Doyle, M., and Walker, R. 2003. "Gaze Stability of Observers Watching Op Art Pictures." *Perception* 32: 1037–1049.

Zeki, S. 1994. "The Cortical Enigma: A Reply to Professor Gregory." *Proc. R. Soc. Lond. B* 257: 243–245.

5 Perceptual Organization in the Visual Cortex

Shinsuke Shimojo

This short chapter describes the author's own studies concerning three distinctive themes. First, transcranial magnetic stimulation (TMS) studies revealed transitional neuronal dynamics from visual input to perception in the visual cortex. Second, visual psychophysics demonstrated various forms of perceptual organization as a result of bottom-up processing and local–global interactions in vision. Third, an analogous processing specific to the resolution of perceptual ambiguity was found in cross-modal integration. These three sets of findings together shed light on how sensory inputs effectively trigger dynamic bottom-up and self-organizing processes in the sensory cortices (the early visual cortex, in particular).

Although seemingly varied in approach and findings, these three studies demonstrate how recent behavioral and neuroscientific research help reveal the aspects of perception that Brentano in the late 19th century felt critical, as is illustrated in the Introduction of this volume.

Transition from Sensory Input to Percept–TMS Studies

The neural transition from retinal input to visual percept should be not merely spatial but rather dynamic (i.e., temporal or spatiotemporal). Whereas the former has been emphasized by functional magnetic resonance imaging (fMRI) studies, the latter has been demonstrated via electroencephalography (EEG), magnetoencephalography (MEG), and other techniques. Among all, TMS is unique partly because of its excellent temporal resolution (<1 ms) and partly because it is an active intervention into, as opposed to passive recording of, neural activity.

For example, we were able to create an artificial scotoma by applying a single-pulse TMS to the visual cortex (Kamitani and Shimojo, 1999). We first presented a large-field patterned stimulus (a black and white grid or striped pattern) for a brief period of time (40 ms typically) and then stimulated the visual cortex from outside of the scalp with a single-pulse TMS via an 8-shaped coil. When the time delay of TMS ranged from 90 to 170 ms, we found an artificial scotoma in the contralateral visual field, in which no

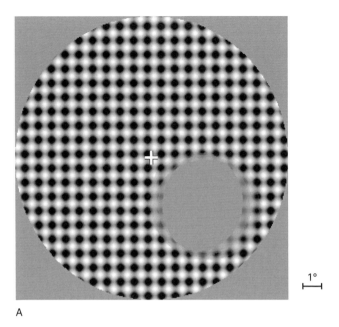

1°

A

Figure 5.1 (plate 3)
Artificial scotoma induced by TMS. (A) Examples of scotoma. The left occipital lobe of the subject
was stimulated by an 8-shaped coil with a monophasic single pulse. The duration of visual stimulus was 40 ms, and the delay of magnetic stimulation from the onset of the visual stimulus was
100 ms in this example. The subjects' own drawing/duplication of the scotoma percept was superimposed over five consecutive trials. (B) Backward filling-in phenomenon. The red (green) homogenous background was presented for more than 1 sec, followed by the black and white stripes
for 80 ms, and then replaced with a green (red) homogenous background for more than 1 sec. The
delay of TMS was 106 ms in this case. The color of the subsequent, but not preceding, background
filled into the scotoma backward in time. (C) A schematic spatiotemporal diagram to illustrate the
backward filling-in phenomenon. The color of the subsequent background "fills-in" to the scotoma in the striped pattern, and is thus perceived earlier and simultaneously with the stripes
surrounding (modified from Kamitani and Shimojo, 1999, figures 1 and 5).

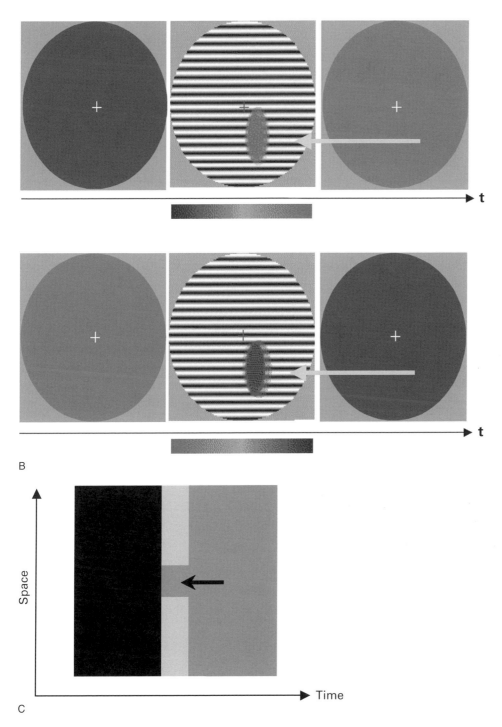

B

C

Figure 5.1 (plate 3)
(continued)

pattern other than a homogenous gray field was perceived (figure 5.1A, plate 3). This indicates a surprisingly wide time window (80 ms or longer) during which vigorous corticocortical interactions, initially triggered by the retinal input, led to phenomenologically the same result (of scotoma). At the phenomenological level, it is intriguing to note that the scotoma, although it is created by neural suppression, is still perceived as a "figure" surrounded by a ground.

To address how the color (feature) within the scotoma was determined, we manipulated the background colors (green or red) before and after the visual pattern presentation while repeating the same experiment. The results were consistent and robust: The color (or texture) of the background *after* the visual pattern presentation "sneaked into" the scotoma backward in time, being perceived simultaneously with the surrounding visual pattern (figure 5.1B). Thus, a vigorous dynamic reorganization of perceptual simultaneity across adjacent areas occurred (figure 5.1C).

In an independent series of studies, we demonstrated an intriguing "replay" effect by a dual-pulse TMS that is again applied to the visual cortex (Halelamien, Wu, and Shimojo, 2007; Wu and Shimojo, 2002; Wu et al., 2001, 2007). A visual stimulus (of almost any kind) was presented briefly with a sustained eye-fixation point, followed by a dual-pulse TMS with a delay of 100 to 1,000 ms. As a result, a vivid percept of the visual stimulus was perceived in a majority of subjects, including naive ones. The optimal range of the TMS delay for this replay effect varies across subjects but mostly within a range of 200 to 800 ms.

When the subject made a saccadic eye movement between the stimulus presentation and the TMS, the replay maintained its location in the retinotopic coordinate system (thus not with regard to the environmental frame; unpublished observation; see figure 5.2). This is an important observation indicating that the effect occurs relatively early in the visual cortical processing. Another intriguing observation was that the background color in the replay was vivid only near the luminance-defined contour but not noticeable father away (figure 5.2). This is consistent with some electrophysiological findings. First, the vast majority of color-coded neurons are orientation tuned as well (Friedman, Zhou, and von der Heydt, 2003). Likewise, whereas there are some neurons in V1 responding even when the receptive field was contained in a homogenous surface, this type of neuron constitutes only one third of the population (Komatsu, Murakami, and Kinoshita, 1996).

Our detailed experimental examinations further revealed that the percept is not always a faithful duplication of the original retinal stimulus, although the effect occurs allegedly in a relatively early cortical level, particularly when there was an illusion involved in the initial percept (Wu and Shimojo, 2007). In a variation of the flash lag effect, for instance, a transiently given feature, such as a color, was mislocalized in the direction of motion in accordance with the general definition of the flash lag effect. However, the replay of the colored arm, in this case, was closer to the physically valid location in most of the subjects.

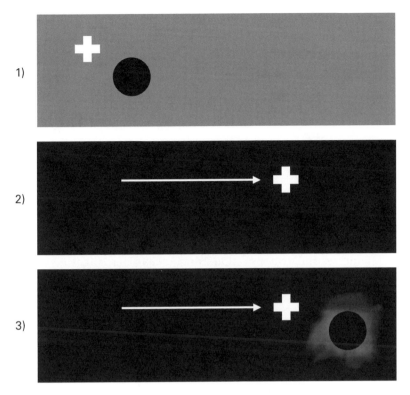

Figure 5.2
Retinotopic nature of the "replay" effect. (1) An object (a red disk) on a colored background was presented briefly while the subject's eyes fixated at a cross. (2) The fixation point jumped, and the subject followed with its eyes. (3) Dual-pulse TMS was applied to yield the replay effect. The object and the background color, but only near the object's contour, were "replayed" precisely in the same retinotopic location regardless of the saccade.

When we compared simple visual stimuli (such as basic geometric shapes) and more complex natural scenes in the replay effect, the latter type of stimuli tended to yield more vigorous replay effects (Halelamien et al., 2007). This somewhat counterintuitive result may be interpreted in accordance with the recent findings (e.g., Mayer, Herrmann, and Geisel, 2001) that the visual cortex is highly tuned to natural scene statistics and thus optimized to encode them most efficiently.

The phenomenology of the replay varied a lot across subjects. Some reported a photopic or Xerox-like duplication of the colorful scene. Some reported the figure (or the background) only in full color but blank in the background (figure). Some reported contours without any filled color. Although varying widely, these reports are yet more or less consistent with the known neuronal selectivity at the early visual cortical areas V1 and V2.

The two TMS studies described here, taken together, provide some rare neurophysiological evidence suggesting that our visual perception is not just "re-presenting" what is already available in the environment or the stimulus but rather a result of extensive dynamic cortical interactions.

Visual Cortex as a Stimulus-Driven Device (or a Field of Local–Global Interactions) for Perceptual Organization

Feature selectivity of individual neurons in the early visual cortex has long been considered the neural basis of visual perception (the "neuronal doctrine") (Barlow, 1972). This approach, however, soon encountered difficulty facing the directly three-dimensional and holistic nature of perception (Nakayama, He, and Shimojo, 1995). To bridge this explanatory gap, one may need to introduce the richer and more perceptually grounded idea of "visual surfaces."

To illustrate this point, see the demonstration in figure 5.3. This is meant to be a stereogram, but to be more specific, we prefer calling it the "minimum filling-in stereogram" (Nakayama and Shimojo, unpublished data). The distinctive difference from the

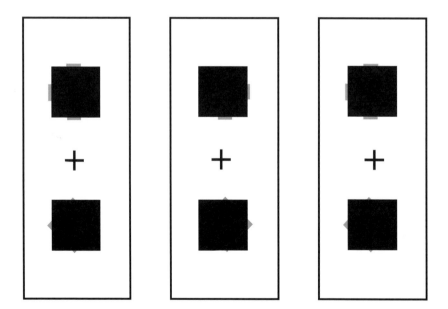

Figure 5.3
Minimum stereogram for filling-in. This stereogram is designed to demonstrate both crossed (front) and uncrossed (behind) disparity cases to both crossed and uncrossed fusers. Try to free-fuse the central crosses, and the observer should be able to see the crossed and the uncrossed cases side by side.

classical stereogram is the following. The binocular disparity is normally expressed in the lateral shift of the corresponding portions between the eyes in the classical stereogram but, in this case only in the presence/absence of the corresponding portion (the gray bar along the vertical edge of the black square). Note, also, that the black squares are entirely homogenous, thus lacking dense local disparity information except along the vertical contours.

Even with such limited local cues, a human observer has no problem perceiving a clear three-dimensional layout with specific surface quality, such as either a gray cross or a gray diamond semitransparent and floating in front of a black square behind. This, however, is only when the implied disparity of the gray portions are crossed (front). When it is uncrossed (behind), then an entirely different three-dimensional surface layout emerges perceptually—an opaque gray cross or diamond partly occluded by the rectangle in front. Note that in both cases, the percept is only one of an infinite number of possible interpretations based on the visual inputs to the eyes.

Davinci stereopsis is yet another example of this kind (Nakayama and Shimojo, 1990), in which only few dots that are interocularly unpaired can yield a vivid perceptual impression of surfaces in depth. We have a series of related demonstrations indicating that the visual system comes up with a consistent three-dimensional surface layout as a solution to what are indicated by a variety of cues, such as collinearity of contour, disparity, motion, relative luminance contrast (called "Metelli's rule"), and so on (Nakayama and Shimojo, 1990; 1992; Nakayama, Shimojo, and Silverman, 1989; Nakayama, Shimojo, and Ramachandran, 1990; Shimojo and Nakayama, 1990a, b, 1994; Shimojo, Silverman, and Nakayama 1988; Shimojo et al., 1989).

Although these perceptual effects are strictly stimulus-driven, they may involve vigorous lateral and top-down interactions at cortical levels (the same may apply to the TMS studies described earlier). More important, the rapidity by which the percept seemingly arises calls to mind a possible computational analogue, namely, some sort of one-shot computation; to resolve innate ambiguity in the visual input and to reach a globally consistent scene interpretation. In this sense, Rudolph Arnheim's interpretation of the historical message from the Gestalt tradition comes to mind (i.e., that perception follows its own organizational principle) (Arnheim, 1984).

This conclusion—that perception reaches a globally consistent scene interpretation—may, however, require a little more specification. First, global consistency should imply consistency across local cues, each of which already indicates which multiple surface interpretations are (im)possible. Consistency of this kind is often violated in the well-known "impossible figures." In these instances, local surface/edge relationships, such as "this surface is more in front," "this surface partly occludes the other," and "these two surfaces form a convex edge" are globally inconsistent along a particular contour. Thus, consistency among such local signals may be tested by some sort of constraint propagation in computational terms.

Second, the concept of global consistency should obey a more probabilistic or statistical constraint that is particularly related to the spatial relationship of the viewpoint with regard to the object. The generic view principle is a classical example. It prefers a scene interpretation that allows the input to be a generic view (i.e., qualitatively unchanging across a wide viewing angle) as opposed to an accidental view.

To begin with, a class of images (topologically the same images) can be obtained from a limited or a broad angle of viewing (figure 5.4A). For example, a square-shaped thin plate in the real world may be seen as a bar image from a limited range of viewing angles but as a rectangular image, as such, from a wider range. Meanwhile, a cube in the real world may be seen as a square-shaped image from a limited angle. Thus, one may call the square-shaped image as a generic view of a square-shaped plate but an accidental view of a cube. Based on this, one may also call a real-world (three-dimensional) interpretation (e.g., cube) of an image input (a square image) *accidental* and another interpretation (thin, square plate) *generic*. The generic view principle states that the brain prefers a more generic scene interpretation of the visual input (i.e., image). We have shown that depth/surface perception by binocular stereogram obeys this principle (figure 5.4B; Nakayama and Shimojo, 1992). In this regard, it is also interesting to note that a variety of impossible figure examples include a violation of this second criterion of the global consistency (i.e., in accordance with the generic view principle; the impossible figures usually include an accidental viewing angle).

If we further include minimum complexity constraints (e.g., minimum numbers of surfaces, simplest configuration, etc.), the list may be considered more or less completed (although how to define "minimum" might be another sticky problem, computationally speaking). We can see such global interactions in some other demonstrations in the literature: Koffka's ring (figure 5.5A), White illusion (figure 5.5B), Adelson's haze illusions (figure 5.5C), and so on. In these impressive illusions, local features (e.g., T and X junctions) interact with contrasts among regions, already providing sufficient information to signal a particular surface relationship. As a result, the attained surface perception is both consistent and stable.

A similar point may be made for illusory contours (Takeichi, Watanabe, and Shimojo, 1992) and neon color spreading (Takeichi, Shimojo, and Watanabe, 1992). Fuse the stereogram in figure 5.6, for instance. All the inducers for the illusory triangle belong to the zero-disparity surface except for the three dots inside the corners. When the dots have a crossed (front) disparity, only these dots appear to float in space closer to the illusory contour. When uncrossed (behind), however, another surface that includes the three dots is formed behind the triangle-shaped illusory window. Thus, in this case, the local but unambiguous disparity interacts vigorously with the perceptually formed contour to yield a stable and consistent impression of surface(s) in depth.

Yet another related point is that such dynamic global organization of perception is mostly independent of knowledge. On top of most of the illusion demonstration

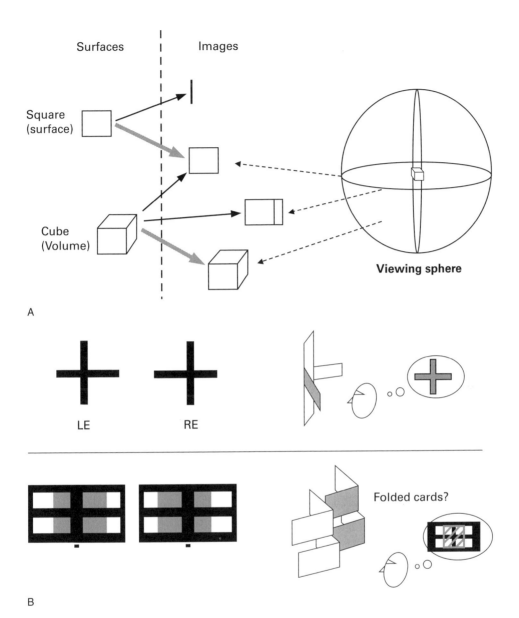

Figure 5.4

Generic view principle. (A) Illustration of the principle. Relations between objects in the real world and their visual images are indicated by arrows (thin: accidental, thick: generic). On the right side is a "viewing sphere," which consists of viewing angles that give rise to categorically the same visual images (i.e., one, two, or three surface[s] visible) as indicated by dashed arrows. (B) The generic view principle applied to stereograms. (Top) The cross-stereogram may appear like the folded arm as illustrated on the right side but rarely presumably because it would be too "accidental." It rather appears as one arm occluding the other with a depth in between. (Bottom) Likewise, the stereogram would not appear as folded cards. Instead, it appears as a semitransparent gray surface in front (in the case when it has a crossed disparity).

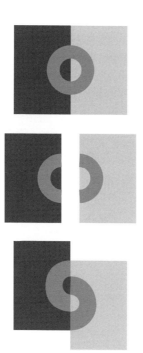

A

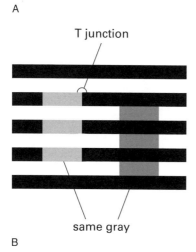

B

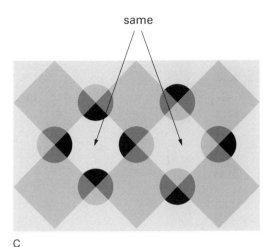

C

Figure 5.5
Some related illusions. (A) The Koffka ring. The brightness of the doughnut-shaped area may appear differently across the top, the middle, and the bottom figures, indicating critical roles of luminance-defined edges as well as T and X junctions. (B) The White illusion. The gray parts appear differently depending on where they are embedded in the stripes, indicating roles of grouping and T junctions. (C) Haze illusion. The diamond-shaped areas appear grossly different in terms of surface quality, again indicating roles of X junctions, luminance contrast, and so on (taken from E. Adelson homepage).

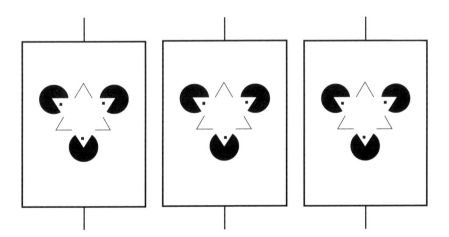

Figure 5.6
This stereogram, just as figure 5.3, is designed to demonstrate both crossed (front) and uncrossed (behind) disparity cases to both crossed and uncrossed fusers. Compare the two depth cases to note the difference in three-dimensional surface formation (modified from Takeichi et al., 1992).

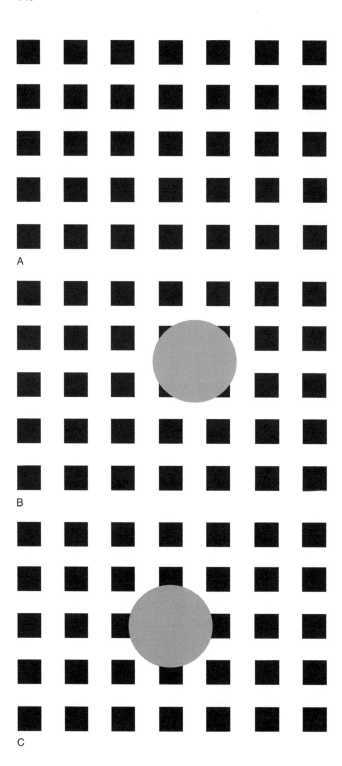

above, the demonstration by Kanizsa (1979) would be another good example (figure 5.7). A gedanken experiment, inspired by Koffka (1935) as well as Kanizsa and extended by the author from their originals, would be as follows: An observer may see the original material (i.e., just a regular array of black squares on a sheet of paper; figure 5.7A). Then an experimenter puts an opaque gray disk either as in figure 5.7B or C. Now the experimenter asks the observer two different questions: "What do you know is behind this disk?" and "How do you perceive the black parts partly occluded by the disk?"

The answer to the former question would be something like, "A regular array of black squares, just like the surround." However, the answer to the second question may more likely to be either "A big black square partly occluded by a gray disk" (in the case of figure 5.7B) or "A big black cross partly occluded by a gray disk" (in the case of figure 5.7C), regardless of his or her own knowledge.

This gedanken experiment eloquently demonstrates independence of perception from abstract knowledge. More strikingly, evidence shows that this type of surface perception is at an early cortical level, early enough to create a corresponding afterimage (Shimojo, Kamitani, and Nishida, 2001). To witness this, fixate at the fixation point in figure 5.8A for at least 20 sec. Then fixate at figure 5.8B. The reader may see a square-shaped afterimage, which is corresponding to the filled-in surface, as opposed to elemental inducers, at least during a part of the adapting period (the demonstration may work better on a computer monitor than on paper, also better when colored as in the original publication). Thus, in short, when we see a visual surface, there is a neural representation of that surface that is strong enough to create an afterimage of the percept not just the input elements.

Stimulus-Driven, Bottom-Up, and Top-Down—Some Clarification on Terminology

It may be better to stop here and ponder our terminology to avoid further confusion.

The concept of "top-down" may have two different meanings. In information-processing and psychology contexts, it may simply mean an inference based on cognitive knowledge. By now it must be obvious to readers that the examples of vigorous global organization in perception described in this chapter are largely independent of top-down processes in this particular sense.

In the physiological or neuroscientific context, however, it may mean something else. It could specifically refer to those feedback pathways from a higher to lower

◄ Figure 5.7

Koffka's/Kanizsa's Gedanken Experiment. (A) One sees this unoccluded pattern first. (B) Then one sees the same pattern partly occluded by a disk at this location or at another location (C). One would be asked what (s)he perceives as opposed to what (s)he knows. See text.

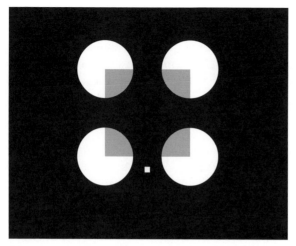

A

B

Figure 5.8
Afterimage of a filled-in surface. (A) Fixate on the white fixation point for 20 sec. (B) Refixate on the blank. Keep fixating for 10 sec, at least, and one may see a whitish afterimage shaped as a large square that corresponds to the filled-in surface during adaptation. The demonstration works better in color on a CRT display (see Shimojo et al., 2001, for more details).

cortical areas/levels, which in fact occupy the majority of visual cortical axons (DeYoe et al., 1994). Considering the local nature of receptive field structure in the early levels of the visual cortex, the type of global perception of concern here obviously requires lateral corticocortical interactions or top-down pathways in this specific sense, or, most likely, both.

This selective usage of the term "top-down" has critical significance with regard to the main message of this chapter. To rephrase, the visual processing attains a three-dimensional surface interpretation of the visual scene as a globally consistent and unique solution. This is accomplished mainly by a process triggered by the retinal stimulus. Although it does not invoke much of the top-down process in the first sense (knowledge-based inference), it most likely involves a massive amount of the top-down pathways in the second sense (feedback pathways).

Ambiguity Solving in Cross-Modal Integration—Similar Principles can Be Applied to Cross-Modal Cases

As mentioned earlier in this chapter, a three-dimensional surface interpretation is attained as a solution to the ambiguity that is intrinsic in the retinal inputs via specific interactions that are both local and bottom-up and global and top-down. Similar principles of neural information processing can be mostly applied to cross-modal situations (see Shimojo and Shams, 2001, for a review). The "double flash" illusion (Shams, Kamitani, and Shimojo, 2000; Shams, Shimojo, and Kamitani, 2001) is just one example.

To see this illusion, a visual stimulus should be briefly presented with two sharp sounds (figure 5.9A). The time range of the two sounds should be ±100 ms approximately from the onset of the visual stimulus (figure 5.9B). As a result, one perceives the physically single flash of the visual object as doubled. Thus, the ambiguity in the visual inputs—caused mainly by the limit of visual temporal resolution in this case—is solved with assistance of auditory processing, but only within this temporal window.

This robust phenomenon is neither explained by some cognitive artifact nor erased by feedback procedure. Moreover, it can be observed even when the two sounds are replaced by two tactile stimuli (Violentyev, Shimojo, and Shams, 2005). When the stimulus parameters are carefully adjusted, the visual perception becomes ambiguous (i.e., the visual stimulus may be perceived as a single or double flash, and this is true within subjects). It may suggest that such ambiguity exists with any parameter combinations, and it may be just that one percept is too dominant in most of the cases. Depending on the signal-to-noise ratio (i.e., clarity/sharpness) of the visual and auditory stimuli, and other factors such as visual eccentricity, the brain attains the most reliable event interpretation consistent with the evidence given from the ears and eyes. Evidence from EEG (Bhattacharya, Shams, and Shimojo, 2002; Shams, Kamitani, et al.,

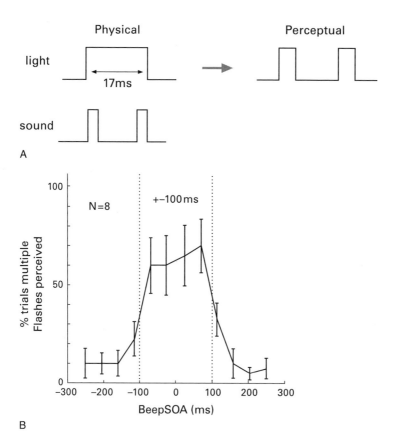

Figure 5.9
Double flash (or illusory flash) illusion. (A) Illustration of the stimulus sequence and the basic illusion. (B) Temporal tuning of the illusion. Percentage of trials in which multiple flashes were perceived is plotted against the beep SOA (stimulus onset asynchrony, i.e., the time delay from the flash onset to the onset of the first sound) (see Shams et al., 2000, for more details).

2001) and fMRI (Watkins et al., 2006) shows that the illusion is caused by auditory stimuli, whereas the critical modulation of neural signals is in the early visual cortices, probably including the primary visual cortex (V1). Such modulation is possibly via the direct projection from the auditory cortex (Rockland and van Hoesen, 1994) or via subcortical structures such as the superior colliculus (SC). Although these findings may be counterintuitive, it is consistent with the idea that the perceptual illusion is phenomenologically in the visual domain (i.e., a single flash appears to be double flashes). Also, according to the EEG studies mentioned earlier, the critical neural process that is responsible for the illusion effect occurs quickly after the stimulus onset, certainly faster than 200 ms from the onset.

Although the results are not inconsistent at some level of description with the max-imum likelihood or the Bayesian theory of cross-modal integration (Ernst and Banks, 2002), it clearly has more implications with regard to the structure of visual percept captured by that of auditory stimuli. Note further that this principle is analogous both mathematically and biologically to that of the generic view in the case of visual perception.

Thus, the brain quickly resolves perceptual ambiguity, which is typically intrinsic to the sensory stimulus, via stimulus-driven, self-organizing mechanisms; both in the case of vision as well as cross-modal interactions. The only minor, although not entirely negligible, difference would be that a three-dimensional surface layout is the result of the process in vision, whereas an object or event generated in perception more generally involves cross-modal integration.

Conclusions

This chapter described three different sets of studies: TMS studies on the visual cortical dynamics, visual psychophysics on the visual surface representation, and cross-modal integration, particularly in the case of the double-flash illusion. Although these topics are seemingly diverse, they all point to the same aspects of perceptual organization. The results together characterize the perceptual processing in the sensory cortices as quick, self-organizing processes designed to generate an unambiguous percept from sensory inputs. Whereas we may follow von Helmholtz' (1856) characterization of such a perceptual process as "subconscious inference," we need to quickly qualify it further as mostly independent of explicit knowledge, strictly stimulus-driven, and yet massively involving top-down/bottom-up and local–global interactions in a specifi-cally neuroanatomical sense.

References

Arnheim, R. 1984. *Art and Visual Perception: A Psychology of the Creative Eye. The New Version.* Berke-ley and Los Angeles, CA: University of California Press.

Barlow, H. B. 1972. "Single Units and Sensation: A Neuron Doctrine for Perceptual Psychology?" *Perception* 1 (4): 371–394.

Bhattacharya, J., Shams, L., and Shimojo, S. 2002. "Critical Role of Gamma Band Responses in the Sound Induced Illusory Double Flash Perception." *NeuroReport* 13: 1727–1730.

DeYoe, E. A., Fellmanm, D. J., Van Essen, D. C., and McClendon, E. 1994. "Multiple Processing Streams in Occipitotemporal Visual-Cortex." *Nature* 371 (6493): 151–154.

Ernst, M. O., and Banks, M. S. 2002. "Humans Integrate Visual and Haptic Information in a Sta-tistically Optimal Fashion." *Nature* 415 (6870): 429–433.

Friedman, H. S., Zhou, H., and von der Heydt, R. 2003. "The Coding of Uniform Colour Figures in Monkey Visual Cortex." *Journal of Physiology-London* 548 (2): 593–613.

Halelamien, N., Wu, D. A., and Shimojo, S. 2007. "TMS Induces Detail-Rich 'Instant Replays' of Natural Images." *Journal of Vision* 7 (9): 276. <http://journalofvision.org/7/9/276/>, doi:10.1167/7.9.276>.

Helmholtz, H. L. F. von. 1856. *Treatise on Physiological Optics*. Translated by J. P. Southall (1924/1925). New York: Dover.

Kamitani, Y., and Shimojo, S. 1999. "Manifestation of Scotomas Created by Transcranial Magnetic Stimulation of Human Visual Cortex." *Nature Neuroscience* 2: 767–771.

Kanizsa, G. 1979. *Organization in Vision*. New York: Praeger.

Koffka, K. 1935. *Principles of Gestalt Psychology*. New York: Harcourt Brace.

Komatsu, H., Murakami, I., and Kinoshita, M. 1996. "Surface Representation in the Visual System." *Cognitive Brain Research* 5 (1–2): 97–104.

Mayer, N., Herrmann, J. M., and Geisel, T. 2001. "Signatures of Natural Image Statistics in Cortical Simple Cell Receptive Fields." *Neuocomputing* 38: 279–284.

Nakayama, K., He, Z. J., and Shimojo, S. 1995. "Visual Surface Representation: A Critical Link Between Lower-Level and Higher-Level Vision." In *Frontiers in Cognitive Neuroscience*, edited by S. Kosslyn and D. N. Osherson. 2nd ed. Cambridge, MA: MIT Press.

Nakayama, K., and Shimojo, S. 1990. "DaVinci Stereopsis: Depth and Subjective Occluding Contours From Unpaired Image Points." *Vision Research* 30: 1811–1825.

Nakayama, K., and Shimojo, S. 1992. "Experiencing and Perceiving Visual Surfaces." *Science* 257: 1357–1363.

Nakayama, K., Shimojo, S., and Ramachandran, V. S. 1990. "Perceived Transparency: Relation to Depth, Subjective Contours, Luminance, and Neon Color Spreading." *Perception* 19: 497–513.

Nakayama, K., Shimojo, S., and Silverman, G. H. 1989. "Stereoscopic Depth: Its Relation to Image Segmentation, Grouping, and the Recognition of Occluded Objects." *Perception* 18: 55–68.

Rockland, K. S., and van Hoesen, G. W. 1994. "Direct Temporal-Occipital Feedback Connections to Striate Cortex (v1) in the Macaque Monkey." *Cerebral Cortex* 4 (3): 300–313.

Shams, L., Kamitani, Y., and Shimojo, S. 2000. "What You See Is What You Hear." *Nature* 408: 788.

Shams, L., Kamitani, Y., Thompson, S., and Shimojo, S. 2001. "Sound Alters Visual Evoked Potentials in Humans." *Neuroreport* 12: 3849–3852.

Shams, L., Shimojo, S., and Kamitani, Y. 2001. "A Visual Illusion Induced by Sound." *Cognitive Brain Research* 14: 147–152.

Shimojo, S., Kamitani, Y., and Nishida, S. 2001. "Afterimage of Perceptually Filled-in Surface." *Science* 293: 1677–1680.

Shimojo, S., and Nakayama, K. 1990a. "Amodal Representation of Occluded Surfaces: Role of Invisible Stimuli in Apparent Motion Correspondence." *Perception* 19: 285–299.

Shimojo, S., and Nakayama, K. 1990b. "Real World Occlusion Constraints and Binocular Rivalry." *Vision Research* 30: 69–80.

Shimojo, S., and Shams, L. 2001. "Sensory Modalities Are Not Separate Modalities: Plasticity and Interactions." *Current Opinion in Neurobiology* 11: 505–509.

Shimojo, S., Silverman, G. H., and Nakayama, K. 1988. "An Occlusion-Related Depth Mechanism Based on Motion and Interocular Order." *Nature* 33: 265–268.

Shimojo, S., Silverman, G. H., and Nakayama, K. 1989. "Occlusion and the Solution to the Aperture Problem for Motion." *Vision Research* 29: 619–626.

Takeichi, H., Shimojo, S., and Watanabe, T. 1992. "Neon Flank and Illusory Contour: Interaction Between the Two Processes Leads to Color Filling-in." *Perception* 21: 313–324.

Takeichi, H., Watanabe, T., and Shimojo, S. 1992. "Illusory Occluding Contours and Surface Formation by Depth Propagation." *Perception* 21: 177–184.

Violentyev, A., Shimojo, S., and Shams, L. 2005. "Touch-Induced Visual Illusion." *NeuroReport* 16: 1107–1110.

Watkins, S., Shams, L., Tanaka, S., Haynes, J. D., and Rees, G. 2006. "Sound Alters Activity in Human V1 in Association With Illusory Visual Perception." *Neuroimage* 31 (3): 1247–1256.

Wu, D. A., Halelamien, N., Hoeft, F., and Shimojo, S. 2007. "TMS 'Instant Replay' Validated Using Novel Double-Blind Stimulation Technique." *Journal of Vision* 7 (9): 275. <http://journalofvision.org/7/9/275/, doi:10.1167/7.9.275>.

Wu, D. A., Kamitani, Y., Maeda, F., and Shimojo, S. 2001. "Interaction of TMS-Induced Phosphenes and Visual Stimuli." *Vision Sciences Society* (*Abstract*), 57.

Wu, D. A., and Shimojo, S. 2002. "TMS Reveals the Correct Location of Flashes in Motion-Mislocalization Illusions." *Vision Sciences Society* (*Abstract*), 15.

II Color, Shape, and Space

6 The Perception of Material Qualities and the Internal Semantics of the Perceptual System

Rainer Mausfeld

The perception of material qualities poses a preeminent challenge for perception theory and provides an instructive study case for probing the soundness and explanatory force of theoretical frameworks for perception. Phenomena pertaining to the perception of material appearances are particularly suited to expose the explanatory gap between the information available in the sensory input and the meaningful categories that characterize the output of the perceptual system. More than seemingly elementary attributes, such as shape or color, material appearances impart objects their meaningful properties of, say, being soft, wet, malleable, silky, juicy, edible, or deformable. We are obviously endowed with a specific perceptual capacity by which we can visually attain aspects of perceptual objects that pertain to their "hidden" dispositional powers and propensities. Due to this capacity, we cannot only identify specific kinds of objects and stuff, but we can also visually grasp an abundant variety of properties of objects that go far beyond purely visual attributes. This capacity is part of our more general perceptual capacity for making causal assignments and for embedding all of our experiences into various kinds of internal causal analyses. The specific kind of dispositional properties and causal ascriptions that are perceptually accessible from the sensory data is subordinated to the type of perceptual object that is activated by the sensory data. In the case of *surfaces*—understood as *perceptual* objects not as physical ones—these dispositional properties pertain to material qualities, and the causal ascriptions to, for example, how surfaces will appear under changes in their orientation and location, which haptic experiences will be elicited by them, and how they will behave under various kinds of interactions, both with an agent and with other objects.

Although the capacity of visually attaining dispositional properties of objects constitutes one of the most remarkable functional achievements of our perceptual system, this capacity has received scant attention in traditional perceptual psychology. Apart from a few exceptions, investigations of the principles underlying the perception of material qualities have been largely neglected in favor of investigations of seemingly simpler attributes, such as shape or color. This situation is peculiar because investigations into the visual perception of material qualities of, say, *surfaces* promises to be a particularly rewarding field for the attempt to identify more abstract principles of perception. The general principles that are brought to bear by this achievement pertain to the perceptual system's capacity to attain the biologically important dispositional properties of its perceptual objects by a "reading-through," as it were, of the available sensory image. A theoretical framework that is general enough to deal in an explanatorily satisfactory way with material qualities of *surfaces*, such as shiny, wet, deformable, or walkable, is, or so I argue, also suited to appropriately deal with corresponding achievements with respect to other types of perceptual objects. With regard to perceptual objects of the type *living animal*, for example, these achievements comprise the capacity to perceptually attain "hidden powers" and "essences" of those types of objects. With regard to perceptual objects of the type *mykind*, they comprise the capacity to read through the object's surfaces to perceptually attain what we can refer to as "mental states of others." This can be strikingly illustrated by the demonstrations provided by Heider and Simmel (1944), which show that certain kinds of motions of simple geometrical objects suffice for eliciting a perceptual ascription of complex internal attributes pertaining to mental states of *mykind* (cf. Scholl and Tremoulet, 2000). Available evidence suggests, or so I claim, that there is no difference of principle with respect to the fundamental mode of operation of the perceptual system, between the perception of material qualities and the perception of, say, mental states of others. Although corresponding theoretical ideas have been widely expressed and elaborated since the seventeenth century, current orthodoxy has pursued a different path of thinking. According to regnant conceptions in perceptual psychology, the perception of material qualities of surfaces is regarded as different in principle from the perception of dispositions of, say, a living object or the perception of mental states of *mykind*. Although the first kind of dispositions are presumed to be attainable more or less "directly" from complex spatiotemporal properties of the sensory input, the perception of the latter dispositions is presumed to rest on alleged "higher order" or "cognitive" processes by which these dispositions were inferred from the sensory data. The fundamental flaws underlying corresponding conceptions have been disclosed again and again, notably by the Gestaltists. Although compelling empirical and theoretical evidence has been accumulated exposing the utter inadequacy of corresponding conceptions, they still dominate the field. However, such a situation is not unusual in the history of the natural sciences. It chiefly emerges when there is a clash between theoretical concepts that are strongly suggested by the available experimental evidence and deeply engrained commonsense notions. In fact, the propensity to cling to conceptions whose inadequacy, in light of the available evidence, stands to reason can be used as an expedient clue for the influence of tacit commonsense intuitions. With respect to physics, it is well known that its entire history can be read as a continuous quarrel with commonsense intuitions. What holds for physics even stronger holds for perception theory. We are held captive by the way perception appears to us.

We are strongly convinced that perceiving keeps us in more or less direct contact with the world and that what we perceive by and large is the world as it really is. Our ordinary conception about perception discounts, on the basis of an important functional achievement of the brain, all the processes that occur between the distal causes and the percept, and thus considers perception an entirely conspicuous process. Of course, we are willing to accept all sorts of sophistications and, under unusual circumstances, exceptions of this account, but otherwise regard it as a kind of truism. We thus have great difficulties in being aware that almost all of our ordinary intuitions about perception become misconceptions when transposed to the field of perception theory. Our brain is not equipped with mechanisms by which we can observe its own machinery, and the most fundamental principles underlying perception are, consequently, not transparent to us. Because of this, our ordinary intuitions about perception are an inapt guide for the endeavor to achieve, within the framework of the natural sciences, a theoretical understanding of the principles on which our perceptual achievements are based. Rather, a theoretical understanding of these principles can only be achieved by standard methodological principles of the natural sciences, which have proved highly fruitful in developing appropriate explanatory frameworks, often at the expense of sacrificing deeply valued commonsense intuitions. In speaking of ordinary or commonsense conceptions about perception, in the present context, I understand the term in the broadest possible way, namely, as the diversity modes in which we conceive of perceptual phenomena and the process of perception in all contexts other than that of the natural sciences. (This usage comprises not only those concepts and ways of world-making that underlie, as part of our biological endowment, our ordinary discourse about the world and our acts of perceiving but also derived concepts and pertaining to perceptual issues that have been developed for other purposes than those of the natural sciences, whether technological, philosophical, or of any other kind.)

Since the historic origin of rational enquiries, commonsense intuitions about perception have constituted the severest and almost insurmountable obstacle for the development of theoretical insights into the abstract principles on which our perceptual achievements are based. Enquiries into the nature of perception naturally have much greater difficulties than physics had to dispense with ordinary intuitions and commonsense classifications of phenomena and to instead follow lines of theorizing that are traced out by the development of successful explanatory accounts. During recent decades, a theoretical convergence of different disciplines such as ethology, research with babies, and perceptual psychology has made more visible the contours of a general theoretical framework for a deeper understanding of perception. These developments, however, have not yet gained wider acceptance because they are grossly at variance with our commonsense conceptions about perception. Yet this sacrifice of commonsense intuitions about perception will repay itself amply by the gain in explanatory width and depth of the theoretical insights into the abstract principles on which the achievements of the perceptual system are based.

In this chapter, I attempt to flesh out the abstract theoretical framework that is currently (re-)emerging in the course of a theoretical convergence of several disciplines. In the first section, I formulate what appears to me to be the fundamental problem of perception theory, namely, the generation, by the perceptual system, of meaningful categories from physicogeometric energy patterns. In the second section, I briefly characterize basic intuitions and assumptions underlying what can be regarded as the current *Standard Model of Perceptual Psychology* and point out why this model is profoundly inadequate for dealing with the fundamental problem of perception theory. In the third section, I suggest a level of analysis that promises to be fruitful for dealing, in conformity with established procedures of the natural sciences, with the problem of perceptual "meaning" and the problem of what constitutes a "perceptual object." In the fourth section, I adumbrate the outlines of the theoretical perspective on basic principles of the perceptual system as it appears to be emerging from the convergence of different disciplines. This approach, which centers on the notions of complex data types and conceptual forms, draws an entirely different theoretical picture of the role of the sensory input than traditional accounts. In the final section, I return to the issue of material qualities and discuss, within the general theoretical framework outlined, some observations and results on the perception of certain material properties, namely, lustrous and glassy appearances.

The Fundamental Problem of Perception Theory

Perception theory, as I understand it here, aims at a theoretical understanding of the basic principles on which our perceptual achievements are based; it proceeds on the assumption that these achievements are brought forth by a specific type of biological system, the perceptual system (which presumably is made up of several subsystems). Although perception theory acknowledges that the full range of our perceptual phenomena results from complex interactions of the perceptual system with other systems of the brain, it assumes that the proprietary mode of functioning of the perceptual system can be abstractly characterized by a set of fundamental principles. Hence, it assumes that a broad range of core perceptual phenomena can be understood from a rather small set of theoretical principles. Perception theory thus proceeds on the standard methodological path of the natural sciences: It assumes that the apparent complexity of a certain set of phenomena derives from simple, and hence more abstract, principles that reflect the fundamental features of the idealised domain of nature under scrutiny. More specifically, perception theory assumes that the perceptual system, like other systems of the brain, can be regarded as a computational system (understood here in a rather loose sense; i.e., as a system that performs specific types of abstract operations on its input and its internal data structures and delivers certain types of outputs to other systems). It furthermore employs the idealization that the perceptual system can, to some interesting extent, be investigated independently of other computational systems of the brain, such as systems comprising motoric or linguistic representations, systems dealing with imaginations, or general interpretative or inferential systems. Because of these assumptions, perception theory will inevitably abstract away from a wealth of phenomena that appear to us striking from the perspective of our ordinary intuitions. As in other domains of the natural sciences, perception theory is willing to trade off descriptive richness for a gain in theoretical understanding, of sufficient widths and depth, of the fundamental principles on which the mode of operation of the perceptual system rests.

If we attempt to formulate what seems to be the fundamental problem of perception theory, we thus have to be aware that we are aiming at an explanatory account of the core principles of a specific system, namely, the perceptual system (rather than providing an account for, say, achievements that are crucially based on the interactions of a variety of different subsystems or even intrinsically pertain to the entire organism). As a computational system, the perceptual system owns, on the one hand, a type of interface that connects it with physical states external to the organism and, on the other hand, several types of internal interfaces by which it connects with the motoric system and higher imaginative, interpretative, or linguistic systems. The standard input to the perceptual system can be characterized by a physical spatiotemporal energy pattern (chemical or interoceptive types of inputs can be subsumed under this abstract characterization). To characterize its output, we first need to specify to which type of internal interface we want to refer. Naturally, all outputs of the perceptual system have to be organized in terms of data formats that can be read by the respective subsequent systems. Among these subsequent systems are ones that make some part of the output of the perceptual system phenomenologically accessible to us. The phenomenal percept and its internal organization is not only the most salient aspect of perception for us, it also mirrors a crucial property of the output of the perceptual system (viz. its organization in terms of meaningful categories). This property of an organization in terms of internally meaningful categories applies to all types of outputs that the perceptual system provides at its interfaces to subsequent systems. By way of example, we can formulate the *Fundamental Problem of Perception Theory* for those types of outputs that are also phenomenally expressed.

As an illustration, take an apparently simple visual scene, such as the one depicted in figure 6.1. Although the visual input can be described as a geometrical luminance pattern on the retina, the output of the perceptual system, as mirrored in our phenomenal percept, is exceedingly rich and goes far beyond the input.

Perception theory thus has to deal with this question: What internal principles do we need to ascribe to the system under scrutiny to account for the finding that physical

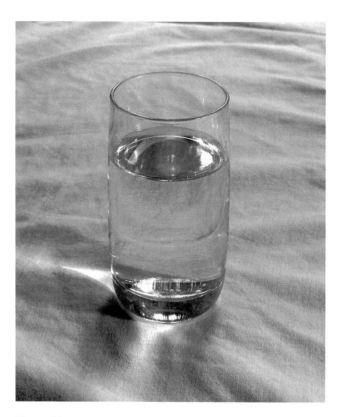

Figure 6.1
Illustration of material qualities.

spatiotemporal energy patterns can yield an organization of the output in terms of all the meaningful categories into which we segment our perceptual world? In the present examples, these categories refer to "container" with the attribute "breakable" or "transparent" and to "water" with the attribute "liquid" or "drinkable."

Figure 6.2 is a first stab at graphically depicting this problem. However, this way of describing the perceptually relevant entities of the external world is dictated by our commonsense conception of perception. What is depicted here as being the input is, at the same time, also the semantically organized percept and, thus, the output of the system. Furthermore, our commonsense intuitions abet us to object to the type of abstract description taken in figure 6.2 to be the output. Rather, we would prefer to describe the output more directly in terms of phenomenal categories. Thus, commonsense intuitions lead us to a formulation by which input and output are basically identified, as allegorized in figure 6.3. This illustration caricatures, not entirely unduly, the naive realism that is deeply built into our commonsense conception of perception: At the

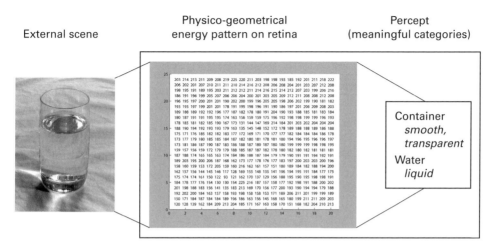

Figure 6.2
Illustration of the explanatory gap in perception theory.

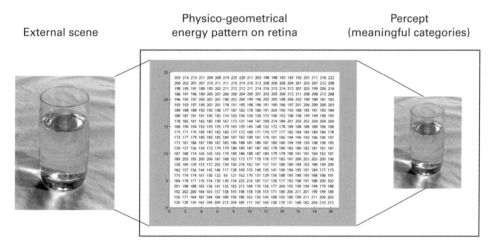

Figure 6.3
How the explanatory gap is trivialized in commonsense conceptions of perception.

core of our quotidian conception of perception is the belief that the external world can be basically characterized by the way it appears to us, and that therefore the categories of our percepts are nothing but categories of the external world. In fact, the predisposition to take perceptual concepts for "things in the real world" is the distinguishing mark of all of our mental activity. Kant thought of it as a "transcendental illusion." The transcendental illusion is the propensity to "take a subjective necessity of a connection of our concepts . . . for an objective necessity in the determination of things in themselves" (*Critique of pure reason*, A297/B354). Due to this propensity, whose influence cannot be remedied by intellectual insight into it, we inevitably tend to mistake our own mental categories to hold "objectively" (cf. Grier, 2001). Scientific enquiry has shown how deep in fact the abyss is between what we take to be the "external mind-independent world" and the world as conceptualized in human perception. Even in cases where our linguistic vocabulary (as also employed in physical discourse) seems to suggest that our perceptual categories have a direct counterpart in the physical world, such as in the case of "illumination" or "surface," a closer examination reveals that physically defined categories and perceptually defined categories do not match, and that, with respect to the functioning of the perceptual system, the occurrence of the former is neither necessary nor sufficient for the occurrence of the latter. The way we perceptually segment our world does not conform to the way we divide up things in the world when we are doing physics, an observation that Ludlow (2003) terms a "type mismatch" (p. 150).

Although naïve realism already founders in the face of the most elementary scientific facts, say about the properties of our sense organs, it intellectually expresses some of our deepest convictions about the mental activity of perceiving, namely, being in direct touch with a mind-independent world. These convictions—which Hume (in his *An Enquiry Concerning Human Understanding*, § 118) regarded as "a natural instinct or prepossession"—are so deeply entrenched in our conception of the world and our interactions with it that it is hardly surprising that they exercise a continuous impact on perception research (where they are particularly explicit in current versions of Bayesian frameworks for perception) (cf. Mausfeld, 2002).

Our built-in conviction that perception represents the way the external world is constitutes itself a functionally important achievement of our brain, and thus ultimately has itself to find a place in an explanatory account of our mental capacities. It becomes detrimental, however, when it is, with respect to perception theory, illegitimately transferred to scientific enquiry. In this case, it goes along with the tendency to use categories of the output for a description of the input. The predisposition to use physical categories from commonsense taxonomies, and thus from the output of the perceptual system, as independent descriptions of the physical world that allegedly need to be "recovered" from the sensory input in the process of perception, pervades perceptual psychology. Thus, by mistaking output categories for input categories, the

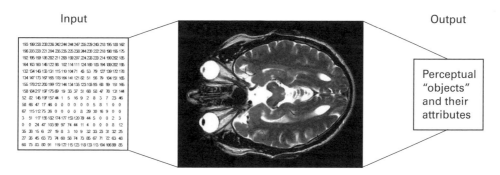

Figure 6.4
The *Fundamental Problem of Perception Theory.*

proper explanatory task of perception theory is trivialized. This was emphasized particularly by the Gestaltists and by Albert Michotte. Michotte (1954/1991) was exceptionally sensitive to the problem of meaning in perception. His experimental work led him to acknowledge that "our sensory experiences . . . are infinitely richer in content than could ever have been anticipated" and that underlying such achievements "seems to be a kind of 'prefiguration' of abstract concepts, the mental 'categories' of substance, reality, and causality" (pp. 44–45).

So as not to succumb to our commonsense preconceptions of perception and for theoretical reasons given in more detail later, we should avoid, in the present context, any reference to an external scene, and thus to the potential external causes of the sensory input, and rather confine the formulation to the actual input of the biological system under scrutiny. The *Fundamental Problem of Perception Theory* amounts then to this question: On the basis of what principles can the perceptual system generate given a specific physical spatiotemporal energy pattern as input, an output that is organized in terms of meaningful categories, as depicted in figure 6.4? The task of perception theory thus is to identify the *internal structure* (i.e., the complex data types and computational principles) of a biologically given computational system on the basis of which the system can generate perceptually meaningful semantic distinctions given certain sensory inputs.

The Standard Model of Perceptual Psychology

Perceptual psychology and psychophysics, in most of their currently prevailing approaches, have framed their enquiries in a way that either bypasses or trivializes altogether the *Fundamental Problem of Perception Theory*. Their underlying conception of perception condenses in what can be called the *sensation-perception model* of perception. This conception is grounded on a distinction between sensations, as the "raw

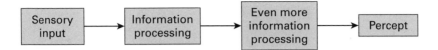

Figure 6.5
The Standard Model of Perception.

material" of experience, on the one hand, and perceptions, which were typically conceived of as referring to objects in the external world, on the other hand. A distinction of this kind, as advanced by Spencer, James, Wundt, or Helmholtz, pervades, in various forms, perceptual psychology. Sensations and perceptions were generally held to "shade gradually into each other, being one and all products of the same psychological machinery of association" (William James, *Principles of Psychology*, chapter XIX) or of some other inferential machinery. The sensation-perception model of perception thus conceives of perceptions as a hierarchy of processing stages within the same set of sensory data types by which the sensory input is transformed into the meaningful categories and distinctions, namely, the "perceptions" whose meanings derive from what they refer to in the external world.

The sensation-perception model, in its many guises, became what may be called the *Standard Model* of perceptual psychology and psychophysics. According to this model, the process of perception can essentially be described as subsequent stages of "information" processing, by which the sensory input is successively transformed into the percept as illustrated (following Neisser, 1976, p. 17) in figure 6.5. (As to the concept of information underlying this scheme, Jackendoff [1987] noted that "sometimes one gets the impression that information is to be thought of as a sort of abstract liquid that is poured from one receptacle into another, that is filtered free of unwanted detail, and that overflows into forgetfulness if the receptacle into which it is being poured is already full" [p. 38].) Although the notion of information, as employed in the context of corresponding conceptions of perception, is notoriously vague and beclouds the actual problems involved, this Standard Model of Perception is mostly regarded in current orthodoxy not as a model but as a self-evident truth.

More specifically, it is presumed that the sensory input provides information about elementary sensory qualities, such as color and motion, and that by so-called lower level processes these elementary qualities are glued together by some associative or inferential machinery (as depicted in figure 6.6). The remaining gap to the percept is then bridged by what is usually referred to as "cognitive processes" or "higher order" processes, which are assumed to account for everything that cannot be explained by the so-called lower level processes.

There are basically two ways to interpret these schemes of perceptual information processing, both equally fatal. On a weak interpretation, the arrows indicate, in a loose

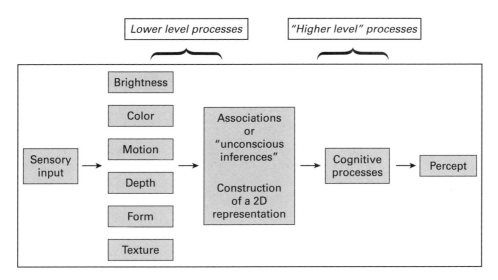

Figure 6.6
More detailed description with respect to vision of the Standard Model of Perception.

colloquial manner, some temporal sequence, leaving the kind of relations between the boxes, particularly in the last step, entirely unspecified. On a stronger interpretation, the arrows are understood as indicating consecutive steps of mathematically definable transformations of the sensory image by which the output of a previous step is transformed to yield the input for the next transformation, by which finally the percept is yielded. While the first interpretation completely bypasses the *Fundamental Problem of Perception Theory*, namely, to explain how semantic perceptual categories can arise from a stimulation by physical spatiotemporal energy patterns, the second interpretation amounts to an alleged solution of this problem that is deeply flawed already on conceptual grounds for reasons addressed earlier.

The key flaw of the Standard Model is that it dodges, by its very conceptualization of perception, an essential task of perceptual research (viz. the identification of the internal conceptual structure of perception and the symbolic objects to which the computational procedures of the perceptual system apply). The Standard Model is, moreover, not even aware of this explanatory deficit because it borrows semantic distinctions, such as "surfaces," "shadows," and "illumination" tacitly from the output of the perceptual system and uses them for a description of the input (particularly when the Standard Model is supplemented by an inverse optics approach of "recovery of world structure"). Thus, the problem of perceptual semantics has not even been recognized by traditional approaches as a serious theoretical challenge because it is concealed precisely by one of the eminent achievements of our brain (viz. the externalization of its own semantic categories into what we regard as the external world).

The gross inadequacy of the Standard Model's way of framing the explanatory task of perception theory has been pointed out since the seventeenth century. By corresponding enquiries, it became evident that the problem of perceptual meaning cannot be resolved by deferring the explanatory duty to the sensory information. Not even the core notion of a "perceptual object" can be derived by whatever mathematical machinery from the sensory input. Hume was well aware of this problem and noted, in his *Treatise of Human Nature*, that the senses

give us no notion of continu'd existence, because they cannot operate beyond the extent, in which they really operate. They as little produce the opinion of a distinct existence, because they neither can offer it to the mind as represented, nor as original. . . . We may, therefore, conclude with certainty, that the opinion of a continu'd and of a distinct existence never arises from the senses. (book 1, part IV, section II)

Therefore it has generally been noticed since the seventeenth century that there was an explanatory gap to be filled. Michotte (1954/1991) was particularly cognizant of the theoretical challenge that the "remarkable case of phenomenal permanence" and the underlying notion of the identity of an object over time and over various classes of transformations poses for perceptual psychology (cf. Casati, 2005; Scholl, 2007; Spelke, Gutheil, and Van der Walle, 1995). Perception theory has to provide an explanatory framework for these kinds of basic phenomena. However, the explanatory task to come to terms with the most fundamental theoretical notion (viz. that of a "perceptual object") is dodged by deriving this notion from a allegedly "corresponding" notion of an "external world object" and by placing the explanatory burden on experience and some inferential machinery. These externalist approaches to the problem of perceptual meaning, which historically were advanced notably by Hume and Helmholtz, came to dominate perceptual psychology. In the context of the Standard Model, various types of mechanisms have been proposed, by which sensory experiences can allegedly be transformed into perceptual categories. For instance, Hume assumed that mechanisms "of compounding, transposing, augmenting, or diminishing the materials afforded us by the senses and experience" (*An Enquiry Concerning Human Understanding*, section II) were at the core of our mental capacities. Von Helmholtz (1856) placed the explanatory burden on experience-based "unconscious inferences," and more recent computational approaches regarded at the core of perception some kind of sensory data-based inferential processes of a recovery of "world structure." The apparent attractiveness of these conceptions of perception predominantly derives from the fact that they accord with our commonsense conceptions of perception. They are, however, profoundly inadequate already on conceptual grounds. Later developments and insights into what can be achieved by inductive procedures made clear that no general inductive machinery, however powerful, can derive from the sensory input, and thus, more generally, from experience, the kind of internal conceptual structure that is explanatorily required (unless it is already based on a conceptual structure as powerful as the one to be inferred). However powerful the inductive machinery is assumed to be, there is no way to arrive at symbolic objects that are logically more powerful in the sense that their structure is not expressible in the logical language in which we describe the bases of the inductive procedure (cf. Fodor, 1980). Because essentially no perceptual object or attribute of our perceptual system is definable in the logical language by which we describe the physical energy pattern that constitutes the sensory input, the internal structure underlying perceptual meaning cannot be attained by inductive procedures (unless we surreptitiously describe the input in terms of the yet-to-be-explained output categories). All the same, prevailing thinking in perceptual psychology and psychophysics is marked by its deep-rooted commitments to a more or less naïve realist metaphysics and an empiricist theory of mind. As Köhler (1947) noted, perceptual psychologists are "so fond of their empiricist convictions" (p. 140). Such detrimental influences of commonsense conceptions are an important factor for why large parts of the field have turned into a data-driven and hence nonprogressive enterprise.

In the history of perceptual psychology, the strongest critique of the Standard Model was advanced by Gestalt psychologists on the basis of accumulating empirical evidence. They furthermore recognized that the Standard Model's emphasis on issues of processing results from mistaking the explanatory task of neurophysiology for the explanatory task of perceptual psychology, and thus from conflating different levels of analysis. However, despite the Standard Model's utter inadequacy, it is almost taken as a truism in much of current perceptual research. It is inherent to truisms that they obviate the conception of any alternatives. Accordingly, the alternative conceptions of perception that fuelled Gestalt psychology, Michotte's "experimental phenomenology," or the approaches of many others who recognized how rich the internal conceptual structure of the perceptual system is have been disregarded. This situation appears to be changing in more recent years, during which ethology and various domains of cognitive science, notably perceptual research with babies, have been providing a wealth of experimental findings in support of a radically different conception. Although the theoretical conceptions underlying these experimental investigations have mostly remained implicit, the distinguishing features of these ways of framing the task of perception theory are clearly discernible. Before I attempt to characterize some core elements of the emergent theoretical framework, I deal, in the following section, with a more general, methodological issue, namely, with the question of what can be regarded as an appropriate level of idealization for dealing fruitfully with the problem of meaning in perception theory.

The Problem of the Internal Semantics of the Perceptual System

A decisive feature of the previous formulation of the *Fundamental Problem of Perception Theory* is that it singles out a specific level of analysis as particularly appropriate for gaining theoretical insights into the nature of perception. This level of analysis pertains to an investigation of the *internal* principles of a specific biological subsystem. It abstracts away from aspects with which other levels of analysis are concerned, for example, aspects pertaining to neural implementation and physical basis or to evolutionary development and adaptive function.

It is a matter of course that the assumption that the perceptual system qualifies as a subsystem of the brain that can, by standard methodological practices of idealization and abstraction, be studied in isolation, in no way implies the denial of dependencies with other systems. With respect to rational enquiry, the question is not how in reality things are related to each other. The nature and functioning of the perceptual system is related to and dependent on various aspects of reality, such as its phylogenetic development, on the metabolic system, the immune system, or a great variety of other internal computational systems, or on the physics of the brain. Rather, the question is what constitutes an appropriate level of idealization for successful explanatory frameworks of perception.

From our commonsense intuitions, an abstraction that focuses on the *internal* principles of the system involved appears to be rather odd because it discards most of what we usually consider important questions about perception. In the context of the natural sciences, however, such an abstraction, which is in line with general methodological principles of multilayered analyses of biological systems (e.g., Tinbergen, 1963), disburdens the explanatory task of perception theory from issues that do not promise to advance theoretical understanding of the internal principles of the system under scrutiny.

Among the issues that should be considered as external to the explanatory task of perception theory proper are also issues that pertain to levels of analyses employed by ecological physics or functionalist evolutionary biology. These fields are primarily concerned with, for example, understanding the kinds of physical regularities of the external world that are taken advantage of by the perceptual system, with functional and adaptive aspects of the perceptual system, or with its evolutionary history. To be sure, the perceptual system, as other computational or noncomputational biological systems, has, in its evolutionary development, taken advantage of external physical regularities in the sense that the way internal mechanisms work is moulded or even determined by specific external physical regularities. However, from this it does not follow that considerations about adaptive purposes or about the "proper" external objects of perception figure in explanatory accounts of the internal principles by which the perceptual system generates its outputs on the basis of specific inputs. As in the case of other biological systems, an understanding of the internal functioning of the perceptual system neither rests on a diachronic analysis of its selectional history nor on considerations of which physical entities should be regarded as the "true" or "proper" antecedents of the sensory input (aside from heuristic purposes and our ordinary or meta-theoretical talk, in which such enquiries are inevitably embedded). Needless to say, perception must structurally mirror or at least not contradict biologically relevant aspects of the external world. This, however, is hardly an insight but rather simply rephrases from a functional point of view the kind of mental phenomena that have been singled out as an object of enquiry. From it, it by no means follows that categories or attributes of perception are categories or attributes of the external world: Even if perception would mirror not even in a single case the true manner of being of the external world (whatever that is supposed to be), it still could provide a coupling to biologically relevant structural aspects of it.

Therefore, the prior formulation of the *Fundamental Problem of Perception Theory* in particular dispenses with considerations about what might be the "proper" objects in the external world that are causally responsible, among the infinite set of potential causal antecedents, for the sensory input. Each sensory input that gives rise to a specific percept can be physically produced in many different ways (think of an object on a CRT screen or in a virtual reality setting). Because it is, for the explanatory purposes of perception theory, immaterial what the distal causes of a certain sensory input are, any reference to the potential distal causes of the sensory input is extrinsic to perception theory. Consequently, notions such as "perceptual error," "veridicality," "reference," or "proper function" have no place in explanatory accounts of the functioning of the perceptual system, and there are no explanatory lacunae in perception theory to be filled by introducing these notions. Particularly, the notion of "perceptual error," which is a distinguishing element of our ordinary discourse about perception, is of no avail for perception theory (cf. Mausfeld, 2002, 2010a, b).

Perception theory rather attempts to theoretically understand the perceptual system and identify its abstract internal principles by which it generates, given specific physical spatiotemporal energy patterns as inputs, outputs that are organized in terms of meaningful categories. The semantic categorizations that the perceptual systems supplies to subsequent systems are not determined by "corresponding" properties of the external world. Rather, they are individuated by the kind of data formats and computational machinery with which the perceptual system is biologically endowed. Perception theory thus places the explanatory burden for an understanding of perceptual categories on the internal structure of the biological system under scrutiny. While the problem of meaning is mostly unrecognized or dismissed as almost trivial in our commonsense conception of perception due to its built-in externalization of "perceptual meaning," perception theory considers this problem as being at the core of its explanatory task. I refer to it as the problem of the *internal semantics* of the perceptual system.

Investigations of the internal semantics of the perceptual system aim to identify the data formats, and thus the symbolic objects, on which the computational procedures of the perceptual systems are based. The form or logical structure of these symbolic objects and the structure of their interrelations define the core "perceptual ontology" of the perceptual system and the type of computational principles that can be applied to these objects.[1] The internal semantics therefore exhaustively characterizes the "world" as conceived of by the perceptual system, and hence the kinds of "perceptual objects" of the perceptual system and the way they are related. The internal semantics of the perceptual system does not capture percept–world relations but only the relation between internal perceptual objects. Although the external semantics of perception (i.e., acts of referring to entities in the external world) is dependent on the complex interaction of the perceptual system with higher interpretative systems, and applies to the level of the entire organism, the internal semantics is an *intrinsic* property of the perceptual system. Because of this, the internal semantics captures those aspects of "perceptual meaning" that are amenable to abstraction and idealization and thus can reasonably be regarded to be within the reach of naturalistic enquiry.

Confining semantic issues to intrinsic properties of the system under scrutiny is often referred to as an *internalist approach* to meaning.[2] From the perspective of our commonsense intuitions of perception, an internalist approach disregards what we, in ordinary context, consider as the most important element of "perceptual meaning," namely, our acts of referring to "objects in the external world." From an internalist view, however, this capacity depends on the intricate interpretative capacities brought forth by the integrative action of the entire system (i.e., of persons). Hence, it does not promise to provide a deeper theoretical understanding of intrinsic properties of the specific system under scrutiny (i.e., of the internal principles of the perceptual system).

What appears, from our ordinary perspective, to be an illegitimate stricture on the study of perceptual meaning turns out to be an eminent methodological advantage for the explanatory task at hand. An internalist approach emphasizes the fact that what we refer to in perception as "objects in the world" are in fact mental objects and, thus, directs attention to the central question of what constitutes a "perceptual object." Furthermore, it makes incontestably clear that explanatory demands compel us to ascribe a rich internal structure to the system, not unexpected for a complex biological system. Because the perceptual system is regarded as a computational system, this means to ascribe to it a rich structure in terms of its internal data formats and computational principles.

Internalist approaches to perception have a long and fruitful tradition in the field. The underlying conceptual frameworks were first laid out during the seventeenth century. They found their most sophisticated and strongest expression in Descartes' sign theory of perception and his idea of a "semantic relation" between the sensory input, on the one hand, and the conceptual forms by which the perceptual system is endowed, on the other hand (cf. Gaukroger, 1995, p. 287; Yolton, 1996, p. 73ff).

An internalist approach has also been, implicitly or explicitly, at the basis of ethological enquires (e.g., Gallistel, 1998; Lorenz, 1941/1982; Tinbergen, 1963). Ethological investigations into the perceptual capacities of different species, which have not been encumbered by our commonsense intuitions about perception, have yielded fruitful explanatory frameworks for dealing with issues of the internal semantics of different perceptual systems. Internalist approaches have also yielded copious and fruitful insights during the history of perceptual psychology. It has long been noted that "the visual system populates 'the world' with all sort of 'objects' that have no physical reality" (Jackendoff, 2002, p. 308; cf. Köhler, 1947, p. 157). Think, for example, of perceptual objects associated with figure-ground segmentations, perceptual groupings, or amodal completions. These observations and phenomena constituted the focus of Gestalt psychology, which was firmly rooted in an internalist perspective. (As is known, the theoretical frameworks of the Gestaltists were critically deficient. However, one has to bear in mind that neither the Gestaltists nor previous thinkers had the conceptual apparatus provided by the theory of computation at their disposal. They therefore could not appropriately formulate the abstract issues involved but rather had to couch their insights in their own and often idiosyncratic terms, which served as makeshift.) The Gestaltists were also aware that our perceptual objects (i.e., the symbolic objects of the perceptual system) cannot, in any meaningful sense, be understood as *representations of* "corresponding" physical categories. However, this insight has almost been lost in perceptual psychology, which, due to built-in preferences for an externalist conception of perception, routinely employs this term "representation" in the sense of a world-mind mapping.[3]

In other areas of cognitive science, notably linguistics and enquiries into lexical semantics, internalist approaches yielded highly fruitful explanatory frameworks for various domains of mental phenomena. The most prominent advocate of an internalist approach is Chomsky (e.g., 1966, 1996, 2000), who has pioneered and elaborated it as a general research program for the study of mental phenomena and adamantly defended it against externalist conceptions.

Perception theory, as the attempt to gain theoretical insight into the principles underlying the mode of operation of the perceptual system, has first and foremost to address the question of what constitutes the minimal meaning-bearing elements and thus the "perceptual objects." In line with the wealth of empirical observations and phenomena that have been accrued in the history of the field, perception theory acknowledges the fact that perceptual meaning cannot be derived from the sensory input or from a description of the external world no matter how sophisticated the mathematical apparatus underlying such attempts is. The available evidence also shows that the biologically given internal semantics of the perceptual system is multifariously rich and variegated, as well as highly intricate and unexpected. Its features are highly idiosyncratic with respect to our physical descriptions of the external world and often strongly deviate from our ordinary intuitions and expectations. They can only be identified by empirical investigations of the internal structure of perceptual objects and their attributes.

In the next section, I attempt to expose a few general principles of perception that I believe to be both well motivated and empirically well supported by the corresponding work in perceptual psychology, ethology, research with babies, and internalist enquires into other domains of the cognitive sciences.

On the Functional Architecture and the Conceptual Forms of the Perceptual System

At the core of the theoretical picture that can be abstracted and distilled from the corresponding empirical[4] and conceptual work is the distinction between (at least) two different subsystems of the perceptual system. Such a distinction with respect to the functional architecture of the perceptual system is required to explanatorily account for the "wide gulf between sensory stimulus and percept" (von Szily, 1921, p. 971). As mentioned before, there is, within the mathematical language employed by physics, no mathematical machinery, however powerful, by which the specific conceptual structure underlying the organization of our percepts can be derived from the physical sensory input. The abstract concepts underlying perception and the "mental categories of substance, reality, and causality" (to use Michotte's words) can only be expressed in a natural way in a logical language that is strictly richer and more powerful than the logical language appropriate for a description of the sensory input. In other words, these abstract concepts are neither reducible to nor expressible by the concepts of the logical language in which we describe the sensory input. Hence, there is no way to derive them within that language (as much as, say, the biological concepts of the "cell" cannot be defined within a purely physical language or as mental concepts cannot be defined by or derived from neural ones).

Needless to say, it is exceedingly difficult to formulate in a precise manner a corresponding distinction between a computational subsystem whose data formats can be expressed in the same logical language that we use to describe the input and computational subsystems whose data formats are not expressible in this logical language. Nonetheless, a distinction of this kind is at the root of a venerable and fertile intuition that, in various guises, pervades the history of perceptual psychology. Using the terminology employed here, this intuition amounts to the idea that the "nature" of conceptual forms is not exhausted by their extensional descriptions in terms of sensory inputs or sensory codes by which these forms can be elicited but rather requires an autonomous level of analysis (employing a suitably rich logical language). With respect to a computational architecture, this idea entails the requirement to make precise how to conceive of computations *between* systems whose internal computations are based on different sets of primitives, respectively.

Accordingly, explanatory needs require us to distinguish (at least) two different subsystems of the perceptual system (or two different levels of abstraction, which are iden-

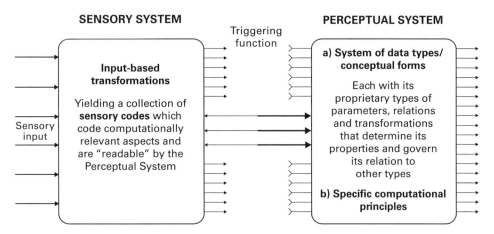

Figure 6.7
Functional architecture of the perceptual system.

tified here with actual idealized subsystems) that mediate between the sensory input and its output. The defining difference between these two subsystems is the expressive power of the logical language by which their respective data formats can be defined. At the front end of the perceptual system, we can single out a subsystem whose operational mode can be completely described in terms of the physicogeometrical language in which we describe the sensory input. Such a logical language is, however, incapable of expressing the core concepts underlying the output of the perceptual system. Therefore, we have to postulate a second system that is based on a more powerful logical language and whose data formats and symbolic concepts yield all the semantic distinctions that characterize the output of the perceptual system. I refer to these two systems as *Sensory System*, on the one hand, and *Perceptual System*, on the other hand (this distinction differs fundamentally from the one associated with the Standard Model). I use the generic term "perceptual system" to refer to the system that is composed of the *Sensory System* and *Perceptual System* as characterized here. The general functional architecture of the perceptual system can be illustrated by figure 6.7.

The *Sensory System* deals with the transduction of physical energy into codes that fulfill the structural and computational needs of the *Perceptual System* and that are, at its interface with the *Perceptual System*, "readable" by it. By definition, the data formats on which the computations of the *Sensory Systems* are based are definable in terms of the same physicogeometrical language by which the sensory input can be described. The operations of the *Sensory System* are, accordingly, purely sensory-based transformations, such as filtering and convolutions, calculation of certain derivatives of luminance distributions, gain control operations, calculations of global statistical features, or any other mathematical operation on the sensory input or on codes obtained from such operations. Considerable insights have been gained by sensory physiology and psychophysics into the operations of the *Sensory System*, which has been the proper object of enquiry of these fields. The *Sensory System* preprocesses the sensory input, in terms of a rich set of input-based symbolic data types, in a way that is dynamically interlocked with the specific requirements of the *Perceptual System*. A more detailed analysis of it would in turn necessitate a distinction of different levels of abstraction (which extend from transduction codes and simple transformations thereof to highly abstract codes in terms of internal symbolic objects of the *Sensory System*).

The conceptual apparatus of the *Sensory System* is highly hierarchically organized. At the top of this hierarchy, and thus at the level of its interface to the *Perceptual System*, this apparatus particularly includes abstract concepts that are highly adapted for the demands of the *Perceptual System*. Among these concepts are ones pertaining to "texture," "connected region," "optical flow," various types of "edges" or "junctions," and so on, or, in Marr's terms, notions by which a "2D representation" can be characterized.

Among the expressions of the *Sensory System* are also those that have been traditionally referred to as "cues" or "signs." Cues or signs are considered to be those features of the sensory input that supposedly stand for and convey information about properties of external objects or relations. Accordingly, they have been regarded, since Alhazen and Helmholtz, as providing the base of evidence in inferential accounts of perception. On such conceptions, the inferential procedures have to embrace methods of "cue integration" and "cue combination" because each single cue is regarded as ambiguous, incomplete, and of limited accuracy with respect to the properties it is supposed to represent. Although the cue concept is among the most popular ones in perceptual psychology, it hovers, in its ordinary usage, theoretically in the air. It is again based on mistaking the output of the perceptual system for its input. It takes for granted what actually has to be investigated, namely, the conceptual structure in which it has to be grounded. Cues do not bear any meaning by themselves. Rather, the notion of a cue is conditional on the conceptual structure by which cues are invested with meaning. Thus, the notion of a cue or sign cannot be detached from explicitly specifying the entire conceptual system with respect to which something can function as a cue. Speaking of cues or signs prior to a specification of the conceptual structure, by which cues or signs are conveyed their meaning, only makes sense within our ordinary discourse about perceiving (which takes for granted what actually has to be part of an explanatory framework of perception theory). In the context of perception theory, however, we need to first identify the core structural properties of the *Perceptual System* before we can reasonably refer to certain symbolic objects and their attributes, relations, and so on of the *Sensory System* as cues or signs. It is important to realize that such notions refer to relations that are entirely mind-internal. What is signified by a cue or sign is not an external object but a concept of the *Perceptual System*.[5]

Correspondingly, taking of cues as being ambiguous or incomplete refers to entirely internal relationships between a whole system of cues provided by the *Sensory System*, on the one hand, and the conceptual forms of the *Perceptual System*, on the other hand. The intricate issues involved cannot be dodged by surreptitiously using the semantic distinctions that are generated by the *Perceptual System* for a description of its input. With respect to perception theory, the main explanatory burden has to be placed on enquiries into the specific structure of the conceptual forms of the *Perceptual System* and their interrelation.

The structure of the data formats and conceptual forms underlying perception have as yet, however, not been the target of systematic investigations in perceptual psychology. Rather, perceptual psychology has largely bracketed the problem of perceptual semantics by focusing on perceptual processing with respect to data formats that are either defined by neurophysiological magnitudes or presumed to mirror what we, in our quotidian description of the external world, consider to be external world categories (such as surfaces, illuminations, shadows, trees, animals, etc.). Among the few conceptual forms whose structure and triggering conditions have been investigated more systematically are the core ones pertaining to "perceptual objects." These studies have already yielded significant theoretical insights into the constitution of a "perceptual object" by a spatiotemporal continuity as paradigmatically illustrated by Michotte's "tunnel effect" (cf. Burke, 1952; Flombaum and Scholl, 2006) and by internal principles of cohesion and solidity, the study of which has been pioneered by Spelke (e.g., 1990, 2000). Apart from these and a few other exceptions, there is, in contrast to the abundance of studies that deal with aspects of processing, almost a complete absence of experimental or theoretical studies that specifically address the "information structure" (Jackendoff, 1987, p. 39) on which any kind of processing by definition is based. Therefore, we have only the most rudimentary ideas about the specific types of its conceptual forms and their structural properties. All the same, we can derive from phenomenological considerations, from findings of ethology, developmental psychology, and, more indirectly, from investigations of the structure of the mental lexicon (e.g., Chomsky, 2000; Jackendoff, 2002; Pustejovsky, 1995) conjectures about the types and structural properties of the conceptual forms that define the internal semantics of the perceptual system.

The conceptual forms of the *Perceptual System* can be understood as those data formats underlying its computations that are "visible" at its interfaces with subsequent systems and thus can be "read" by those systems. As in the prior formulation of the *Fundamental Problem of Perception Theory*, I deal here, by way of example, only with the conceptual forms on which the semantic distinctions and categories of our phenomenal percept are grounded. In focusing exemplarily on the phenomenal output, it is, however, important to be aware that the structure of the conceptual forms of the *Perceptual System* is only partly visible at the surface of the phenomenal percept. In particular, we do not notice in our phenomenal experience that the conceptual forms involved are highly underspecified by a given input provided by the *Sensory System*. Rather, the systems that use the outputs of the *Perceptual System* for constructing the phenomenal percept seems to be furnished with specific computational means to fill in the blanks, as it were, and thus to completely specify, on a certain level, a phenomenal appearance at each moment.

The output of the *Perceptual System* is not exhausted by the semantic distinctions and categories of our phenomenal percept. Nevertheless, the conceptual forms underlying these phenomenal distinctions and categories provide the basis for our perceptual ontology and thus constitute the realm of "perceptual objects."[6] Among the exceedingly rich set of complex conceptual forms in terms of which we perceive the "external world" are conceptual forms pertaining to, for example, "surface," "physical object," "food," "tool," "event," "potential actor," "self," "other person," or "event," with their associated attributes such as "walkable," "manipulable," "edible," "color," "shape," or "emotional state" and their appropriate relations such as "ausation" or "intention." Conceptual forms *create*, as it were, what we perceive as the world out there. They define the way in which we perceptually make sense of the world. It is a distinctive feature of the conceptual forms of the *Perceptual System* that they are not tied to a specific sensory channel and moreover cannot be expressed in terms of purely sensory concepts. This has been emphasized ever since the beginning of systematic enquiry into perception, notably by the Gestaltists. Only on the presumptions underlying the *Standard Model* can one be surprised about the "evidence for vigorous interaction among sensory modalities" (Shimojo and Shams, 2001). However, the specific qualitative and quantitative type of interaction can provide important theoretical insights into the internal structure of the conceptual forms involved. These conceptual forms are intrinsically transmodal in character (cf. Köhler's [1947] characterization of the spatial and temporal perceptual relations of "disturbance," "beginning," "edge," "hole," "piece," "part," "open," "incomplete," "proceeding," "deviating," and "interrupting").

We can conceive of the conceptual forms of the *Perceptual System* as abstract structures, each of which has its own proprietary types of parameters, relations, and transformations that govern its relation to other conceptual forms and to sensory codes. Furthermore, the available experimental evidence (cf. footnote 2) indicates that the *Perceptual System* can be regarded as a hierarchically organized typed domain (of possibly unlimited depth). Thus, its symbolic objects belong to different classes of data types, each of which is characterized by specific structural properties and by the type of computations that are applicable to it.[7] With respect to the conceptual forms considered here, each type defines a set of perceptual objects with uniform behavior, which, in our ordinary language, normally can be named (e.g., "surface," "illumination," "artefact," "animal," "mykind"). The hierarchy of types constitutes the biologically built-in "knowledge" about "entities" and "situations" and their properties of our perceptual world and about our potential "perspectives" on these. The *Perceptual System* can therefore be understood as a self-contained system of "perceptual knowledge," which is coded in the structure of its conceptual forms. The meaning of these conceptual forms is entirely determined by their intrinsic structure and their systematic relations to each other (i.e., by the internal semantics of the *Perceptual System*). Also, the *Perceptual System* can reasonably be assumed to have its own computational principles, in particular ones that pertain to an evaluation metric, the satisfaction of internal constraints, or a more global coherence. In particular, perceptual phenomena suggest that it possesses a rather idiosyncratic evaluation metric (as mirrored in phenomena traditionally discussed under the heading of "cue integration") and likewise idiosyncratic principles by which it glues together fragmented structures of partially activated conceptual forms into a globally more coherent structure (as witnessed, for example, by phenomena pertaining to so-called impossible objects or the so-called dual nature of picture perception).

Conceptual forms have their own properties, which can be rather surprising when viewed exclusively from the perspective of an adaptive coupling to the external world. Clearly, the organism *as an entirety* must be adapted to the specific circumstances and biologically relevant properties of the environment in which it has evolved. From this, however, no substantial constraints—beyond the weakest ones of some structural consistency—can be derived as to the data formats or conceptual forms underlying perceptual computations. These forms can neither be reasonably assumed to mirror "corresponding" aspects of the external world nor to be "optimally" adapted to specific features of the physical environment. Our most complex perceptual achievements (e.g., seeing dispositional properties of objects [e.g., pertaining to material qualities], intentional properties of objects [e.g., tools], or mental states of others) were, in the evolutionary development of the functional architecture of the perceptual system, only made possible by *decoupling* the data types of the *Perceptual System* from the given sensory information and by furnishing the *Perceptual System* with conceptual forms that go far beyond anything expressible in sensory terms. Theoretical considerations and findings of evolutionary biology (e.g., Gould, 2002; Webster and Goodwin, 1996) suggest that, just like other biological traits and design features of the organism, the structure of the conceptual forms, on which the computations of the perceptual system are based, cannot simply be derived from alleged adaptive requirements. Rather these conceptual forms will, in their evolutionary development, most likely be essentially codetermined by constraints that stem from the fact that only certain physical and computational channels were open as feasible evolutionary paths (cf. Carroll, 2005). The conceptual forms of the *Perceptual System* must not only be adequate with respect to the external world (however one understands such a requirement), they must also be computationally adequate (i.e., they have to fit into the entire computational architecture).

With respect to the functional architecture of the brain, the *Perceptual System* possesses interfaces to various other systems, notably to higher order interpretative systems, where meanings are assigned in terms of "external world" properties. It generates options for patterns of activated conceptual forms given a sensory input, which are interpretable by these external systems. At present, we still have only the most rudimentary ideas and theoretical speculations about the higher order systems that take advantage of the outputs provided by the *Perceptual System*. Much more is known, however, about what is regarded here as the *Sensory System* and its computational principles. Hence, more specific conjectures about the relation between the *Sensory* and the *Perceptual System* can be inferred from the available experimental evidence. I again attempt to abstractly characterize a few fairly general principles that appear to me well motivated and empirically well supported in the light of findings that have been accrued in various fields.

On the present account, the *Sensory System* and the *Perceptual System* have their own types of data formats. Most importantly, the conceptual forms of the *Perceptual System*, over which its computations are performed, cannot be derived within the computational apparatus of the *Sensory System*. Conceptual forms are logically autonomous in the sense that they cannot be achieved by mathematical transformations of the sensory input. The relation between these two systems can therefore only be mediated by some interface function. Such an interface function has to take the output of the *Sensory System* as an argument and call a set of conceptual forms. The notion of an interface function thus captures and makes more precise the intuitions that are usually expressed by the locutions that a certain "sensory information triggers, or is a cue or sign for" some semantic categorization. I therefore refer to such an interface function also as a triggering function. Although not much is presently known about the specific properties of the conceptual forms of the *Perceptual System* and their triggering functions, certain features can be tentatively derived from computational considerations within the rich constraints provided by perceptual phenomena.

Computational considerations suggest that the codes provided by the *Sensory System* at its interface with the *Perceptual System* serve a dual function. First, they activate appropriate conceptual forms and thus determine the potential data formats of the *Perceptual System* in terms of which input properties are to be exploited. Second, they assign concrete values to the free parameters of the activated conceptual forms. Thus, with regards to the *Perceptual System*, the sensory codes serve as "instructions" for the activations and specification of conceptual forms. The sensory input opts, as it were, for the activation of a system of conceptual forms with which the system is biologically endowed. This process is constrained by internal requirements of the *Perceptual System* that pertain to the more global coherence of the activated conceptual forms. Therefore, it is reasonable to regard it as a dynamic bidirectional process geared toward achieving some state of optimal global stability in terms of the internal constraints of the *Percep-

tual System. Presumably, we can account for the "creative forces" (von Szily, 1921, p. 971) of perception, as described and emphasized by Descartes, the Gestaltists, Michotte, and many others, already by properties of the *Perceptual System*. In a sense, conceptual forms can be regarded as actively seeking the kind of sensory codes (and thus the sensory information) by which they are most completely activated. Structurally, these "creative forces" could have their basis in an underspecification of the conceptual forms with respect to a given input. Underspecification means that the elements that figure in the logical structure of a conceptual form are not fully specified by a given input. Such a semantic underspecification can serve as the structural basis of special computational mechanisms to computationally handle problems of ambiguity and vagueness. The system can achieve a higher degree of flexibility and global stability if changes, following small variations in the input, in the conceptual forms triggered, and in the values of their free parameters are, intuitively speaking, kept at a minimum, particularly at the interfaces of the *Perceptual System* with subsequent systems. Such a strategy would protect the system from settling, under "impoverished" situations, on some definite interpretation that would have to be changed to an entirely different interpretation following a small variation in the input. In addition, and independent from issues of the handling of impoverished input situations, underspecified conceptual forms boost the potency of generative processes and enhance the conceptual versatility of the *Perceptual System*. By routinely operating with underspecified conceptual forms, the *Perceptual System* can simultaneously provide different layers of semantic "interpretations," a remarkable capacity that pervades our perceptual and cognitive domains (Mausfeld, 2010b).

The theoretical perspective tentatively and abstractly outlined earlier attempts to condense and make more explicit certain theoretical intuitions that have fruitfully guided systematic investigations of perception since their historic origins and that have, more recently, been reinvigorated by a wealth of convergent findings from perceptual psychology, ethology, and developmental psychology. Nevertheless, our theoretical understanding of the principles underlying perception still barely scratches the surface. Thus, this theoretical perspective is, needless to say, still skeletal and in need of precision and specification. However, in comparison with currently prevailing approaches to perception, which are imbued by deeply entrenched commonsense conceptions about perception, much has already been gained if one takes seriously the besetting foundational question that any successful explanatory account of perception eventually has to answer: What are the abstract internal principles by which a specific biological system, namely, the perceptual system, can generate on the basis of physical spatiotemporal energy patterns, outputs that are organized in terms of semantic categories? The theoretical perspective outlined previously enables us to ask novel and promising questions about the principles underlying perception and hence opens up new lines of enquiry. This can be strikingly illustrated by a unique perceptual attribute, namely, the attribute of "realness." On traditional accounts, this attribute is not considered as providing a serious theoretical challenge for perceptual psychology because it is usually regarded as a description of the input or underlying scene. In fact, however, the assignment of the attribute "realistic" to an input is an *achievement* of the perceptual system and thus in need of theoretical explanation. This idea was emphasized by Metzger (1941) and particularly by Michotte (1948/1991), who conceived of "phenomenal reality" as a "dimension of our visual experience," which he regarded as being closely linked to the internal attribute "potential for being manipulated" (p. 181). On the prior account, this global attribute of "phenomenal reality" seems to be based on special principles of the *Perceptual Systems* by which it evaluates, in a given input situation, the internal global coherence of a system of activated conceptual forms, the degree to which these forms are specified by the input and other criteria. Because the criteria for an assignment of the attribute "real" to an entirety of a situation (which also pertains to the experience of a spatiotemporal continuity as a person) are entirely determined by the internal semantics of the perceptual system, the properties of this attribute and its triggering conditions are unpredictable and surprising from our ordinary perspectives on perception. Instructive examples can be found in the field of computer graphics rendering, where one attempts to construct computer models of perceptual environments or scenes by which images on a screen can be generated that appear realistic, either globally, as in the case of a virtual reality setting, or with respect to certain aspects, such as the material appearances of the depicted objects. These problems of rendering have an interesting counterpart in art history. The simulation of material appearances on a canvass had been regarded as a particular challenge in painting, notably in Dutch renaissance art (cf. Gombrich, 1976). Although already Alberti, in his *Trattato della pittura* (1435/1972), recognized that by a proper juxtaposition of white and black only the impressions of gold, silver, and glass can be elicited, a realistic impression of material colors in painting turned out to be exceedingly difficult to achieve.

The Perception of Material Qualities

Our perceptual system is evidently endowed with a rich internal vocabulary, as it were, for "material qualities." This vocabulary, which is, on the present theoretical perspective, coded in the conceptual forms of the *Perceptual System*, pertains to types of material such as "skin," "soil," "stone," "metal," "wood," "water," and a copiousness of attributes associated with it, such as "malleable," "rigid," "soft," and "taut" (these terms function only as linguistic makeshift descriptions for the internal attributes). The perception of types of material and material qualities, whether visual, haptic, or auditory, cannot be understood as simply mirroring corresponding external world properties and hence as being derivable from the sensory input. Of course, as any other

perceptual attribute, they have a physical basis in the sense that their triggering conditions are tied to a set (or rather a medley) of external physical regularities. However,
the particular perceptual attribute has to be internally available as part of the structure
of the type of "perceptual object" to which it pertains. The attribute and its specific
structural properties cannot be understood by extensionally describing it by its triggering conditions. This is generally acknowledged for attributes such as "color" or, in the
auditory domain, attributes referred to as "tonal volume" or "sound spaciousness" (cf.
Blauert, 1997). Nonetheless, we are usually inclined to believe that perceived material
qualities mirror corresponding world properties more than colors do.

Of course, material appearances, as any other perceptual attribute, are tied to structural regularities of the external world. From this, however, nothing follows as to
whether the specific classes of regularities that are tied together by the organism to
perceptual categories correspond to organism-independent "natural classes" of physics.
The claim that our perceptual system has evolved under rich physical regularities is a
truism (in fact, infinitely many physical regularities of any degree of "oddness" can be
formulated). However, there is, trivially, no a priori notion of what constitutes an
organism-relevant physical regularity. With respect to perception theory, what can be
regarded as a relevant regularity of the world entirely depends on the structure of the
organism under scrutiny, such as its size, the spatial and temporal integration properties of receptors and other neural structures, the properties of its memory, and its conceptual capacities. Consequently, it is in particular the biologically given conceptual
endowment of the perceptual system that determines which regions of the parameter
space of the physical world are regarded as "environment" and hence can function as
triggering conditions for perceptual categories. Thus, the kind of image properties by
which specific material appearances of "perceptual objects" can be elicited will most
likely depend as much on the structure of the conceptual forms involved as on external
world regularities.

Issues pertaining mainly to ecological physics and rendering recently have revived
investigations of material appearances. These investigations revealed that material appearances, such as luster, silk (e.g., Koenderink and Pont, 2002), translucency (e.g.,
Fleming and Bülthoff, 2005), or gloss (e.g., Fleming, Dror, and Adelson, 2003; Wendt,
Faul, and Mausfeld, 2008), have exceedingly intricate triggering conditions. They can
be invoked by a multiplicity of combinations of specific ranges of image parameters. As
expected, some subsets of the triggering conditions, by which a given material appearance can be elicited, can be related to regularities of the ecological physics of the "corresponding" type of material (i.e., to regularities in the way light interacts with certain
types of physical surfaces). Yet the entirety of triggering conditions for a certain material appearance (i.e., the equivalence classes of input properties that are tied to a certain
material appearance) cannot be derived from or reduced to external physical regularities. These equivalence classes, which extensionally describe the internal semantic

categories for material qualities of perceptual objects, are determined by the structure of the conceptual forms of the *Perceptual System*. Because of this, the triggering conditions for material appearances are given by a rather motley conglomerate of physical conditions, which has about the same degree of "naturalness" as metameric color classes have with respect to the wavelength composition of lights. Unsurprisingly then, material appearances can also be evoked by input conditions that are physically incorrect or incoherent (e.g., Fleming and Bülthoff, 2005) with respect to a generation process caused by a "corresponding" type of material. For the endeavour to gain insights into the structure of the conceptual forms in which material appearances figure as an internal attribute, it is therefore an essential task to identify the complex triggering conditions by which they can be evoked. The more idiosyncratic with respect to external physical regularities the triggering conditions turn out to be, the more likely they will shed some light on the logical form of the "perceptual objects" to which these attributes, as part of their conceptual form, belong.

In perceptual psychology, investigations of perceptual attributes pertaining to material qualities have been, apart from a few exceptions, almost entirely neglected. This was predominantly due to its theoretical preoccupation, notably in psychophysics, with elementary attributes (in particular, attributes that appear to be directly related to specific elementary coding processes of a single sensory modality and that are not too difficult to be manipulated experimentally). Attributes for material qualities or the type of perceptual object to which they belong, however, are intrinsically transmodal in character and thus go, in particular, far beyond purely visual attributes. Therefore, they defy, more than seemingly elementary attributes, traditional attempts to understand them in terms of sensory input properties and properties inferentially derived from these (unless one tacitly presumes the internal availability of corresponding semantic categories). This was recognized not only by Gestaltists but also by many thinkers outside prevailing lines of thinking. For instance, in his dissertation supervised by Husserl, Schapp (1910) emphasizsed: "The *things as perceived* own a surplus of properties which are not simply coloured surfaces and which cannot be obtained by associations or inferences from other sensory properties. One directly sees tenacity, brittleness, obdurateness, bluntness and many other attributes for which we lack linguistic descriptions." Similar insights were expressed with respect to the complex attributes of perceptual objects that pertain to perceived possibilities for actions, notably by Jakob von Uexkuell, Wolfgang Köhler ("requiredness"), Kurt Koffka ("demand character"), Egon Brunswik ("intentional object"), or James Gibson ("affordances"). (Gibson, however, differed from the other ones in that on his conception of affordances "meanings" are externalized altogether.)

However, two interesting exceptions to this traditional neglect of material appearances can be found in the classic literature, namely, investigations, notably by Helmholtz, of stereoscopic luster and Katz's enquiries into modes of appearances.

Modes of Color Appearance

The preoccupation with apparently elementary attributes that can allegedly be investigated more or less in isolation had a particularly detrimental effect on enquiries into color perception. Traditional color science has almost exclusively been based on a notion of "pure" color or "color per se," which can be studied independently from the conceptual structure or internal semantics of the perceptual system and hence independently from the type of "perceptual object" to which a corresponding attribute belongs. Consequently, perceptual attributes pertaining to material qualities have been regarded not as primordial attributes but rather as derivative ones that can be inferred from certain combinations of colors, luminance textures, and so on. In fact, however, empirical as well as theoretical evidence strongly suggests that material qualities are primordial and the attribute of "color per se" is predominantly based on cultural and technology-driven abstractions (cf. Mausfeld, 2003).

The perceptual primacy, as it were, of material colors is also mirrored in the way we linguistically exploit the output of the perceptual system. For instance, Hochegger (1884) found it "remarkable that etymological investigations on abstract colour names always find the roots in words that mean shiny, glowing, burning, shimmering, dingy, burnt, etc. Even the expressions for colours which seem to be abstract are, in fact, not primordial but rather emerged from paleness, brightness, glossy, matt, dingy etc" (p. 36). In the transition from the ancient Greek's emphasis on forms of light, such as brightness, luster, and the changeability of colors, to the subsequent culturally shaped progression toward an increasingly abstract color vocabulary, we can observe a shift from color appearances as material properties and "forms of light" to an abstractive notion of "color per se" as an intrinsic object property. (Of course, the fact that our perceptual and cognitive capacities provide us with the means to arrive at an abstract notion of "color per se" is of theoretical interest and in need of explanation itself.)

Katz (1911), following Hering, was clearly aware that "color" is intimately interwoven with the organization of "space"—in his felicitous terms, a "marriage of color and space"—and thus cannot be studied in isolation. By his "modes of appearance," Katz provided a descriptive account for the fact that qualities of color intrinsically depend on the way in which the "perceptual objects" to which "colors" are attached are organized in perceptual space. Accordingly, Katz distinguished various categories of phenomenal appearance, such as "surface colors," "volume colors," or "illumination colors," each of which exhibits distinctive phenomenological characteristics and different coding properties with respect to other perceptual attributes. The guiding idea behind this classification is that the appearances of color phenomenally segregate into mutually exclusive categories because they mirror, as Gelb (1929) put it, internal processes or states of "essentially different nature" (p. 600) (whereas on the *Standard Model of Perception*, the different "modes of appearance" are simply regarded as context-dependent modifications of "color per se"). Accordingly, "color" does not constitute a

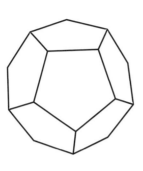
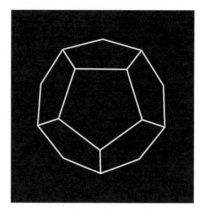

Figure 6.8
Von Helmholtz's display for stereoscopic luster.

unitary or homogenous attribute. Rather, color-related parameters figure, with different coding properties, in the structure of different types of conceptual forms (cf. Mausfeld, 2003). Katz's classification of modes of color appearance already captures basic intuitions underlying investigations of material appearances.

Lustrous Appearances and Their Triggering Conditions

The other exception to the traditional neglect of material appearances are investigations of the phenomenon of stereoscopic lustre, which was recognized as of great theoretical importance by Helmholtz, Brücke, Wundt, Kirschmann, Bühler, and many others. The phenomenon in point can be easily demonstrated by the stimulus used by Helmholtz (1867) and displayed in figure 6.8.

Under stereoscopic viewing conditions, the binocular combination of the two line drawings of inverted luminance contrast yields a vivid lustrous appearance. Similar appearances can be produced by a variety of different highly reduced stimulus configurations, both under binocular and monocular viewing conditions. It is of particular theoretical interest that lustrous appearances can be elicited by highly impoverished stimulus conditions that do not contain cues pertaining to texture, luminance gradients, or specular highlights. The classic literature comprises a range of studies that attempted to identify critical image parameters for lustrous appearances and that showed that the kind of image properties by which luster can be elicited is exceedingly variegated and can consist of relatively simple input features. There are also instructive similarities with respect to the auditory perception of material qualities. Corresponding experiments (e.g., Carello, Wagman, and Turvey, 2005; Klatzky, Pai, and Krotkov, 2000) show that also in this domain relatively elementary features act as a triggering basis for assigning complex material properties to the "auditory objects" involved.

Furthermore, material properties of "auditory objects" are intrinsically transmodal in character as well. This again suggests that the perception of material properties critically depends on structural properties of the conceptual forms involved.

Lustrous Appearances and the Internal Segregation of Accidental and Essential Components

The attribute of luster pertains to a property of perceptual objects of the type "surface" that captures a specific structural relation with respect to another type of conceptual form, namely, "illumination." This structural relation is, in turn, part of the entire organization of perceptual space, into which "surfaces" and "illumination" are embedded. The attribute of luster apparently denotes an intrinsic property of a special class of "surfaces," namely, those that can make visible, via their spatial relations to an "illumination," intrinsic properties of the "illumination" as well as certain aspects of the spatial relation between the specific instances of "surface" and "illumination." In the local sensory input, both types of triggering conditions are inextricably entangled. Thus, special computational means are required to disentangle them. As in the cases of related achievement, such as disentangling color-related properties of "surfaces" and "illumination," the latter functions primarily as a medium to attain intrinsic properties of the former. Thus, the computational task, as it were, that the *Perceptual System* faces is to perform a causal analysis in terms of its conceptual forms, by which it can disentangle what is regarded, in the internal semantics of the system, as *accidental properties* of "surfaces" and what is regarded as *essential* or *intrinsic properties*.

The internal causal analysis, which underlies a segregation of intrinsic and accidental aspects of "surfaces," seems to go along with, or probably is even based on, an internal segregation of both causal components into different spatial layers. This idea is in particular suggested by the phenomenological observations that lustrous appearances, both for monocular and binocular viewing conditions, exhibit some kind of phenomenal segmentations into two different (shallow) depth layers. This observation has been extensively reported and discussed in the classical literature on this topic (e.g., Bixby, 1928). The shallow depth segmentation involved in almost all material color appearances is again evidence for the "marriage of color and space" in the internal structural organization of corresponding attributes.

Hering (1879), who clearly recognized how intimately the attribute of color is interwoven with the internal organization of perceptual space, therefore places, in line with his internalist inclinations, lustrous appearances entirely within his discussion of the organization of perceptual space. According to Hering (1879), lustrous appearances arise as a consequence of a shallow depth segmentation with respect to the percept of a surface by which an "essential" and an "accidental" color component of a surface are disentangled. Such a "cleavage of sensation" into shallow depth layers arises when there is a "surplus of light" with respect to the acceptable values for "surfaces" and "ambient illuminations." The sensory input pattern is, on Hering's account, internally sliced into perceptual layers, which pertain to internal representations of different types, namely, to a "surface" type and an "illumination" type, the specific interrelations of which result in the activation of the kind of "surface"-type attribute that codes a specific internal "material quality." The components represented by the different perceptual layers involved are taken to be related to the functional achievement of causally disentangling, with respect to the sensory input, from illumination properties an intrinsic surface attribute, namely, luster that cannot simply be captured by descriptions in terms of geometrically homogenous spectral reflectance distributions of matte surfaces. Although Hering's account of lustrous appearances as part of the organization of perceptual space remained highly sketchy, it draws attention to important aspects of the conceptual forms involved (including those for global spatial aspects) and their organization.

Glassy Appearances and the Internal Organization of Space

Material appearances, of which Katz' "modes of appearance" are a special case, seem to intrinsically depend on the way in which the "perceptual objects" to which corresponding attributes are attached are organized in perceptual space. Because of this, the triggering conditions for the attribute "luster" and its structural properties can only be understood in intimate connection with the structural and computational organization of spatial aspects. This becomes even more apparent in the case of another attribute for material appearance, namely, "glassiness."

In the classic literature, several observations were reported that, for certain stimulus configuration that typically involve static presentations of stereoscopically fused images of three-dimensional objects or three-dimensional scenes, a filling of space in between the objects seems to occur. Karpinska (1910) reported that, under certain conditions, in stereoscopic viewings of line drawings the space in between the lines appears to be filled with something that has no other material quality than solidity. Schumann (1920) attached to Karpinska's observations a particular importance for a theoretical understanding of the organization of space. Schumann reported that under his stereoscopic viewing conditions, the empty "interspace" appears as if it is filled with a certain kind of material that his subjects described as "vitreous and tangible" (p. 228), reminding them of "glass," "ice," "gelatine," or "frozen air" (p. 232). His subjects also reported that, with respect to the discernible depth layer that is nearest to the observer, this glassy appearance looks as if it belonged to a frontoparallel surface. Subjects, however, differed to the degree to which they see this layer as extending in spatial depth. While some saw the glassy layer as rather thin, others reported it as filling the entire space. Möller (1925) followed up Schumann's investigations and performed an extensive range of observations into this phenomenon, using a great variety of different stimulus conditions. Since then, corresponding phenomena, albeit occasionally reported, have not received systematic theoretical or experimental interest.

Unlike lustrous appearances and their triggering conditions, the occurrence of glassy appearances under these viewing conditions does not seem to be easily amenable to interpretations in terms of internal causal analyses (and, to an even lesser extent, to interpretations in terms of external world regularities). Rather these occurrences seem to mirror internal properties of the way attributes are attached to conceptual forms pertaining to surfaces and the organization of space. Within the theoretical framework outlined here, the occurrence of glassy appearances under highly impoverished input conditions can be understood as the result of a constitutive property of the perceptual system (viz. its capability to computationally operate on semantically underspecified conceptual forms) (Mausfeld, 2010b). On this conception, glassy appearances occur under input conditions by which conceptual forms for "surfaces" are activated whose parameters for lightness, color, or texture cannot be assigned values by the sensory input.

The phenomenon of a glassy appearance that fills the entire "spatial medium" can be illustrated by the stimulus configuration displayed in figure 6.9. The stereoscopically combined stimulus consists of a random array of white dots on a grey background. In the first stimulus configuration (upper row), the white dots of the two monocular half-images have different disparities, which were randomly chosen for each dot. The dots therefore appear, in the fused image, as lying in different depth planes. In the second stimulus configuration (lower row), the two monocular half-images are identical and

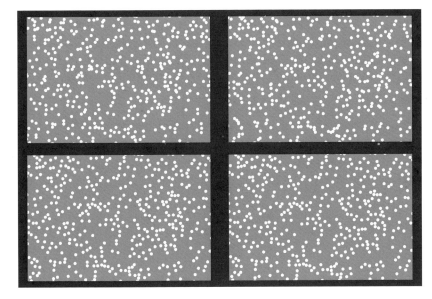

Figure 6.9
Two stereo pairs of "snow flurry" (upper row: white points have different disparities; lower row: all points have the same stereo disparity).

thus appear as lying in a frontoparallel plane. For the images in which the dots appear as occupying different positions in three-dimensional space, observers in the experiment that Gunnar Wendt and I conducted described the situation as showing a "snow flurry" and reported that the "snowflakes" are embedded in a block of "solid glass." No such material appearance of the "interspace" was reported for the lower row half-images, in which the dots do not have different disparities. The appearance of the points being embedded in solid glass did not even disappear when each point moved along its own trajectory during the presentation. Rather, observers reported that the snowflakes moved freely through a block of solid glass.

These and other experiments on the triggering conditions of certain material appearances illustrate that the triggering conditions for material appearances and the structural and computational properties of their internal organization are surprising and often highly unexpected from a perspective that focuses predominantly on external regularities. However, a system that is as complex and has an evolutionary history as long as our perceptual system is not solely constrained by the adaptational requirement of coupling the organism as an entirety as best as possible to its environment. Its functional architecture, including the kind of data formats or conceptual forms over which its computations are performed, will strongly be codetermined by a great variety of internal constraints, ranging from physical to computational ones, that arise during the evolutionary development of a system of this complexity. The nature of the conceptual forms underlying perception will most likely be formed and shaped by powerful internal constraints within the apparently rather broad latitude of design options that are left open by global, adaptational restrictions. Investigations of phenomenal material qualities seem to be particularly rewarding for the endeavour to better understand the structural form of our "perceptual objects" and, along with that, some of the abstract principles of perception on which the achievements of our perceptual system are based.

Acknowledgments

I thank Reinhard Niederée for stimulating conversations and Franz Faul for valuable probing comments from a dedicated externalist's perspective. I also thank the editors for helpful suggestions. This work was supported by BMBF-grant 01GWS060 and DFG grants MA 1025/10-3 and MA 1025/10-4.

Notes

1. Corresponding intuitions have a long history in perception theory. They also find their expression in Brentano's conceptions. With his *Psychology From an Empirical Standpoint* (1874/1995), Brentano intended to develop, as Albertazzi (2006, p. 335) aptly put it, a *"general theory of inner form."*

2. Brentano, who famously held that the true method of philosophy is nothing other than that of natural science ("*Vera philosophiae methodus nulla alia nisi scientiae naturalis est*," Albertazzi, 2006, p. 314), also exhibits a strong internalist inclination. As Albertazzi (2006) said: "If we look at the relation between the thought and the primary object in Brentano's doctrine, we must remember that the real thing to which this thought refers cannot exist outside of the mind" (p. 111).

3. The widespread acceptance of this term, which has yielded tremendous philosophical confusion, historically seems to have been enhanced by the French translations of Descartes' (1642/1985) profound and deep analyses of perception. Descartes had used (e.g., in his Third Meditations) the Latin verbs "exhibeo" and "repraesento" interchangeably, in the sense of something that is internally presented to the mind. In seventeenth-century French, both Latin verbs were translated by "representer" so that the meaning of the term shifted from denoting a predominantly mind-internal presentation to denoting a mind–world relation. Although Descartes had an internalist meaning in mind, the French translation tacitly was guided by our ordinary preference for an externalist interpretation of the term.

4. The contributions of Gestalt psychology and of Michotte may vicariously stand for the overwhelmingly rich amount of findings of perceptual psychology that are in support of this theoretical picture. With respect to color, in Mausfeld (2003) I have given a more detailed account of relevant findings. From the plenitude of relevant experimental findings that have been contributed by other domains, I only mention here, in a rather eclectic way, a few examples. Examples for pertinent contributions from developmental psychology are: Baillargeon (1993), Bonatti, Frot, Zangl, and Mehler (2002), Hamlin, Wynn, and Bloom (2007), Spelke (2000), Spelke, Gutheil, and van der Valle (1995), Trevarthen (1998), or Wang and Spelke (2002). From ethology, I mention, by way of example, Gallistel (1998), Hare, Call, Agnetta, and Tomasello (2000), Hauser, Pearson, and Seelig (2002), Premack and Premack (1995, 2003), Santos, Hauser, and Spelke (2001), or Wehner (2003). Evidence that is of relevance with respect to this conception also comes from linguistics (Chomsky, 2000; see also Pustejovsky, 1995; Yang, 2002) and neurophysiology (e.g., Caramazza and Shelton, 1998). Furthermore, the conception outlined is consonant with well-supported broader meta-theoretical perspectives on the nature of mental phenomena (e.g., Hinzen, 2006; Strawson, 2003). To be sure, no single experiment and no set of experiments can ever be regarded as conclusive evidence for the perspective outlined or any other theoretical framework. My confidence in this conception derives as much from theoretical considerations as from empirical findings. Furthermore, it is, as always in the natural sciences, fortified by the fact that this conception is suggested by a theoretical convergence of quite different disciplines.

5. Descartes clearly recognized that any reference to "external objects" in sign conceptions of perception would lead, within scientific enquiry, to conceptual incoherences. Descartes explicitly identified what I refer to as the *Fundamental Problem of Perception* and the deep explanatory gap that is associated with it. In his attempts to provide, in entirely naturalistic terms, an explanatory framework for bridging this gap, Descartes (1642/1985) formulated a purely internalistic version of a sign theory of perception. Yolton (1984, 1996) referred to Descartes' conception as "inverse sign relation" because, for Descartes, the physical motion, as expressed by neural activity, is the sign, and what is signified is what is expressed in the percept (cf. Gaukroger, 1990). For Descartes,

there are "two reactions operating in perception: the causal, physiological reaction and the signi-fication reaction" (Yolton, 1996, p. 74). The significatory or semantic relation "replaces the *causal* relation between physical motion and ideas, but the *representing* relation goes, as it were, outward from awareness" (Yolton, 1996, p. 190). Descartes thus recognized the explanatory need for pos-tulating a "semantic relation" in perception. "The connection between the signs and innate ideas is clearly more intimate than any causal connection would be, for it is the innate ideas that make the signs what they are, whereas effects can never make causes what they are" (Gaukroger, 1990, p. 25). Descartes' intuitions about this "semantic relation" between what is provided by the senses, on the one hand, and the conceptual forms or "ideas" that give rise to meaningfully orga-nized percepts, on the other hand, were far ahead of anything that could be expressed in terms of the conceptual apparatus available at his time. Unsurprisingly, Descartes' vacillating and tenta-tive usage of terms, due to which he is notoriously hard to interpret, mirrors this lack of an ap-propriate conceptual framework, as provided much later by computation theory.

6. Remark on terminology: I do not regard the symbolic objects or conceptual forms of the *Sensory System* as providing "perceptual objects." However, certain aspects (such as gradient, texture, line) of the conceptual forms of the *Sensory System* can also be captured by the *Perceptual System*. The question as to which aspects are accessible by the conceptual forms of the *Perceptual System* is intricate and is intimately related to the classical problem of the so-called proximal mode. In pres-ent terminology, the *Sensory System* does not comprise "perceptual objects" proper.

7. I use the notion of "data type" in an informal way. Note, however, that a data type, together with its associated operations, can be regarded as a computational module. In this sense, the availability of conceptual forms can be regarded as an extreme variant of modularity. Also from the perspective of evolutionary biology, abstract data types and modularity are intimately con-nected. Modularity presumably is, at all levels of biological organization, the basis for the evolv-ability of complex systems and a driving force in their evolution (e.g., Kirschner and Gerhart, 1998; Wagner, Mezey, and Calabretta, 2005). An increase in modularization with respect to sen-sory input systems and internal systems that take advantage of the sensory information results, however, in an increasing number of interface problems that the system has to solve. Accord-ingly, we can reasonably speculate that the biological emergence of abstract data formats has its evolutionary origin in the requirement of solving these interface problems (cf. Mausfeld, 2010b). More specifically, it emerges from the computational needs to tie together an increasing number of subsystems in a data format that is sufficiently abstract for an integration of the information provided by different subsystems. In this sense, the biological tendency for an increasing amount of modularization spurs and enforces, with respect to computational systems, an increase in data abstraction.

References

Albertazzi, L. 2006. *Immanent Realism. Introduction to Brentano.* Berlin: Springer.

Baillargeon, R. 1993. "The Object Concept Revisited: New Directions in the Investigation of In-fant's Physical Knowledge." In *Visual Perception and Cognition in Infancy*, edited by C. E. Granrud. Hillsdale, NJ: Erlbaum. 265–315.

Bixby, F. L. 1928. "A Phenomenological Study of Luster." *Journal of General Psychology* 1: 136–174.

Blauert, J. 1997. *Spatial Hearing: The Psychophysics of Human Sound Localization.* Cambridge, MA: MIT Press.

Bonatti, L., Frot, E., Zangl, R., and Mehler, J. 2002. "The Human First Hypothesis: Identification of Conspecifics and Individuation of Objects in the Young Infant." *Cognitive Psychology* 44: 388–426.

Brentano, F. 1874/1995. *Psychology from an Empirical Standpoint.* London: Routledge.

Burke, L. 1952. "On the Tunnel Effect." *Quarterly Journal of Experimental Psychology* 4: 121–138.

Caramazza, A., and Shelton, J. R. 1998. "Domain-Specific Knowledge Systems in the Brain: The Animate Inanimate Distinction." *Journal of Cognitive Neuroscience* 10: 1–34.

Carello, C., Wagman, J. B., and Turvey, M. T. 2005. "Acoustic Specification of Object Properties." In *Moving Image Theory: Ecological Considerations*, edited by J. D. Anderson and B. F. Anderson. Carbondale, IL: Southern Illinois University Press. 79–104.

Carroll, S. B. 2005. *Endless Forms Most Beautiful: The New Science of EvoDevo.* New York: W. W. Norton and Company.

Casati, R. 2005. "Common-Sense, Philosophical, and Theoretical Notions of an Object: Some Methodological Problems." *The Monist* 88: 571–599.

Chomsky, N. 1966. *Cartesian Linguistics. A Chapter in the History of Rationalist Thought.* New York: Harper and Row.

Chomsky, N. 1996. *Power and Prospect. Reflections on Human Nature and the Social Order.* London: Pluto Press.

Chomsky, N. 2000. *New Horizons in the Study of Language and Mind.* Cambridge, UK: Cambridge University Press.

Descartes, R. 1642/1985. *Meditations of First Philosophy.* In *The Philosophical Writings of Descartes*, translated by J. Cottingham, R. Stoothoff, and D. Murdoch. Vol. 2. Cambridge, UK: Cambridge University Press.

Fleming, R. W., and Bülthoff, H. H. 2005. "Low-Level Image Cues in the Perception of Translucent Materials." *ACM Transactions on Applied Perception* 2: 346–382.

Fleming, R. W., Dror, R. O. and Adelson, E. H. 2003. "Real-World Illumination and the Perception of Surface Reflectance Properties." *Journal of Vision* 3: 347–368.

Flombaum, J. I., and Scholl, B. J. 2006. "A Temporal Same-Object Advantage in the Tunnel Effect: Facilitated Change Detection for Persisting Objects." *Journal of Experimental Psychology: Human Perception and Performance* 32: 840–853.

Fodor, J. A. 1980. "Fixation of Belief and Concept Acquisition." In *Language and Learning: The Debate between Jean Piaget and Noam Chomsky*, edited by M. Piatelli-Palmarini. Cambridge, MA: Harvard University Press. 142–149.

Gallistel, C. R. 1998. "Symbolic Processes in the Brain: The Case of Insect Navigation." In *Methods, Models and Conceptual Issues. An Invitation to Cognitive Science*, edited by D. Scarborough and S. Sternberg. Vol. 4. Cambridge, MA: MIT Press. 1–51.

Gaukroger, S. 1990. "The Background to the Problem of Perceptual Cognition." In *Arnauld: On True and False Ideas*, translated by S. Gaukroger. Manchester: Manchester University Press. 1–41.

Gaukroger, S. 1995. *Descartes: An Intellectual Biography*. Oxford: Clarendon Press.

Gelb, A. 1929. "Die 'Farbenkonstanz' der Sehdinge." (The Color Constancy of the Objects of Vision). In *Handbuch der normalen und pathologischen Physiologie*, edited by A. Bethe, G. V. Bergmann, G. Embden, and A. Ellinger. Berlin: Springer. 594–678.

Gombrich, E. H. 1976. *The Heritage of Apelles. Studies in the Art of the Renaissance*. Ithaca, NY: Cornell University Press.

Gould, S. J. 2002. *The Structure of Evolutionary Theory*. Cambridge, MA: Harvard University Press.

Grier, M. 2001. *Kant's Doctrin of Transcedental Illusion*. Cambridge, UK: Cambridge University Press.

Hamlin, J. K., Wynn, K., and Bloom, P. 2007. "Social Evaluation by Preverbal Infants." *Nature* 450: 557–559.

Hare, B., Call, J., Agnetta, B., and Tomasello, M. 2000. "Chimpanzees Know What Conspecifics Do and Do Not See." *Animal Behavior* 59: 771–785.

Hauser, M. D., Pearson, H. M., and Seelig, D. 2002. "Ontogeny of Tool Use in Cotton-Top Tamarins *Saguinus oedipus*: Innate Recognition of Functionally Relevant Features." *Animal Behaviour* 64: 299–311.

Heider, F., and Simmel, M. 1944. "An Experimental Study of Apparent Behavior." *American Journal of Psychology* 57: 243–249.

Helmholtz, H. von 1856. "Ueber die Erklärung der stereoskopischen Erscheinung des Glanzes." (On the Explanation of Stereoscopic Luster) *Verhandlungen der naturhistorischen Vereinigung der Rheinlande*, 28–40.

Helmholtz, H. von 1867. *Handbuch der physiologischen Optik*. (Handbook of Physiological Optics) Hamburg: Voss.

Hering, E. 1879. "Der Raumsinn und die Bewegungen des Auges." (The Spatial Sense and Movements of the Eye) In *Handbuch der Physiologie der Sinnesorgane*, edited by L. Hermann. Leipzig: Vogel. 343–601.

Hinzen, W. 2006. *Mind Design and Minimal Syntax*. Oxford: Oxford University Press.

Hochegger, R. 1884. *Die geschichtliche Entwicklung des Farbensinnes*. (The Historical Development of the Color Sense) Innsbruck: Wagner'sche Universitätsbuchhandlung.

Hume, D. 1748/2007. *An Enquiry Concerning Human Understanding*. Oxford: Oxford University Press.

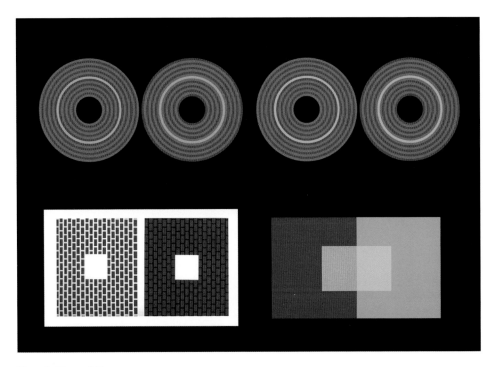

Plate 1 (figure I.2)

Top panels: The perceived color of the rings in the left pair appear different (pink and orange) as do the rings in the right pair (blue and green) but in each pair the physical reflectance of the rings is identical. The patterned background of purple and lime-green circles causes the illusion (Monnier and Shevell, 2003; images and permission courtesy of P. Monnier). Bottom left panels: Given a grid of interlaced red and black stripes, and a grid of red and white stripes, the red perceived is very different though physically identical in both cases. Lower right panel: The proximal stimulus on the retina, consisting of four spatial regions, is given by light radiations specified in terms of intensity, wavelength, area, and time. Perceptually, what one sees is a transparent rectangle over two others, with the emergent property of a yellowish light spreading on the whole appearance; items that do not exist at the level of stimuli (Da Pos, 1989–1991; Metelli, 1941; see also Da Pos, Devigili, Giaggio, and Trevisan, 2007).

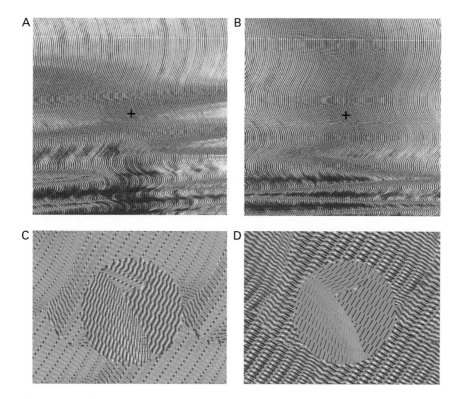

Plate 2 (figure 4.2)

Pseudocolor presentation of cone model simulations for (A) rotation and (B) scaling of figure 4.1. Blue indicates high-contrast regions, red denotes lowest luminance contrast. Figure-ground segmentation in the Ouchi illusions (figure 4.4) is enhanced when moving the figure slightly. For example, during (C) vertical and (D) oblique linear motion, different degrees of blur in the figure and ground may play a role in the perceived relative motion between figure and ground. Visual transduction in cones seems a proper candidate, albeit at a low level of vision for this selective blur.

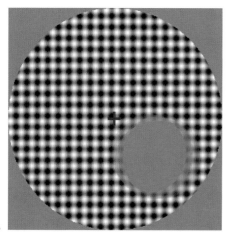

1°

A

Plate 3 (figure 5.1)

Artificial scotoma induced by TMS. (A) Examples of scotoma. The left occipital lobe of the subject was stimulated by an 8-shaped coil with a monophasic single pulse. The duration of visual stimulus was 40 ms, and the delay of magnetic stimulation from the onset of the visual stimulus was 100 ms in this example. The subjects' own drawing/duplication of the scotoma percept was superimposed over five consecutive trials.

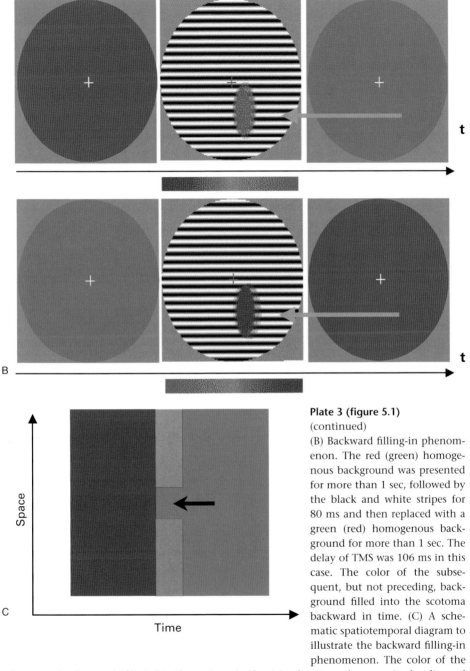

Plate 3 (figure 5.1)
(continued)
(B) Backward filling-in phenomenon. The red (green) homogenous background was presented for more than 1 sec, followed by the black and white stripes for 80 ms and then replaced with a green (red) homogenous background for more than 1 sec. The delay of TMS was 106 ms in this case. The color of the subsequent, but not preceding, background filled into the scotoma backward in time. (C) A schematic spatiotemporal diagram to illustrate the backward filling-in phenomenon. The color of the subsequent background "fills-in" to the scotoma in the striped pattern, thus perceived earlier and simultaneously with the stripes surrounding (modified from Kamitani and Shimojo, 1999, figures 1 and 5).

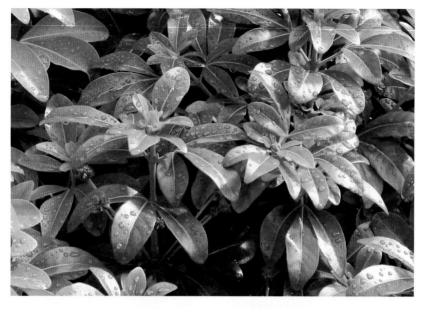

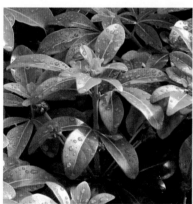 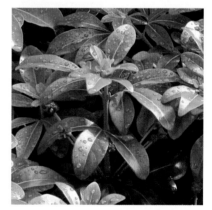

Plate 4 (figure 7.3)
Image of a plant. Top: Compare the perceived depth, viewing with both eyes, and then with one eye only through a small aperture (1–2 cm diameter) that occludes the edges of the picture. The image should look "stereoscopic" (plastic effect) through the aperture. The individual leaves should appear to be clearly defined in depth and appear "touchable". The percept may initially take a few seconds to develop. Observers also report enhanced perception of color (e.g., saturation, dynamic range), material properties (e.g., glossiness) and image sharpness accompanying the plastic effect. Bottom: Cross or parallel fuse the pair of images below. Again, the plastic effect should be apparent despite the fact that there are no disparities between the two images (the images are identical).

Jackendoff, R. 1987. *Consciousness and the Computational Mind.* Cambridge, MA: MIT Press.

Jackendoff, R. 2003. *Foundations of Language.* Oxford: Oxford University Press.

James, W. 1890/1983. *The Principles of Psychology.* Cambridge, MA: Harvard University Press.

Kant, I. 1781/1929. *Critique of Pure Reason* (trans. N. Kemp Smith). New York: St. Martin's Press.

Karpinska, L. V. 1910. "Experimentelle Beiträge zur Analyse der Tiefenwahrnehmung." (Experimental Contributions to the Analysis of Depth Perception) *Zeitschrift für Psychologie* 57: 1–89.

Katz, D. 1911. *Die Erscheinungsweisen der Farben und ihre Beeinflussung durch die Individuelle Erfahrung.* (The Modes of Color Appearance and Their Modification by Individual Experience) Leipzig: Barth.

Kirschner, M., and Gerhart, J. 1998. "Evolvability." *Proceedings of the National Academy of Sciences of the United States of America* 95: 8420–8427.

Klatzky, R. L., Pai, D. K., and Krotkov, E. P. 2000. "Perception of Material From Contact Sounds." *Presence: Teleoperators and Virtual Environments* 9: 399–410.

Koenderink, J. J., and Pont, S. C. 2002. "The Secret of Velvety Skin." *Machine Vision and Applications; Special Issue on Human Modeling, Analysis and Synthesis.* 14: 260–268.

Köhler, W. 1947. *Gestalt Psychology.* New York: Liveright.

Lorenz, K. 1982. "Kant's Doctrine of the a Priori in the Light of Contemporary Biology." In *Learning, Development, and Culture: Essays in Evolutionary Epistemology*, edited by H. C. Plotkin. Chichester: Wiley. 121–143. (Original work published 1941)

Ludlow, P. 2003. "Referential Semantics for I-Languages?" In *Chomsky and His Critics*, edited by L. M. Antony and N. Hornstein. Oxford: Blackwell. 140–161.

Mausfeld, R. 2002. "The Physicalistic Trap in Perception." In *Perception and the Physical World*, edited by D. Heyer and R. Mausfeld. Chichester: Wiley. 75–112.

Mausfeld, R. 2003. "'Colour' as Part of the Format of Two Different Perceptual Primitives: The Dual Coding of Colour." In *Colour Perception: Mind and the Physical World*, edited by R. Mausfeld and D. Heyer. Oxford: Oxford University Press. 381–429.

Mausfeld, R. (2010a). "Colour Within an Internalist Framework: The Role of 'Colour' in the Structure of the Perceptual System." In *Color Ontology and Color Science*, edited by J. Cohen and M. Matthen. Cambridge, MA: MIT Press. 123–147.

Mausfeld, R. (2010b). "Intrinsic Multiperspectivity: On the Architectural Foundations of a Distinctive Mental Capacity." In *Cognition and Neuropsychology: International Perspectives on Psychological Science,* Vol. 1, edited by P. A. Frensch and R. Schwarzer. London: Psychology Press. 95–116.

Metzger, W. 1941. *Psychologie. Die Entwicklung ihrer Grundannahmen seit Einführung des Experiments.* (Psychology: The Development of Its Core Assumptions Since the Adoption of the Experiment) Darmstadt: Steinkopff.

Michotte, A. 1991. "The Psychological Enigma of Perspective in Outline Pictures." In *Michotte's Experimental Phenomenology of Perception*, edited by G. Thinès, A. Costall, and G. Butterworth. Hillsdale, NJ: Erlbaum. (Original work published 1948)

Michotte, A. 1991. "Autobiography." In *Michotte's Experimental Phenomenology of Perception*, edited by G. Thinès, A. Costall, and G. Butterworth. Hillsdale, NJ: Erlbaum. (Original work published 1954)

Möller, E. F. 1925. "The 'Glassy Sensation." *American Journal of Psychology* 36: 249–285.

Neisser, U. 1976. *Cognition and Reality: Principles and Implications of Cognitive Psychology*. New York: W. H. Freeman.

Premack, D., and Premack, A. J. 1995. "Intention as Psychological Cause." In *Causal Cognition*, edited by D. Sperber, D. Premack, and A. J. Premack. Oxford: Clarendon. 185–199.

Premack, D., and Premack, A. 2003. *Original Intelligence. Unlocking the Mystery of Who We Are*. New York: McGraw-Hill.

Pustejovsky, J. 1995. *The Generative Lexicon*. Cambridge, MA: MIT Press.

Santos, L. R., Hauser, M. D., and Spelke, E. S. 2001. "Recognition and Categorization of Biologically Significant Objects by Rhesus Monkeys (*Macaca mulatta*): The Domain of Food." *Cognition* 82: 127–155.

Schapp, W. 1910. *Beiträge zur Phänomenologie der Wahrnehmung*. (Contributions to the Phenomenology of Perception) Halle: Max Niemeyer.

Scholl, B. J. 2007. "Object Persistence in Philosophy and Psychology." *Mind and Language* 22: 563–591.

Scholl, B. J., and Tremoulet, P. 2000. "Perceptual Causality and Animacy." *Trends in Cognitive Sciences* 4: 299–309.

Schumann, F. 1920. "Die Repräsentation des leeren Raumes im Bewußtsein. Eine neue Empfindung." (On the Representation of Empty Space in Phenomenal Experience. A New Sensation) *Zeitschrift für Psychologie* 85: 224–244.

Shimojo, S., and Shams, L. 2001. "Sensory Modalities Are Not Separate Modalities: Plasticity and Interactions." *Current Opinion in Neurobiology* 11: 505–509.

Spelke, E. S. 1990. "Principles of Object Perception." *Cognitive Science* 14: 29–56.

Spelke, E. S. 2000. "Core Knowledge." *American Psychologist* 55: 1233–1243.

Spelke, E. S., Gutheil, G., and van der Walle, G. 1995. "The Development of Object Perception." In *Visual Cognition. An Invitation to Cognitive Science*, edited by S. M. Kosslyn and D. Osherson. Vol. 2. Cambridge, MA: MIT Press. 297–330.

Strawson, G. 2003. "Real Materialism." In *Chomsky and His Critics*, edited by L. Antony and N. Hornstein. Oxford: Blackwell. 49–88.

Tinbergen, N. 1963. "On Aims and Methods of Ethology." *Zeitschrift für Tierpsychologie* 20: 410–433.

Trevarthen, C. 1998. "The Concept and Foundations of Infant Intersubjectivity." In *Intersubjective Communication and Emotion in Early Ontogeny*, edited by S. Bråten. Cambridge, UK: Cambridge University Press. 15–46.

von Szily, A. 1921. "Stereoskopische Versuche mit Schattenrissen." (Stereoscopic Experiments with Silhouettes) *Gräfes Archiv für Ophtalmologie* 105: 964–972.

Wagner, G. P., Mezey, J., and Calabretta, R. 2005. "Natural Selection and the Origin of Modules." In *Modularity. Understanding the Development and Evolution of Complex Natural Systems*, edited by W. Callabaut and D. Rasskin-Gutman. Cambridge, MA: MIT Press. 33–49.

Wang, R. F., and Spelke, E. S. 2002. "Human Spatial Representation: Insights From Animals." *Trends in Cognitive Sciences* 6: 376–382.

Webster, G., and Goodwin, B. C. 1996. *Form and Transformation. Generative and Relational Principles in Biology*. Cambridge, UK: Cambridge University Press.

Wehner, R. 2003. "Desert Ant Navigation: How Miniature Brains Solve Complex Tasks." *Journal of Comparative Physiology A* 189: 579–588.

Wendt, G., Faul, F., and Mausfeld, R. 2008. "Highlight Disparity Contributes to the Authenticity and Strength of Perceived Glossiness." *Journal of Vision* 8: 1–10.

Yang, C. D. 2002. *Knowledge and Learning in Natural Language*. Oxford: Oxford University Press.

Yolton, J. W. 1984. *Perceptual Acquaintance from Descartes to Reid*. Minneapolis: University of Minnesota Press.

Yolton, J. W. 1996. *Perception and Reality. A History from Descartes to Kant*. Ithaca, NY: Cornell University Press.

7 Visual Information in Surface and Depth Perception: Reconciling Pictures and Reality

Dhanraj Vishwanath

Pictures are a special class of surfaces that are planar and have a complex non-random reflectance pattern (sometimes referred to as "surface markings"). What is unusual about such surfaces for the human visual system is that they automatically engender an illusory percept of depth and three-dimensional (3D) layout contrary to the physical two-dimensional (2D) picture surface. They present, in a sense, the ultimate visual illusion: We see depth and 3D structure where there clearly is none. This fact has given pictures a privileged role in the scientific study of depth and form perception ever since the discovery of perspective during the Renaissance (Hagen, 1980; Hecht, Schwartz, and Atherton, 2003; Kubovy, 1986; Pirenne, 1970; Wade, Ono, and Lillakas, 2001). Pictures present a window into the interpretive and constructive capacity of the human visual system, as well as pose a conceptual challenge to the understanding of depth and 3D form perception in general. Consider the example shown in figure 7.1, where one clearly perceives a 3D space with 3D objects arrayed at different depths. An easy way to *explain away* this phenomenon is to say that it happens because the objects depicted in pictures are things familiar to us from the real 3D world, and we have "learned" to recognize them in 2D images. But examples such as the "picture" in figure 7.2, belie such simplistic, "cognitivist" explanations, and current scientific research in visual perception rarely entertains them; seeking, rather, to understand picture perception phenomena from the viewpoint of the working of visual mechanisms (see Cutting, 2003; Hagen, 1980; Koenderink and van Doorn, 2003).

A scientific explanation of pictorial depth based on current models of depth perception poses two serious and unanswered questions: (1) Why do we see depth in pictures even when the predominance of visual information suggests otherwise? (2) Why does pictorial depth appear qualitatively different from "real" depth?

The current model of 3D form and depth perception argues that the visual system is tasked with *faithfully recovering* the 3D structure and layout of the visual world from the various sources of visual and nonvisual information available: the retinal and extraretinal *depth cues*. Specifically, the visual system acts to recover and represent two distinct properties of 3D surfaces: (1) their *geometric structure and layout*, and (2) their

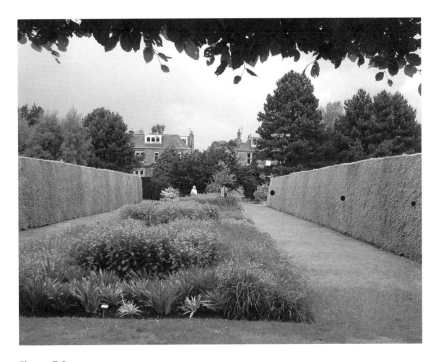

Figure 7.1
Photo of a scene from the Edinburgh Royal Botanical Gardens. Viewing the image with two eyes, 3D surface shape, metric relative depth relations (the farther depth interval between the black dots appears larger than the closer interval), and depth order (what is in front and behind) are clearly perceived. However, the qualitative vividness of depth perceived when viewing a real scene with both eyes is not experienced. Note that there are no visual cues to egocentric distance (actual distance of objects from the observer) within pictorial space (see text). The only indication of egocentric distances is the familiar size of objects (human figures, houses). Absent these objects, absolute size, absolute depth, and distance in the image would be ambiguous.

associated *pattern of reflectance* or *markings* (Adelson and Pentland, 1996; Marr, 1982). In other words, the visual system's internal representation of a surface reflects the physical reality of surfaces in the external world: They have some sort of geometric shape and some *pattern of reflectance* or *markings*. This seems problematic for picture perception. If the visual system has the capacity to represent a planar surface with a pattern of reflectance/markings, why doesn't the visual system do just that when confronted with a picture? Why engender a percept of 3D surface layout when there is none? This question becomes even more problematic when one considers that the predominance of depth information available to the visual system in images such as figure 7.2 correctly specifies a flat 2D surface (table 7.1). There is only one available cue (shading) that potentially specifies a 3D object.[1]

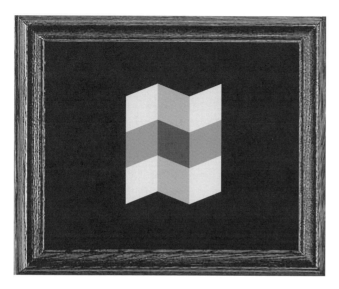

Figure 7.2

An object in the "picture" appears to most observers to be a bent rectilinear 3D surface. In the typical interpretation, the right bent edge appears toward the observer. In another interpretation it appears away from the observer. The percept can switch between the two. For most observers, it is nearly impossible to see the object as a flat 2D surface without considerable effort. Adapted from Adelson and Pentland (1996).

Table 7.1

Depth "cues" available to the visual system listed as being consistent with either the 2D or 3D interpretation

Cues consistent with a flat 2D surface with markings	Cues consistent with 3D object
Binocular disparity	Perspective cues (not available)
Motion parallax (head motion)	Texture (not available)
Vergence	Shading
Accommodation	Aerial perspective (not available)
Blur gradients	Interposition (not available)
Picture surface microtexture	Motion (not available)

Note that all cues on the left column are present under normal binocular viewing of a picture regardless of its pictorial contents. Cues on the right side may or may not be present in a specific picture. For example, in figure 7.2, the only 3D consistent cue available is shading (one might say that there is a rectangularity assumption at work too, but this would strictly not be a "cue" under current definitions).

One possibility is that the aforementioned concerns are too simplistic, and that if one takes into account more sophisticated computational constructs such as nonaccidentalness, ecological Bayesian priors, statistical robustness, and so on, the combination of cues will reveal that the perceived 3D surface structure in pictures is indeed the optimal interpretation given the cue information.

Even if such explanations can work (and we will see why they don't), it still leaves unanswered the second crucial question: Why does the perception of 3D structure in pictures seem to lack a sort of *qualitative vividness* present under natural viewing of real scenes with two eyes? The striking difference is easy to demonstrate in stereo-normal observers by looking at an object that has a complex depth structure, such as a tree or a vase of flowers, and then comparing it to a picture of the same scene. A similar difference is seen when viewing the real object with one or both eyes. When one looks at the real scene with both eyes, the different branches, leaves, and petals appear to be more distinctly separated in depth, unlike in pictures. Observers report that the "space between objects is perceived," that "objects are volumetric," that "things stick out into space," and "that things appear touchable or graspable" (e.g., Sacks, 2006). Pictorial depth, in contrast, seems somehow "detached" from us. The perceptual vividness of depth under binocular viewing has historically been referred to as the "plastic effect" (Ames, 1925; Judge, 1926; Schlosberg, 1941). A simple explanation (and the traditionally favored one) is that such effects can be attributed to binocular processing, and that the perceived vividness essentially *is* stereoscopic depth perception. This could explain why we should not see the plastic effect when viewing pictures because binocular cues do not specify depth within the depicted scene (they specify the location of the picture surface).

Unfortunately, such an explanation fails to explain some other striking visual effects (Ames, 1925; Judge, 1926; Koenderink, 1998; Schlosberg, 1941). For example, if one views figure 7.3 (plate 4) with one eye through a small aperture, such that the frame of the picture is obscured, the plastic effect is clearly seen; observers use essentially the same words to describe this situation as in binocular viewing of real scenes even in the absence of binocular information (this can also be seen in figure 7.1). The plastic effect is also observed when viewing conditions make disparities essentially zero (synoptic viewing). This can be approximated by cross or parallel fusing identical images (figure 7.1 or 7.3). Moreover, the plastic effect is not always present when a real scene is viewed with two eyes; it reduces with viewing distance and is essentially absent at far viewing distances (what Cutting and Vishton [1995] refer to as vista space), and perceived 3D layout at such distances (e.g., a distant landscape) appears almost *pictorial*. These qualitative observations raise the following question: *Why do we seemingly have two types of depth perception when viewing pictures and real scenes?*

Intriguingly, both of these problems—the difficulty in providing a mechanistic explanation for why we see illusory depth in pictures and the fact that this perceived depth appears different from real depth—in most cases seem to support the naïve idea

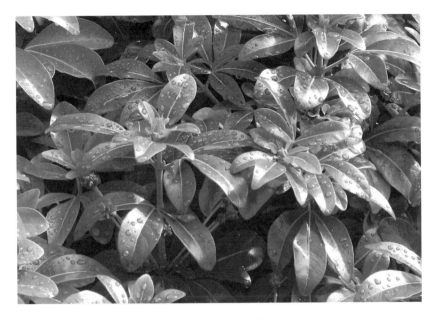

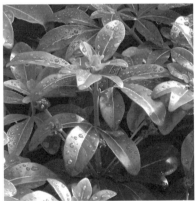 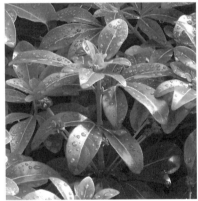

Figure 7.3 (plate 4)
Image of a plant. Top: Compare the perceived depth, viewing with both eyes, and then with one eye only through a small aperture (1–2 cm diameter) that occludes the edges of the picture. The image should look "stereoscopic" (plastic effect) through the aperture. The individual leaves should appear to be clearly defined in depth and appear "touchable." The percept may initially take a few seconds to develop. Observers also report enhanced perception of color (e.g., saturation, dynamic range), material properties (e.g., glossiness) and image sharpness accompanying the plastic effect. Bottom: Cross or parallel fuse the pair of images. Again, the plastic effect should be apparent despite the fact that there are no disparities between the two images (the images are identical).

that picture perception is, after all, just a cognitive phenomenon. Pictures merely *signify* the real world.

In this chapter, I make a different argument. I suggest that pictorial depth is indeed a predictable outcome of the normal visual processing of surface and depth (e.g., Cutting, 2003; Koenderink and van Doorn, 2003; Mausfeld, 2003). The puzzles described previously will appear more tractable once we correctly understand visual perception as the *presentation* of causally efficacious visual information rather than an *inference* to objective external reality. Specifically, I make the following propositions:

1. A perceptual surface is an informational structure that is essentially a complex observer-centric motor plan. It is not a re-presentation of some objective external physical entity. Surfaces, *as we see them*, do not exist in the external world. Their imputed objective existence is based on our perceptual, proprioceptive, and cognitive integrations and categorizations.
2. A perceptual surface does not have "reflectance patterns" or "markings" as a property, in the way we cognitively ascribe "real surfaces" in the external world to have. Perceived surface lightness change is not an inference or re-presentation of reflectance change in the external world; rather, it is the perceptual presentation of *change in surface identity*.
3. The perception of relative depth (depth order, surface slant, 3D shape) and the perception of absolute depth (egocentrically scaled depth separation) are dissociable and distinct. The distinction is revealed in the qualitative differences in depth perception between pictures and real objects/scenes, between monocular and binocular viewing, and between vista space and peripersonal space.
4. The vivid qualitative richness observed in binocular viewing of real scenes but lacking when viewing pictures (namely, *the plastic effect*) is not an epiphenomenon of stereoscopic depth processing, neither is it primarily a function of depth-cue conflict. Rather, it is the perceptual presentation of the *precision* (statistical reliability) of egocentrically scaled depth information.[2] Its salience varies as a function of the availability and reliability of egocentric distance information (required to scale perceived relative depth); whether in pictures or the real world.

The idea of perception as the *presentation* of subjective information was the cornerstone of Brentanian approach and implicit in later Gestalt psychology. More recently, it is mainly Albertazzi's work that has revived the usage of the term *presentation* (Albertazzi, 1998). The idea that perception is the presentation of causally efficacious information, while implicit in the Brentanian approach, has been explicit and computationally motivated in Leyton's (1992) group theoretic model of shape. This notion is crucially different from the more empiricist claims of causal efficacy as sensorimotor contingency that is present in Gibsonian ecological perception and more recent "enactive" theories of perception (see the introduction to this volume).

Aspects of proposition 2 were made in an earlier article (Vishwanath, 2006). Proposition 3, the potential for distinct representations of relative and absolute depth, has been made by several researchers (Cutting and Vishton, 1995; Marr, 1982; Mausfeld, 2003; Niederée and Heyer, 2003; Stevens and Brookes, 1988; Zimmerman et al., 1995) but has not been extensively explored within the psychophysical literature; although neurophysiological work has supported such a distinction in terms of the locus of cortical processing (e.g. Neri, 2005; Neri et al., 2004). Proposition 4 constitutes a novel theory.

The Cue Combination Approach to Depth Perception

The standard model for the perception of 3D surface shape assumes that it is a quantitative outcome of the assessment of the various depth and shape cues available to the visual system (e.g. Buckley and Frisby, 1993; Bülthoff and Mallot, 1988; Clark and Yuille, 1990; Cutting and Vishton, 1995; Landy et al., 1995; Marr, 1982; Norman et al., 1995), an approach usually referred to as cue combination. This assessment leads to the inference of a surface whose properties include geometry (i.e., shape, slant, tilt) and a reflectance pattern or surface markings (Adelson and Pentland, 1996; Marr, 1982). Current approaches to cue combination can be roughly categorized as being consistent with one of two models: (1) Linear weighted averaging (sometimes also referred to as maximum likelihood estimation, weak fusion, or modified weak fusion) (Adelson and Pentland, 1996; Hillis et al., 2004; Landy et al., 1995). (2) Strong coupling/modal priors approaches (Richards and Jepson, 1991; Richards et al., 1996; Yuille and Bülthoff, 1996).[3]

Both approaches can be understood within a generic inverse-optics and perception-as-Bayesian-inference framework, where perceived metric quantities (e.g., 3D surface shape, depth, and slant) are those that are statistically most probable given the available sensory information. More specifically, the perceived scene interpretation (S) is that with the highest posterior probability given the sensory image (I).[4] This, in turn, is proportional to the product of the likelihood of the image given the scene interpretation and the prior probability of that interpretation in the interpretation space. The scene interpretation (e.g., depth or surface layout) favored by the visual system should be the one with the highest joint likelihood and prior probability

$$p(S \,|\, I) \sim p(I \,|\, S) \cdot p(S)$$

In words, the probability of the scene interpretation (S) given the sensory image (I) is proportional to the probability of the image given the scene interpretation multiplied by the prior or intrinsic probability of such scenes in the world. The sensory image is considered to be a set of statistically independent image measures or "cues" (e.g., "pictorial cues" such as texture and shading, disparity, motion parallax, etc.). The

interpreted quantity (e.g., slant) or scene is one of an infinite number of possible interpretations (inverse optics is an ill-posed problem). Because the cues are typically
considered to be a set of statistically independent measures, the likelihood then is simply assumed to be the product of the individual cue likelihoods. So that the posterior
can be written as

$$p(S \mid I) \sim p(i_p \mid S) \cdot p(i_d \mid S) \cdot p(i_m \mid S) \cdots p(S)$$

where the subscripts represent different image measures. To evaluate these probabilities in viewing pictures, we consider two possible perceptual interpretations (S) given
the picture in figure 7.2. The first is the interpretation of a 3D folded object (i.e., the
one that is normally perceived when viewing such a picture [S_{3d}]). The second (S_{2d}) is
the interpretation that would be perceived if the picture were seen exactly as what it is,
namely, a flat 2D surface with pattern of reflectance. The 2D coplanar reflectance interpretation is indicated diagrammatically in figure 7.4; it is not possible to create a pattern on the page that would appear to the reader as the true S_{2d} interpretation (telling,
in itself, the power of illusory depth!). (A good visual exercise for the reader, before
continuing with the rest of the chapter, is to try to visually force a 2D percept on the
object in figure 7.2.)

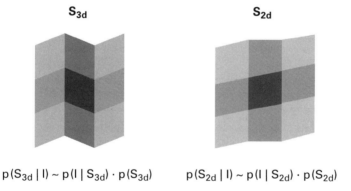

$$p(S_{3d} \mid I) \sim p(I \mid S_{3d}) \cdot p(S_{3d}) \qquad p(S_{2d} \mid I) \sim p(I \mid S_{2d}) \cdot p(S_{2d})$$

Figure 7.4
Two possible interpretations of the pictorial image in figure 7.2. The left is the 3D interpretation,
which appears like a folded 3D surface with rectangular faces (actually, two such possible interpretations can be seen if the image is fixated for several seconds). The right is a "symbolic" representation of the 2D or "flat" co-coplanar reflectance interpretation. Naturally, the correct one
should not appear in any way 3D. However, it is impossible to create an image that would reflect
it accurately. (With effort, some observers are able to see the "true" flat interpretation momen-
tarily in the left image or in figure 7.2). The expressions below the images indicate the respective
posterior probabilities.

Statistical Cue Combination and Picture Perception

The weighted-averaging model is based on the idea that a quantitative perceptual esti-mate (e.g., 3D surface shape, slant, depth) is a weighted linear combination of esti-mates arising from individual cues, where the individual cue weights are inversely proportional to their statistical reliability. So, for example, if slant were to be estimated via two cues, disparity and texture, then the perceived slant would be some combina-tion of the slant estimates derived from each cue individually, where the more reliable cue's estimate would be weighted more heavily. The strong coupling and modal priors models suggest that perceptual interpretations cannot be predicted from simple linear combination of weighted cues because the assumption of statistical independence of cues does not hold; cues are often strongly interdependent, and/or cue estimates alone do not suffice to generate unique perceptual interpretations, and must be augmented by internal assumptions regarding the structure of the external world. These assump-tions are expressed computationally as prior probability functions within a Bayesian probabilistic framework (modal priors approach). Here we only consider the weighted-averaging and modal-priors approach.

An explanation of picture perception under the weighted-averaging approach would need to show that under typical picture-viewing conditions, image measures signalling change in depth (cues such as texture and shading) are more reliable and robust than image measures signalling no change in depth (e.g., cues such as disparity and parallax). An explanation under the modal-priors approach would require a model of the prior assumptions that in combination with actual image measures (cues) results in the per-ceived illusory 3D effect.

Linear Weighted Averaging in Pictorial Interpretation
The most straightforward statistical model for depth cue combination assumes a linear weighted averaging of available cues. Specifically, the rule that results in an unbiased and minimum variance depth estimate is one where each estimator (cue) is weighted by its relative reliability, expressed as the reciprocal of the variance of the estimator, and assuming estimator variance to be statistically independent Gaussian noise (Hillis et al., 2004; Landy et al., 1995). Under a Bayesian framework, this is equivalent to the maximum likelihood estimate (MLE) (Clark and Yuille, 1990; Hillis et al., 2004).

Empirically derived relative reliabilities of depth cues indicate that it will be difficult to explain pictorial depth under a linear cue-weighting model because the cues that seem to be down-weighted (disparity and motion parallax) are often the most reliable. Depth from disparity or motion parallax is exquisitely sensitive. Depth relief discrimi-nation thresholds are equivalent to detecting depth contrasts of less than 0.001 for disparity and less than 0.002 for motion parallax (Rogers and Graham, 1982), consis-tent with reported stereo thresholds of a 2- to 6-second arc of disparity (see Howard and Rogers, 1995). Cutting and Vishton (1995) reported only one ordinal pictorial cue (interposition) that is comparable to disparity and motion parallax at less than a meter viewing distance. In direct comparisons on slant judgment, Hillis et al. (2004) found disparity and texture to be comparable at viewing distances of less than 50 cm (distances at which we routinely view pictures), making it unclear which should be favored in picture viewing based on an MLE strategy.

Moreover, weighted averaging predicts large changes in perceived 3D shape depending on whether a picture is viewed binocularly or monocularly because disparity is absent in the latter viewing condition. Weighted averaging also predicts that perceived 3D shape should be modulated by viewing distance because reliability of disparity and motion parallax is inversely related to viewing distance, with disparity being significantly less reliable at 1 m compared with 30 cm (Cutting and Vishton, 1995; Hillis et al., 2004). Yet such changes are not typically apparent when viewing pictures (see figures 7.1 and 7.2). The shape of the 3D object does not appear to change when one closes and opens an eye or when one changes the viewing distance. The distance modulation of disparity would also predict that we should experience bistability between 2D and 3D interpretations at distances where reliability of disparity, motion parallax, and pictorial cues are comparable (near viewing less than 50 cm). Results with cue conflict stimuli have not been consistent with this: Bistability has been reported at distances of 93 cm (van Ee et al., 2003) but not at 40 cm (Stevens et al., 1991).

Although these foregoing observations confound a weighted-cue based explanation, there is some important evidence of modification of pictorial depth relief judgements consistent with changes in the availability of depth cues. Koenderink and collaborators have examined how surface shape and depth relief judgments for objects represented in pictures are modulated by different viewing conditions (monocular, binocular, synoptic) and different psychophysical tasks (Battu et al., 2007; Doorschot et al., 2001; Koenderink, van Doorn, and Kappers, 1992, 1994; Koenderink et al., 2001; Todd et al., 1996). Koenderink et al. (1992, 1994, 2001) examined local depth relief or surface orientation judgments obtained for predefined locations on the object surface and then interpolated them to obtain a global response surface representing the perceived depth relief. Consistent with weighted-averaging type explanations, perceived depth relief appeared to depend on the level of conflict in cue. The shallowest depth relief was obtained when disparity conflicted with the pictorial cues (a picture viewed binocularly). However, the results do not seem to comport with our normal perceptual experience with pictures (e.g., closing or opening one eye when viewing figure 7.1 or 7.2 does not seem to change perceived shape to the degree suggested by these results).

Moreover, the fact that these studies used local measures to infer global shape, and did not explicitly measure cue reliabilities (that was not the focus of these experiments), complicates interpretations of these results and leaves open alternative explanations. We return to discuss these studies in more detail in a later section.

Robust Estimation in Pictorial Interpretation

An alternative approach to cue integration in the presence of cue conflict is to augment linear weighted averaging with statistically robust strategies where highly disparate signals are disregarded (akin to using the median of the cue responses rather than a simple linear average) (see Landy et al., 1995). However, in picture perception, the fact that at least six cues (disparity, motion parallax, vergence, accommodation, blur gradient, and surface microtexture) contradict the 3D interpretation, and that some of these are reliable (disparity, motion parallax), poses a serious challenge to any explanation based on statistical robustness. Moreover, although emphasis in modified weighted averaging models is on the robustness of the combined estimator, one should also consider the statistical robustness of each cue as an estimator in its own right (i.e., whether changes in scene-independent aspects such as viewpoint produce small or large changes in the estimator likelihood distribution). Viewing pictures can involve multiple glances and viewing positions. In this regard, motion parallax, disparity, vergence, and accommodation are more robust under picture viewing because they signal the same planar 2D surface regardless of viewpoint, whereas the retinal image, and consequently the scene specified by the pictorial cues, changes with viewpoint.

Finally, most cue combination studies, such as those cited earlier, have looked at the interaction of cues for viewing times in the order of hundreds of milliseconds to 1 or 2 seconds. Such conditions should actually favor the pictorial cues, whereas natural viewing of a picture (typically for several seconds to several minutes) should favor the disparity cue. In ambiguous stimuli such as random dot stereograms, shape from disparity can take on the order of several seconds to disambiguate (Howard and Rogers, 1995). Anecdotal evidence also indicates similar temporal effects for stereograms of complex shapes displayed on flat display surfaces, where there are inherent depth cue conflicts. Thus, if anything, staring at a picture should slowly diminish the perceived pictorial depth, an observation that does not obtain (figure 7.2).

Suppression of Disparity and Motion Parallax in Pictorial Interpretation

Regardless of whether it implies a statistically robust strategy, evidence and observations seem consistent with a suppression of disparity and motion parallax during the perception of pictorial depth. A principled reason for disparity suppression proposed by Stevens and Brooks (1988), is that disparity information is only integrated with other cues when the second spatial derivative of disparity is nonzero (disparity gradient is constant); namely, when there is surface curvature, a break in surface attitude, or at surface edges. This could explain why disparity appears to be discounted within a planar picture surface where the disparity gradient is constant. The evidence supporting their claim is not extensive, and though findings on the linkage between disparity processing and surface representation (e.g., Glennerster et al., 2002) appear to provide some support for this theory, other observations appear to question their applicability to pictorial depth. First, other results (Vishwanath et al., 2005) are consistent with the robust recovery of local slant of a planar picture surface via disparity. Second, the proposal would imply that the visual system discounts reliable disparity information from a planar surfaces (e.g., from regular surface markings) even if it could, in principle, provide a more reliable depth/slant estimate for such surfaces. Third, it implies that pictorial depth will not obtain when viewing a smoothly curving picture surface (disparity will no longer be discounted), a prediction that is challenged by taking a picture and bending it backward or forward into a partially cylindrical form.

Summary

The review of the previous empirical studies seems to suggest that weighted averaging models, robustness models, or ones that propose suppression of disparity signals due to other factors will find it hard to explain why we see depth in pictures such as figures 7.1 and 7.2.

A different type of argument suggests that the reason we see 3D structure in pictures is because the visual system makes intrinsic computational assumptions. For example, the visual system prefers "rectangular" interpretations to nonrectangular ones, causing us to see 3D rectangular shapes in figure 7.2, or, it makes interpretations that are probabilistically "nonaccidental" (i.e., that it avoids interpretations where the observed retinal image would be unlikely given that interpretation). For example, it would not interpret a square to be the image of a cube because it is unlikely that the image of a square would obtain from a cube; the most likely image from a cube would be one that shows two or three of the faces of the cube. Although such arguments seem promising, on closer inspection, they fail to be legitimate because such intrinsic assumptions are already part of the definition of the various so-called depth cues. For example, assumptions of parallelism are intrinsic to the definition of the perspective convergence cue, whereas isotropy is intrinsic to the texture cue.

This is precisely the point that Richards and Jepson's (1991) modal priors framework highlights. They explain that a cue or visual "feature" is not a viable inferential tool unless it is combined with intrinsic assumptions of the nature of the external world or viewing conditions. In the next section, we examine this class of explanations. Although weighted cue combination approaches such as MLE generally only take into consideration likelihoods, more recently, such models also incorporate prior assumptions of the inference space (e.g., Ernst, 2005).

Modal Priors Approach to Depth and 3D Shape Perception

In the modal priors approach (Jepson et al., 1996; Richards and Jepson, 1991; Richards et al., 1996), we consider the ratios of probabilities for the scene interpretation S to the probabilities of the complement of S (i.e., all interpretations other than S), indicated by ¬S. For example, for the interpretation S_{3d}, we have:

$$\frac{p(S_{3d} \mid I)}{p(\neg S_{3d} \mid I)} = \frac{p(I \mid S_{3d})}{p(I \mid \neg S_{3d})} * \frac{p(S_{3d})}{p(\neg S_{3d})}$$

The left-hand term (the posterior ratio) will be very large (significantly greater than 1) if the interpretation (in this case, S_{3d}) is more likely given the image than any other interpretation given the image. The interpretation selected by the visual system should therefore be the one with the highest posterior ratio. For any interpretation to have a large posterior ratio, Richards, Jepson et al. have argued that two conditions must be met as the resolution of the image measures or cues (I) improves (i.e., as the associated error (ε) of any image measurement or cue (e.g., disparity) tends to zero). Specifically, (1) the joint likelihood ratio (the first term on the right of the previous equation) must become unbounded (i.e., tend to infinity), and (2) the prior ratio (the second term on the right of the previous equation) must be nondiminishing (i.e., remain bounded away from zero as the resolution of the image measure gets progressively better) (Richards and Jepson, 1991; Richards et al., 1996).

Intuitively, these criteria address the validity of the image measure ("cue" or "feature") for the inference at hand, as well as the validity of the specific interpretation that we make (in this case, 2D or 3D). The *likelihood* criteria essentially says the following: If we have a particular definition of an image measure ("cue" or "feature") that we believe the visual system uses to make interpretations, the measured values of the cue obtained in the image (at theoretically high resolution) must be almost *guaranteed* if what is out there in the world is the interpretation we have made (this is a variant on the non-accidentalness constraint). Let us take the example of figure 7.1 to make this intuition clear. If we consider (for argument's sake) only the disparity cue in isolation along with the interpretation S_{3d}, the following is what the likelihood condition says: As the resolution of the disparity measure improves,[5] the actual disparity values we have in the image must become increasingly closer to those that would obtain if the observer was in fact looking at the object that matched the interpretation in question (S_{3d}). Indeed, at the limit of infinite resolution, they must be exactly the same. We can already see that for the picture in figure 7.2, this does not hold. This is because the disparity that would be generated if we had an actual folded object in front of us will not be the same as that which obtains when looking at a flat picture (figure 7.2), regardless of how close to our face we brought it. In other words, the probability $p(I_d \mid S_{3d})$ will not become larger as the resolution of I_d gets better. On the contrary, it will tend to zero. Thus, disparity does not satisfy the likelihood ratio condition under picture viewing and can therefore be considered an "invalid" image measure in the interpretation domain we are interested in, namely, picture perception.

The second criteria, that of a nonzero discrete prior, is an additional constraint. It states that, even if the likelihood condition is met, it must still be the case that the posterior interpretations that we obtain are *generic* in the world in which we are make the inference. It is a requirement that such configurations have to be more common (in the external world being inferred) than in a purely random world. In the case of the picture in figure 7.2, this would be the requirement for a discrete nonzero prior for the folded card interpretation (S_{3d}) configuration. This may take the form of a discrete prior for "rectangular configurations." By a nonzero discrete or delta prior, we imply that, above and beyond the possible existence of all manner of 3D configurations in the world, the visual system assumes that S_{3d}-type configurations have a special status; the probability distribution of all possible 2D and 3D interpretations is continuous, while there is a discrete positive probability mass for S_{3d}-type interpretations (Jepson et al. 1996). In other words, there must be something *special* or *nongeneric* about such configurations. Note that this seems to suggest that the nonzero prior criteria is just an internal assumption regarding the external world *independent* of the cue. However, we discuss later that this criteria also boils down to a statement of the validity of the cue (Richards and Jepson, 1991).

It is unlikely in practical terms to expect the error of sensory measures to tend to zero. Nevertheless, as Richards, Jepson et al. (1991, 1996) explain, for a collection of image measure (such as disparity, texture, etc.) to count as "key features" that can be used to make an interpretation (S), these two conditions must *in theory* hold.

Picture Interpretation under the Modal Priors Formulation
Figure 7.5 shows the likelihood ratios of three primary image measures or cues for the two possible interpretations S_{3d} and S_{2d}. For both interpretations, the likelihood ratio of the pictorial cue (shading) is very high and becomes unbounded as the resolution of the cue gets better. This is because physical configurations consistent with either interpretation will generate brightness values that match those values obtained in the retinal image (we ignore perspective cues here as the image is an orthographic projection, and contains no perspective convergence cues). For binocular disparity and motion parallax cues, however, only the likelihood ratio given S_{2d} becomes unbounded, whereas that given S_{3d} will tend to zero. The actual values of disparity and motion parallax obtained from viewing a flat painted 2D object (S_{2d}) will be the same as that generated by viewing the picture in figure 7.2. But it is unlikely, or rather impossible, that the values of disparity and motion parallax that obtain from viewing a 3D folded object (S_{3d}) will be the same as that from viewing a picture assuming a high enough resolution.

The likelihood ratio of all cues combined (product of likelihoods) will, therefore, tend to be much smaller for the S_{3d} interpretation than for the S_{2d} interpretation.[6] Based on likelihood ratios alone, we should not expect to perceive 3D structure when viewing a 2D reflectance pattern.

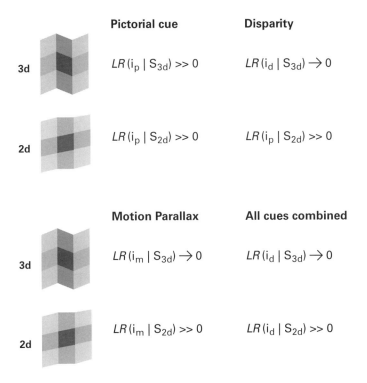

Pictorial cue   **Disparity**

3d $LR(i_p \mid S_{3d}) \gg 0$ $LR(i_d \mid S_{3d}) \rightarrow 0$

2d $LR(i_p \mid S_{2d}) \gg 0$ $LR(i_p \mid S_{2d}) \gg 0$

Motion Parallax   **All cues combined**

3d $LR(i_m \mid S_{3d}) \rightarrow 0$ $LR(i_d \mid S_{3d}) \rightarrow 0$

2d $LR(i_m \mid S_{2d}) \gg 0$ $LR(i_d \mid S_{2d}) \gg 0$

Figure 7.5
Likelihood ratios for three image measure or cues. Note that in this example, "pictorial cue" implies the shading cue, because neither the standard cues of texture or perspective are present in this image. The likelihood ratio for the shading cue will be very large regardless of the interpretation because the shading values we would expect at the retinal image given an actual folded object or a flat pattern of coplanar reflectance would match those in the image of the picture. This is not the case for disparity and motion parallax because the values we would expect from images of a folded 3D object are very different from those obtained from the image of the 2D picture. The "all cues combined" *LR* is simply a product of the other ratios.

What about the prior ratios? A reasonable assumption would be that *no* interpretation should be *a priori* favored by the visual system. We should, therefore, have a continuous prior distribution (possibly uniform) over all possible scene interpretations. For such a distribution, as the resolution of the cues increases, the prior probability support for any particular interpretation diminishes (figure 7.6). In other words, as the possible space of interpretations becomes smaller and tends to a single interpretation, the probability (area under the curve) will also tend to zero. The greater the resolution of the cue, the more specific the interpretation it will support, and thus the smaller the prior probability support for that interpretation. According to Jepson, Richards et al. (1996), given any continuous distribution, no *unique* interpretation of any

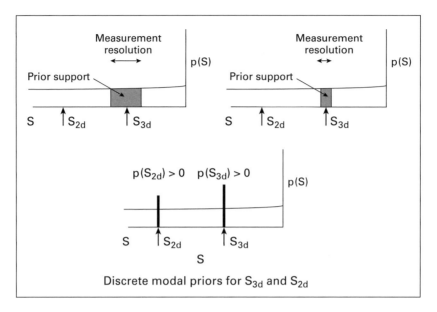

Figure 7.6
Prior distributions for scene structure. (Top left) The graph shows a roughly uniform distribution for all possible scene interpretations in the interpretation space. The shaded region represents the prior probability support for a range of interpretations consistent with the measurements. The larger the range we are willing to consider, the greater the prior ratio. (Top right) As we constrain the possible range of interpretations, e.g., because of the higher resolution of measurements, the prior support for that class of interpretations diminishes. (Bottom) A mixed prior distribution model that also includes discrete probability masses for certain interpretations will have nondiminishing prior support even if we are constrained to that single interpretation. Richards and Jepson suggest that under a Bayesian probabilistic inference model, the interpretation space should be considered to just be a collection of such discrete priors. In other words, the model of the world is already in the observer's head. (Adapted from Richards, Jepson, and Feldman (1996).)

kind is supported due to this diminishing probability. In order for an interpretation to be supported it must have a nonzero discrete probability mass in the prior distribution of possible interpretations, such that its prior probability remains non-diminishing with higher resolution.[7] Such "modes" in the prior distribution are, in essence, the observer's *model* of the world intrinsic to the cue or feature. These modes probabilistically constrain perceptual interpretations to those specified by the cue or feature.

For example, if the visual system had a special preference or expectation for 3D rectangular objects (i.e., parallelism and orthogonality), then we would say that a nonzero discrete probability mass exists for such interpretations in the prior distribution. In that case, the prior ratio for the S_{3d} interpretation will no longer be diminishing as cue resolution gets higher, and the interpretation S_{3d} can be supported. However, by the same argument, if we accept the surface representation models of Adelson and Pentland (1996) and Marr (1982), which claim that the visual system's internal model of surfaces supports coplanar reflectance change (or in Marr's terms, "surface markings"), then we must posit a nonzero discrete probability mode for coplanar reflectance as well; in effect, a nonzero discrete probability mass for the S_{2d} interpretation. We are back to square one: Both prior ratios are now, as required, nondiminishing, but only one of the likelihood ratios is unbounded, the one associated with S_{2d}. All else being equal, S_{2d} should still be the preferred percept. If we don't assume a discrete prior for the S_{2d} interpretation, we would still be left in an ambiguous situation because only one of the conditions is satisfied by each interpretation.[8] But when we look at figure 7.2 there is no ambiguity between 2D and 3D interpretations and no bistability either. The only bistability one might observe is between two possible 3D interpretations that are essentially just variants on the S_{3d} interpretation. As mentioned previously, it is essentially impossible to see the object as a flat painted 2D surface for any sustained period even with effort.

A Coplanarity Prior for Explaining Pictorial Perception

How can we explain the preferred interpretation S_{3d} when we view the picture? One way might be to altogether eliminate S_{2d} from the interpretation space. We can do this if we set the discrete probability mass for the 2D coplanar interpretation (S_{2d}) to be *exactly zero*. Now, when we look at the posterior ratios, S_{2d} will no longer be in contention because it will be zero regardless of the size of the likelihood ratio. *Any* other interpretation with a nonzero posterior ratio, however small, should be favored. This is essentially saying that in "interpreting" 3D surface shape in the presence of coplanar reflectance, the visual system considers disparity (or motion parallax) to be an ineffective or undesirable "feature" (Richards and Jepson, 1991).

Note that this constraint also effectively predicts the percept one sees in the picture shown in figure 7.7. For both objects, the zero prior for coplanar reflectance would predict that the visual system forces a percept of noncoplanarity (even if only infinitesimally). For example, it would imply that the visual system interprets the left object as patches of square whitish surfaces lying infinitesimally separated from an underlying larger dark surface (or vice versa). In the right object, it predicts a percept that is readily perceived; a dark translucent strip lying over another dark strip which together lie on top of (and infinitesimally separated from) a whitish square.[9] In other words, the coplanarity prior would predict that even when the overall interpretation is "flat," the individual patches of different lightness are actually being perceived as separate (if only infinitesimally) from the other patches. This constraint then captures the basic phenomenology of *figure-ground*, where it is essentially impossible to see two adjacent coplanar patches with different lightness as being in the same depth plane.

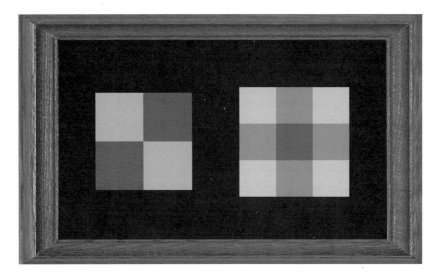

Figure 7.7
Two objects in a picture, both of which appear "flat." The coplanarity prior would imply that, in both cases, surface patches of different lightness are actually perceived to be different surfaces patches that are infinitesimally noncoplanar with adjacent surface patches of different lightness. In the right object, this "scission" into separate surfaces (Anderson and Winawer, 2008) is more apparent, in that one of the dark stripes typically appears as a translucent surface lying on top of the other stripe, although it is ambiguous which one. These examples represent the perception of near coplanarity. Any introduction of shadows and so on to the 2D shape of the objects should make the depth separations between patches more perceptually clear.

Coplanarity Prior and Weighted Cue Combination
Incorporating the coplanarity prior in the weighted averaging framework would result in eliminating the coplanar reflectance interpretations of 3D surface shape indicated by disparity (or other) cues; a similar result to the proposal by Stevens and Brookes (1988) in the case of planar surfaces. However, the prior being proposed here should more correctly be thought of as a co-tangency prior since it does not allow the perception of reflectance patterns regardless of the shape of the underlying surface. Unlike the Stevens and Brookes proposal, it predicts that a pictorial interpretation of 3D surface shape will obtain even for smoothly curving surfaces.

Summary
In trying to find a solution to explaining pictorial depth in the Bayesian inference/ cue-combination approaches, we have arrived at a proposal that corresponds to proposition 2 in the Introduction; namely, that in the interpretation space of 3D surface shape, surfaces do not have, as a property, coplanar reflectance patterns (surface

markings) as traditionally suggested (Adelson and Pentland, 1996; Marr, 1982). The significant difference between the original proposition and the inference-based formulation we have arrived at is that, in the latter, the coplanarity constraint is an assumption that the visual system makes about an *objective external world*. For the purposes of probabilistic inferential models, this assumption is fine (and it works) because such models are essentially naïve realist, externalist models whose main efficacy is in assessing sensorimotor calibration.

However, the proposition in the introduction is actually stronger. It is not that the visual system makes assumptions about, or has an internal model of, the external world. Rather, it is a consequence of the nature of *perceptual surfaces*. The intrinsic property of perceptual surfaces is that perceived lightness change *is* a presentation of change in the identity of surfaces. In other words, the fact that we see depth in pictures is not because we have internalized a model of the world, one in which surfaces have no coplanar patterns (implausible given that coplanar patterns are ubiquitous in the natural world). Rather, it is because of the intrinsic link between lightness and surface identity. The ubiquity of camouflage suggests that animals do not see reflectance change as such either.

The way in which we cognize, attribute, and catalogue surfaces (including pictures) in the external world is determined by *perceptual surfaces* and not the other way around. Although this analysis suggests a new understanding of the relationship between the perception of 3D surface shape and lightness, and the basis for perceiving pictorial depth, it still leaves open the second major puzzle we described in the Introduction: Why are there vivid *qualitative* differences between the experience of pictorial and real depth perception, if the same perceptual mechanisms give rise to them?

Relative and Absolute (Egocentric) Depth in Pictures and Real Scenes

I briefly mentioned in the previous section some significant data on pictorial depth perception (Koenderink et al., 1992, 1994, 2003) that appear to support the idea that perceived depth varies as a function of conflict among depth cues (consistent with the cue-combination framework). But, I also pointed out some observations that complicate such interpretations of those data. I deliberately avoided discussing these studies in more detail because the results and analysis that these researchers report have important implications for linking the two problems posed at the outset of this chapter: Why we perceive depth in pictures and why pictorial depth appears so qualitatively different from real binocular depth.

These studies examined how surface shape judgments in pictures are modulated by different viewing conditions (monocular or binocular) and different psychophysical tasks. Surface shape judgments were obtained for predefined locations on the object surface. These locations represented a tessellation of the object surface into local (triangular) surface patches. Judgments included simple depth comparisons among patch locations (ordinal judgment), judging the aspect of local surface patches using a "gauge figure," and estimates of surface cross-section (magnitude estimation of depth relief of predefined sets of points on the surface). Global perceived surface shape for the object was then obtained by interpolating these local values to obtain a depth map representing a response surface. One of the findings of these studies is the large inter-subject and intertask differences in estimated depth relief, indicating that observers may not have access to unambiguous veridical depth information, and that depth ambiguity is resolved specific to the observer and task. Yet a significant outcome was that once *absolute and relative* metrics are discounted (by making depth scaling and affine distortion free parameters), correlation in surface shape judgements between tasks, and among observers, was extremely high (Koenderink et al., 1992, 1994, 2003). Their results provide compelling evidence that pictorial images can generate consistent percepts of 3D surface layout and suggest that perceived 3D surface shape is consistent across various viewing conditions and observers *up to* some simple transformation such as viewpoint or depth scaling.

Specifically relevant to the immediate discussion, the overall 3D surface shape judgments under binocular viewing of 2D pictures showed significant reduction in depth scaling compared with monocular viewing of the pictures or simulated stereoscopic versions of such pictures (Doorschot et al., 2001; Koenderink et al., 1994). These studies found that the 3D configuration derived from local slant judgments (gauge figure task) was indeed significantly "flatter" when disparity information specified the flat picture surface. For example, figure 7.8 (right panels) shows depth relief judg-

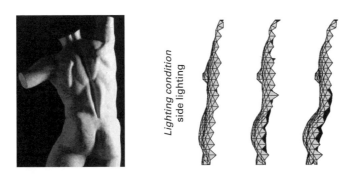

Figure 7.8
Photo on the left indicates the stimulus tested for depth relief judgments. The figures on the right are, respectively, response surface obtained for binocular viewing with stereo base 0 cm (equivalent to binocular viewing of the picture, disparity consistent with a flat surface), base pair 7 cm (disparity consistent with pictorial relief), and base pair 14 cm (disparity exaggerating depth relief) (from Doorschot et al., 2001).

ments obtained for photographs of a real 3D object taken with different disparity bases, where base zero corresponds to "a disparity field with zero depth" (i.e., the same as when viewing a picture; leftmost response surface). Similar results were obtained for a photo of a torso done under binocular, monocular, and synoptic viewing conditions. Taken together, they appear to indicate that conflicting disparity information (as is present in pictures) leads to a reduction in depth relief implied in the judgment of 3D surface shape. Judged depth relief decreases in the following order: (1) binocular viewing of stimuli with consistent disparity information (viewing a real object), (2) monocular viewing of a picture (pictorial cues only, no conflicting disparity information), and (3) binocular viewing with disparity consistent with a flat surface (viewing a picture with two eyes). These results appear to support the idea that disparity information in viewing pictures significantly affects perceived surface layout and relative depth and, therefore, may be viewed as supportive of the probabilistic cue-combination prediction for picture perception. Specifically, it suggests that disparity information leads to a *flattening* of perceived surface layout and depth relief, consistent with the role of disparity in estimating depth. I suggest that there is an alternative interpretation of the results which has a fundamental implication regarding the distinction between *perceived 3D surface layout* and *perceived egocentric (absolute) depth*.

Pictorial Shape and Relative Depth

When we look at figure 7.2, it is clear that the object appears bent with dihedral angles close to 90°.[10] Closing an eye does not appreciably change the overall shape of the perceived object or perceived angles. Viewing the image from a closer or more distant vantage point does not appear to change its perceived shape noticeably either, although the reliability of binocular disparity increases with reducing viewing distance, predicting a flattening at closer distances.[11] Similarly, looking at the image of the torsos (figure 7.8), the perceived 3D surface shape or layout does not seem to change when closing one eye. Most significantly, the depth relief judgments obtained in the experiment in the binocular picture-viewing condition (leftmost response surface) imply a 3D surface shape that seems clearly less than what is naturally perceived in the picture (even with two eyes). If anything, the response surfaces representing disparity consistent with a real object or exaggerated disparity (the rightmost surfaces) appear closest to a correct depiction of the percept of the object in the photo. Indeed, we routinely see pictures of objects we have never seen before and in the subsequent encounter with the real object, we seldom notice any significant difference in depth scaling (i.e., we do not have the impression that objects appear considerably flatter [or sheared] in pictures than they do in real life [apart from possible distortion due to projective parameters used to construct the picture; e.g., wide angle distortion, keystone effects; see Pirenne, 1970; Vishwanath et al., 2005]). Moreover, we can all agree on whether a depiction of a 3D object matches the real 3D object—precisely what separates good drawings from not so good ones! Such judgments do not seem to depend significantly on whether the depiction is viewed with one eye or both.[12] If binocular viewing of pictures did create perceived depth compression or shape distortions in objects, we would not rely on pictures so much because they would not provide a generally true perception of 3D object/surface shape (we are quite sensitive to distortions, typically in the range of 5% change of an object dimension [Vishwanath et al., 2005]).

Pictorial Space and Egocentric (Absolute) Depth

To what can we attribute the psychophysically measured differences in the studies just described? The answer to this question, I believe, lies in proposition 3 in the Introduction; namely, that relative depth and absolute (egocentric) depth are separate dissociable perceptual constructs, both phenomenally and psychophysically. By relative depth, I imply that an observer has an understanding of *metric* relative depth relations within and among objects, including 3D surface shape, slant, depth order, and so on, all of which imply an understanding of the *ratios* of distances or depths among points in the visual field (e.g., knowing that in figure 7.1, the depth separation between the left and center dot on the hedge is greater—and how much greater—than that between the right and center dot). Note that this definition also includes what the cited studies imply by *depth relief*. In other words, the depth reliefs of surface shape indicated by, say, the left and center response surfaces in figure 8, would imply different percepts of relative depth even if we can find a linear transformation that can equate the two.

On the other hand, *egocentric depth* implies that the observer has knowledge of the depth relations scaled in some meaningful way to the actions of the observer. Note that this neither implies knowledge in terms of some "objective" units (there are none) nor does it imply objective knowledge or measures of the "real objects" in the "external world"; in other words, absolute depth is not about a naïve sense of "veridicality" (see also Koenderink and van Doorn, 2003). Rather, what is correctly implied by absolute depth is an internal perceptual estimate of a spatial parameter in terms of the consequences of potential motor actions (that the observer can carry out in the visual field of its operation). For example, I have a precise perceptual estimate of the absolute distance of the monitor I am looking at, not because there is encoded in my brain some number that matches physical reality (say, 28.4 cm), but rather, that I have a precise and accurate estimate of the consequences of my actions, such as reaching out to it.[13]

There is already sufficient reason to believe that relative and absolute depth representation has to be different from a cue-combination standpoint. This is because depth cues generally only provide relative depth information, and this information has to be scaled by egocentric distance information to derive absolute depth. If our perception of relative depth (3D surface shape, slant, depth order) is distinct and phenomenally separate from our perception of absolute depth, then it is plausible to think that perceptual tasks used to measure 3D surface shape or depth will selectively access one type of depth encoding over another. The fact that different depth measurement tasks may access different aspects of perceived depth is one of the important points raised by Koenderink and van Doorn (2003) as well as other authors (e.g., Glennerster et al., 1996).

What I propose here is that the specific *local judgment* tasks that were used in these studies likely depended on the availability and reliability of perceptual estimates of egocentrically scaled depth (absolute depth), and that such estimates are dependent on the concurrence of different sensory signals as predicted by cue-combination models. Importantly, this access to absolute depth information depends on perceptual access to *egocentric distance*. Although the tasks appear to be testing *perceived 3D surface shape,* it is possible that the results (changes in relief across conditions) are actually indicative of the change in perceptual access to absolute depth relations required to do the local magnitude estimation. This perceptual access appears to be affected by the internal consistency of sensory signals to depth and distance and should vary across observers. The more ambiguous the access to absolute metric depth becomes, the greater the regression of simple *local* quantitative magnitude estimates to the frontal plane and the flatter the overall depth relief implied by those local judgments. Analogously, if we probed *local* surface aspect judgments for the object in the picture in figure 7.2 (under binocular viewing), we might find the same pattern of results. The surface depth relief reconstructed from local aspect judgments should appear to be significantly "flatter" than the overall object we clearly see when we look into the picture. It will also likely be flatter than the depth relief derived from the same task under monocular viewing of the picture, or viewing of an identical "real" object.

Pictorial Space and the Distinction between Relative and Absolute (Egocentric) Depth

The results of the Koenderink et al. studies (1992, 1994, 2003) suggests that, although pictorial relief is consistent across observers, depth scaling of this relief differs in idiosyncratic ways among observers and viewing condition up to an affine transformation. This could be taken to imply that relative depth relations (3D surface shape) perceived among observers and among viewing conditions (within an observer) are idiosyncratic and potentially significantly different. The distinction I make here is different in the following way.

I suggest that the percept of relative depth (3D surface shape, slant, layout) when viewing a picture (monocularly or binocularly) is *more or less veridical* in normal picture viewing, although it may not be *metrical in the absolute sense.* What do I mean by veridical? I mean that for any given normal observer, what he or she perceives as the depicted 3D surface layout (relative depth) in a picture is *more or less* the same 3D surface layout he or she would see when looking at the real object with both eyes[14]. For example, the surface layout and relative depth relations perceived for the object depicted in figure 7.2 should appear relatively unchanged compared with what is perceived when looking at the actual "real" object. Similarly, the percept of a real object under monocular viewing should also be veridical (in the relative sense) because the 3D surface shape or layout perceived remains unchanged in important ways when one opens the second eye. What appears different among these cases is the percept of absolute depth. In pictorial space, we have no real sense of absolute depth because we have no sensory information of absolute distance. Distance signals such as vergence, accommodation and so on, specify distance of the picture surface and not its pictorial contents. The only distance information available is that afforded by familiar objects in the scene. Evidence thus far suggests that familiar size does not operate as a normal visual cue (Predebon, 1993).

In other words, observers' percepts of "veridical" relative metric depth information *mostly* obtains regardless of whether the domain is pictorial[15] or real objects, and appears to depend primarily on aspects of the perceptual presentation that have to do with pictorial information. It is only the perception of egocentrically scaled metric depth that appears to vary significantly depending on the viewing conditions and coherence of signals (all else being equal).[16] What I propose is that the tasks used in the experiments described are possibly measuring *some* aspect of the perception of absolute depth. Because absolute depth is by definition a *calibrated* quantity, we should find that judgments vary depending on the co-calibration of sensory information (e.g., binocular vs. monocular retinal signals), as well as the reliability of that calibration; a calibration that cue-combination models correctly predict has to be statistically optimal.

This brings us to a point where we can finally answer the second crucial question: "Why does pictorial depth appear so qualitatively different from real stereoscopic depth?" The answer lies in proposition 4, that this qualitative difference, a.k.a "the plastic effect," (Ames, 1925; Schlosberg, 1941) is in fact the perceptual presentation of the reliability or precision of internal estimates of absolute depth. We now look at evidence that supports this proposition. So as not to belabor the analysis, I revert to using standard terminology about "depth cues," "distance information," and so on, as used in cue-combination models.

Depth Appearance and the "Plastic Effect"

A standard understanding of the plastic effect is that it is a purely nonfunctional epiphenomenon (quale) of binocular depth processing (see Koenderink, 1998, for a historical analysis of this misplaced belief). There have been no formal investigations to support this assertion, but one basic observation disputes it: Controlled monocular viewing of 2D pictures shows evidence of the plastic effect (Ames, 1925; Judge, 1925; Koenderink, 1988; Schlosberg, 1941). This can be demonstrated by viewing a high-resolution photographic image (figure 7.1 or 7.3) through a small oval aperture (1–2 cm diameter[17]) that occludes the picture frame while holding the head steady. Under such viewing conditions, observers spontaneously report essentially the same qualities used to describe stereoscopic viewing of real 3D objects or simulated stereoscopic images.

To explain this observation, Ames (1925) suggested that the perception of the plastic effect was based on the relative conflict among depth and distance cues. This theory is based on the fact that the plastic effect is perceived under binocular viewing of real scenes or monocular aperture viewing of pictures where there is *no conflict* in the depth cues available. This is in contrast to the binocular viewing of pictures, where there is clear conflict between the cues specifying the flat picture surface and those specifying the pictorial 3D scene (see table 7.1).

However, this theory does not explain a range of other observations. For example, the plastic effect appears to diminish with viewing distance under *binocular* viewing of real scenes, although conflict among cues does not change with viewing distance under these conditions. This can be easily demonstrated by going outdoors to a location that affords visible objects ranging in distance from less than a meter to more than several hundred meters, as well as an unobstructed view of more distant objects beyond (in so-called vista space). When one compares the difference in "plasticity" between monocular and binocular viewing for successively farther object clusters, the differences appear quite marked at near distances but diminish with increasing distance and are essentially absent in vista space beyond.[18] This occurs despite any changes in cue conflict. In fact, observers comment on how distant landscapes often appear "pictorial." Widespread empirical evidence indicates that the reliability of various sources of egocentric distance information (vergence, accommodation, disparity) reduces with increasing distance, which suggests a link between the reduction of the plastic effect and the reduction in reliability of egocentric distance information; and, in turn, the reliability of absolute depth estimates that rely on distance estimates.

The Plastic Effect under Monocular Viewing and Apparent Micropsia

Another crucial observation (one that appears not to have been previously reported) is that when a picture is viewed monocularly through an aperture, the evident plastic effect is also accompanied by changes in perceived size and distance; things appear closer and smaller than they do under normal binocular viewing (see figures 7.1 and 7.3). This too suggests an effect of change in perceived egocentric distance, but why would such an effect occur? Under binocular viewing of a picture, all sensory information related to estimates of distance (accommodation, vergence, blur) specify the distance to the visible picture surface, and, thus, depth within pictorial space remains unscaled. When visual access of the picture surface is eliminated by viewing monocularly through an aperture, any remaining distance cue (e.g. accommodation) would have to accrue to the only perceptually available surfaces (the pictorial objects). In other words, this could be some form of accommodation-related micropsia (Hollins, 1976; McReady, 1965) of pictorial contents. Note that based on this explanation, if we continue to view the picture with one eye but take away the aperture so that the frame and the context of the display is visible, the picture surface is again perceptible, and accommodation-based distance information should accrue correctly once again to the picture surface. We should therefore expect the plastic effect and the micropsia effect to diminish, which is indeed what appears to happen (figures 7.1 and 7.3).

The Plastic Effect and the Retinal Blur Gradient

The previous observations support the idea that the plastic effect appears to depend on the availability of distance information required to scale perceived relative depth to obtain absolute depth. If this is true, we can make an unusual prediction. If it is possible to introduce reliable egocentric distance information into pictorial space even under binocular viewing (where the picture surface *is* visible), we should predict that egocentric scaling of pictorial space can occur and the plastic effect might obtain. Our recent results have confirmed that retinal blur gradients are a robust source of distance information and that the blur gradient operates in quantitative way; where perceived distance varies with the magnitude of blur, as well as the availability and reliability of other sources of distance information such as vergence and accommodation (Vishwanath, 2007, 2008). We have found that the distance perceived in images of natural textures without blur gradients appear up to five times more distant compared with the same image with a simulated blur gradient (see figure 7.9).

Consistent with our prediction, pictorial images with a simulated blur gradient are anecdotally reported by naive observers to have heightened plastic quality compared with similar no-blur images; even under binocular viewing where there is conflict between disparity and monocular cues. This can be seen by comparing the images in figure 7.10. This observation provides further support that the plastic effect is linked to egocentric distance information and, in turn, to the reliability of absolute depth perception. Interestingly, the effect of blur gradients and monocular aperture viewing are similar, showing a distance, scaling, and plastic effect (compare the images in figure 7.11). (The miniaturization that is seen in the blurred version is also apparent under monocular viewing of the unblurred image.)

Realism, Absolute Depth, and Egocentric Distance

The fact that the plastic effect may be linked to perceptual estimates of egocentrically scaled depth relations makes imminent sense. The plastic effect is in essence the qualitative perceptual experience that makes objects appear "real," "touchable" or "graspable" and where one feels a visual "immersion" and "embodiment" in space. Each of these experiences is crucially linked to the vivid sense that we can successfully interact and manipulate things in the visual field through motor action. Successful motor in-

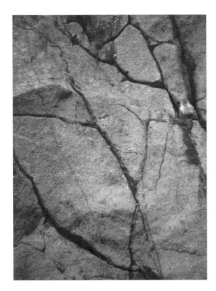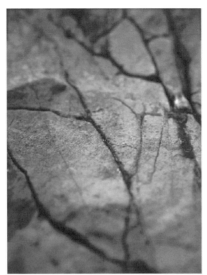

Figure 7.9
Photograph of a rock face with and without a simulated vertical blur gradient. Right image looks significantly closer.

teraction has a singular prerequisite: reliable egocentrically defined perceptual estimates of spatial properties such as direction, size, distance, and absolute depth. Although direction is precisely given in the "local signs" of the retina, the other spatial estimates will depend crucially on the availability, consistency, and reliability of sensory information for egocentric distance. Thus, we should expect the terms that describe the plastic effect, such as "realism," (Michotte, 1991) "immersion," "touchable and graspable," and "embodiment," to vary as a function of this information.

Because reliability of absolute depth estimates depends on both relative depth information and the information on egocentric distance, the theory would predict that there would be two ends of the scale of the qualitative magnitude of the plastic effect. The highest possible level of the plastic effect should be seen at near viewing distances under binocular viewing and self-motion. There should be a complete absence of the plastic effect in the binocular viewing of pictures (without intrinsic blur gradients). In all other conditions, the degree of the plastic effect will depend (in real scenes and pictures) on whether there in self-motion, how distant the objects are, whether viewing is monocular or binocular, and so on.

Disparity and motion parallax signals should give rise to the plastic effect regardless of the "correctness" of the distance information as long as the distance information is relatively reliable. To see depth from disparity, these signals have to be scaled with

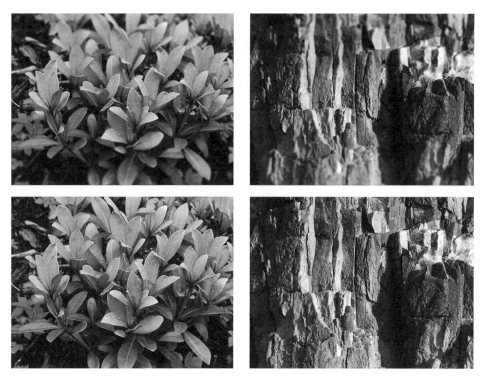

Figure 7.10
Photographs of a plant and a rock face with and without a simulated vertical blur gradient. Observers report a heightened plastic effect for the leaves in the central region in the blurred version, and for the ridges and clefts of the rock face (best seen in full-screen mode).

whatever distance information is available, correct, or incorrect. It is only when such information is entirely unreliable that no plastic effect is seen. In the case of motion parallax, this can be readily observed when looking out of the window of a moving vehicle; the plastic effect is clearly apparent within nearer distances, but far objects appear to "slide past" each other in an apparent lack of phenomenal separation. Thus, the plastic effect appears independent of the *accuracy* of absolute depth or distance information in any *objective* sense.

Moreover, the theory implies that the very aspect of depth perception that makes things appear "real" (the plastic effect) is actually based on the value of an internal *subjective* quality. Reliability of perceptual estimates, as described here, has nothing to do with the "real world" but is a purely internal construct about how well the perceptual presentation of visual surfaces predicts the success of any imminent motor action.

The theory and analysis here suggests, intriguingly, that the local depth judgment tasks used in previous studies (Koenderink et al., 1992, 1994) might be used as a

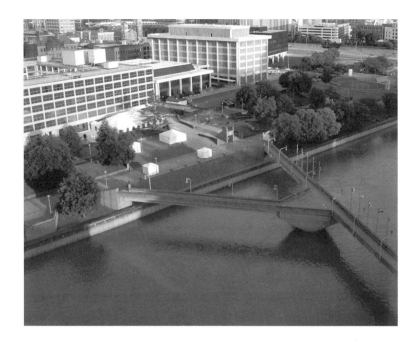

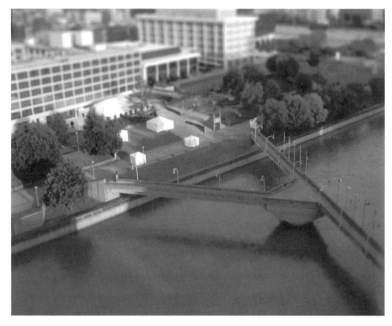

Figure 7.11
Photograph of a city scene with and without blur gradients. The blurred image demonstrates the so-called tilt-shift miniaturization effect, which was discovered by photo artists and was the first evidence of the potential role of blur in distance perception. Viewing the nonblurred image with one eye through an aperture (1–2 cm) results in a similar scaling/miniaturization effect. A heightened plastic effect is typically reported in both cases.

measure of the plastic effect. The fact that the depth reliefs obtained in those studies were highest precisely for those conditions in which the authors informally reported a heightened plastic effect, e.g., synoptic viewing, (Koenderink et al., 1994) appears to support this. The crucial test will be to measure depth judgments for real objects and pictures of objects using the same tasks but systematically varying the availability and reliability of distance information (e.g., by changing viewing distance). We are currently conducting these studies.

Duality of Pictorial and Real Depth

The fact that the plastic effect appears dissociable from the perception of 3D surface structure further supports the notion that there are two ways in which we can experience depth. But the distinction appears to not be between pictorial and real space, but rather, between relative and egocentrically scaled depth; the latter which can be reliably present or absent in pictures and real scenes depending on the available egocentric distance information.

In pictures, individual surfaces seem vividly distinct from the supporting surface and unambiguously arrayed before us. Even the various buttons, windows, toggles, and so on, that I am looking at on my computer monitor seem clearly identifiable as different surfaces at different depths; what seems a little less distinct is the actual metric difference in depth between them. It is only when we wilfully neglect attending to the reflectance patterns on the surface, such as when we pick up a picture, that we may become unaware of changes in pictorial 3D surface identity and attitude (Mausfeld, 2003).

The previous analysis suggests that a standard inferential cue-combination model of surface perception that assumes a representation of a metric surface geometry and a pattern of reflectance (e.g., Adelson and Pentland, 1996; Marr, 1982) will find it difficult to explain both the quantitative outcome and qualitative phenomena underlying the perception of depth in pictures. Two important notions have been suggested to build a more comprehensive model of surface representation and depth perception, under which probabilistic inferential models of depth perception may be subsumed.

The first is the proposal that perceptual surfaces do not have, *as a property*, reflectance patterns (a.k.a. surface markings). Rather, reflectance change—or, more correctly, lightness change—is the perceptual marker of change in surface identity. Indeed, change in surface identity can be perceived even in the absence of change in physical reflectance (e.g., Kanizsa Triangle, Kanizsa, 1979). Interestingly, difference in lightness in this case is perceived simultaneously with the perception of these illusory surfaces, where the illusory surface for example appears brighter than the background despite the fact that they are supported on identical physical reflectance backgrounds. These observations suggest that surfaces are truly internally generated and are not simple inferences to external "surfaces" with different reflectance patterns; and that perceived lightness change is primarily a phenomenological property of the *presentation* of these internally generated surfaces. This idea also finds some sympathy in work that has championed an early encoding of surfaces in the visual stream (Nakayama, He, and Shimojo, 1995) and the primary role of surface decomposition in lightness effects (Anderson and Winawer, 2008).

The idea of surfaces as internally generated and lacking the property of coplanar patterns may be made compatible with probabilistic inferential approaches to depth perception by assuming that *the prior for coplanar reflectance change and coplanar surfaces is zero*. To extend this notion to the MLE/cue-combination approach, we would need to configure the definition of the disparity and motion parallax cue such that they have embedded priors that do not allow the inference of coplanar surfaces, similar in vein to how the texture cue has embedded priors regarding the uniformity of texture patterns or, for example, that the perspective cue has embedded priors regarding parallelism of lines. Models based on such cues and priors (including the coplanarity prior) do not provide a model for the "recovery of 3D surface shape." Rather, their domain of application is in evaluating the calibration of the perception of 3D surface shape with stimulus measures (see below), including the calibration and reliability of estimates of egocentric distance.

The evaluation of the calibration of perceived egocentrically scaled depth will likely have to be modelled separately from that of relative depth or 3D surface shape within cue-combination regimes. Such a model—to predict the variability of estimates of absolute depth—will likely involve combining all depth and distance cues, regardless of the nature of the surface layout. This model should also directly predict under what viewing and stimulus conditions we will perceive plastic depth.

What Is a Surface?

If the perception of surfaces cannot be considered an inference to objective surfaces that exist out there in the real world, then what is a surface?

Our "objective," naïve-realist, definition of a surface might be that surfaces are "smoothish" things with a particular geometry and reflectance pattern and usually constitute the boundary of objects. More sophisticated physical theories might say that surfaces are the interface between phase changes in matter. Under an inverse-optics cue-based model, perceptual surfaces are then an inference to these real surfaces. The real surface's existence in the world is established via measurements of their geometry (depth, slant, curvature, etc.) and perhaps a measurement of their reflectance function. The information contained in the perceptually inferred surface (under a naïve-realist model) is parasitic on this "real" measurement-based definition of external surfaces.

Yet we are able to perceive 3D surface layout in the absence of consistent metric information (pictures) and appear to identify unique, oriented surfaces when there are none (pictures). More important, our percepts of surfaces are not exhausted merely by the definition of their geometry and reflectance. What we see is a vivid, smoothish, colored entity, rather than a collection of measurements and reflectance values. We are able to make perceptual-motor measurements of these smoothish, colored things at will (by touching, moving, etc.), and nothing constrains what type of, or how many such, measurements we may choose to make. In other words, *a perceptual surface is never informationally exhausted by any set of psychophysical measures we may use to define it.*

More important, such measures do not capture the most perceptually immediate property of surfaces, their *continuity*. In inferential models, continuity is absorbed into the regularity assumptions (e.g., standard AI-style smoothness constraints) or by the fiat definition of cues (e.g., texture is assumed to be generated from a single continuous surface). In other words, in inferential models, the information content (smoothness/continuity) resides in the inferential machinery rather than in the percept itself (Vishwanath, 2005). The percept is reduced to the actual measures (location and direction of points in space) and higher order geometrical constructs derived from them (such as curvature, slant, etc.) (Mausfeld, 2003; Vishwanath, 2005). But when we look out into the world (or into pictures), we don't "see" a discrete series of points, nor do we "see" numbers representing curvature, distance, reflectance, or what have you. What we see are vivid, smoothish, colored entities, *from which* we can define certain psychophysical measures such as slant, distance, and so on. In other words, the external measures (cues) are the ones that are parasitic on the perceived smoothish entity we call a surface not vice versa (Vishwanath, 2005).

Perceptual Surface as Motor Plan
Thus, a surface in perception is not a mere collection of geometric, electromagnetic, or neural measures, nor is it an inference to a geometry and reflectance pattern in the external world. Rather, a surface is a peculiar informational structure that shapes the sensory flux into something most likely to be captured by the following definitions:

- Surface structure is the presentation of a complex motor plan.
- Lightness is the perceptual presentation of surface identity.

We see continuity and smoothness when presented with this information structure because that perceived smoothness is the signature of the potentiality for a continuous motor act. In other words, the table surface in front of me appears smooth because smoothness is the perceptual indicator that I can run my finger along the entity without interruption. Wherever I see a sudden change in lightness, it is an indicator that my continuous motor action will be interrupted. It is not—as far as the brain is concerned—*primarily* a signal indicating change in reflectance. The notion of reflectance is more likely a cognitive construct—part of our higher order cognitive ontology of the external world (Vishwanath, 2006).

Naturally, I can test the validity of this "presentation" of a complex motor plan (perceived surface) via precisely such motor action. In the preponderance of situations, my motor actions and sense of touch calibrate with the presented plan, and I declare my perception to be veridical. In other situations, the presentation and action do not calibrate (e.g., a picture), and I declare it to be an illusion. In still other situations, I can artificially *extend* my mode of motor measurement by using sophisticated devices such as tape measures, laser range finders, time-of-flight devices, or what have you, and I then declare that the motor plan (perceived surface) is metrically *biased* in some way for large distances, for high slants, or what have you (distance and slant most correctly defined, by the way, in terms of this motor presentation). Conveniently, my perceptual system has given me a way of being implicitly weary of putting all faith in the 3D presentation before me: by modulating the perceived plastic quality of that 3D presentation.

As mentioned in the Introduction, this idea of surfaces as a motor plan is not consistent with models that assume that perception is the encoding of sensorimotor contingency (Gibson, enactive perception) because such models need to assume an objective structure external to the observer to which the sensorimotor contingencies have to calibrate. Here, instead, is proposed an entirely internal perceptual structure that presents the possibility for action and whose metrics can be calibrated by motor action. Thus, it is not the contingencies that are perceived but a perceptual object that may have associated qualities related to sensorimotor contingency (the plastic effect).

Surfaces and Inference

Inferential models of perception are not designed to understand the nature of surfaces at this level of description. Inferential models are designed to examine the nature of metric calibration of the plan with motor and *extended* motor measures, perhaps to uncover potential metric biases in that calibration. This assessment of calibration requires the fiat definition of modes of motor or extended motor measurements, otherwise known as *cues*. Naturally, because these cues are defined by fiat within an inverse-optics framework, it is neither useful not coherent to say that the visual system "recovers" surfaces using such cues (Mausfeld, 2003; Vishwanath, 2005). Nevertheless, quantitatively probing the motor plan (perceived surface) to examine sensory and motor co-calibration (the domain par excellence of cue-combination approaches) is essential—essential as a diagnostic of when the plan is deficient, to provide hints to the underlying informational structure of the plan, and to begin to map out the related neural signatures. More generally, identifying breakdowns in co-calibration not only helps refine a previously established cue or inferential framework but it also provides hints for a richer understanding, and more viable theory, of the information content of perception.

Conclusion

An analysis of the primary effect of picture perception suggests the limitations of models of visual perception based on an inverse-optics cue-based conceptualization of perception: They reduce the information contained in visual perception to essentially metric estimates of distance and direction whose important and primary relevance is limited to the assessment of the co-calibration of the sensorimotor system. Although such assessment is essential for various areas such as physiological optics, diagnosis of defects in the visual and motor apparatus, and, to some degree, the mapping of neural pathways and specificity, the analysis here suggests that they do not on their own provide a theory or framework for understanding how external stimulation is converted into the perceptual reality that we see. I have proposed that the core quantitative aspect of cues—statistical reliability—appears in itself to be *qualitatively* expressed in perception.

Development of a more realistic framework of other aspects of information structure of surface and depth perception will likely show most promise in light of theories that have taken *non-metric* informational content and semantics as central to a computational description. For example, the notion of surfaces as a motor plan appears to be most readily subsumed under Leyton's symmetry-based group theoretic construct, where shape, most generally construed, is considered a nested machine and where the causal information content is embedded in the definition of this nested machine as successively more symmetric states (Leyton, 1992, 2001).

Notes

1. Some readers might object, saying that there are available "non-accidentalness" cues or "rectangularity/orthogonality" cues. However, these are not strictly depth cues, since they are not measures on the image, but assumptions (priors) underlying depth cues (e.g. perspective foreshortening) and their interpretation.

2. Note that precision is not dependent in any way on the accuracy or "veridicality" of absolute depth.

3. An alternative approach to cue combination is the intrinsic constraint model for depth perception (Tassinari, Domini, and Caudek, 2008). This approach, in contrast to the others, does not see depth perception as the recovery of veridical depth structure, but rather considers perceived depth magnitude in terms of subjective reliabilities where depth cues are considered to be strongly interdependent.

4. The term "image" or "I" refers generically to the retinal image or, more specifically, the retinal image construed as a collection of image measures, such as luminance, disparity, texture, motion parallax, and so on, also referred to as "cues."

5. Disparity resolution gets better at nearer viewing distances, so it would be equivalent to bringing the picture closer to the eyes.

6. In figure 7.3, the product of likelihoods $LR(I|S_{3d})$ is indicated to be diminishing as resolution becomes better. Although actual geometric analysis is not presented here, analogous to Jepson's and Richards' (1991) approach, the product of likelihoods is expected to have at least a squared error term in the numerator, which will tend to zero as error becomes small (high resolution).

7. Note that Jepson, Richards, et al. establish the nonzero prior criteria by looking specifically at the measurement space for the type of interpretation in question (e.g., co-location, motion or rest, etc.) and how the specific ratios behave as the error (e) of measurement becomes smaller (cue resolution gets better). Readers are directed to those articles for a better understanding of the derivation of the criteria.

8. One might argue that, in such a scenario, a full computational analysis of the cues involved would perhaps show that the S_{3d} interpretation prevails. In a sense, such an argument is moot because the thrust of Jepson and Richards' argument is essentially that neither percept should prevail if each is unable to satisfy the required criteria. The assumption that surfaces have a property called reflectance change is, however, a strong claim that should under this formulation stipulate a nonzero modal prior for coplanar reflectance interpretations.

9. In the lightness perception literature, this separation into surfaces of different lightness and/or translucency has been referred to as "layered representations" or "scission" (Anderson & Winawer, 2008). While this work is generally relevant to the issue regarding the link between lightness and surface identity, Anderson & collaborators work is primarily aimed at understanding how lightness and lightness constancy is affected by surface decomposition.

10. In one of the two possible 3D interpretations, the folded object appears to be standing upright. In the other interpretation it appears as a folded object lying down and the angles appears to be about 120°.

11. Note that there may be bistability between two possible 3D percepts (see previous note), but I focus on the predominant one here for ease of description.

12. The fact that an artist might close one eye when creating the depiction is a different issue related to what we discuss later in the chapter.

13. Direct realists please beware that this does not imply a Gibsonian or "Enactive" view. It is only related to them insofar as such perceptual encoding (absolute or relative depth) is *calibrated* by the actual contingencies experienced by the observer over time.

14. There may of course be idiosyncrasies across observers based on visual dysfunction, or other factors, as suggested by the Koenderink et al. (1992, 1994, 2003) data.

15. A "rich" picture such as a photograph (i.e., one providing the same pictorial information as the real objects) is assumed here.

16. I am not implying that relative depth judgments such as slant are not affected by the availability and reliability of monocular information to 3D shape. I am only suggesting that when all such information is equivalent, there may be little difference in perceived relative depth relations among different viewing conditions. Moreover, actual psychophysical measurement may indeed reveal a small effect of viewing conditions on relative depth judgments because there is no reason to believe the two representations are entirely independent.

17. The effect is best seen with the image shown on a full screen. Note the use of an aperture and not a pinhole.

18. This occurs even if one informally considers clusters of objects such that their depth dimension scales with viewing distance (D) or with scaling of disparity (D^2).

References

Adelson, E. H., and Pentland, A. P. 1996. "The Perception of Shading and Reflectance." In *Perception as Bayesian Inference*, edited by D. Knill and W. Richards. New York: Cambridge University Press. 409–423.

Albertazzi, L. (Ed.). 1998. *Shapes of Form: From Gestalt Psychology to Phenomenology, Ontology and Mathematics*. Dordrecht: Kluwer.

Ames, A. 1925. "The Illusion of Depth in Pictures." *Journal of the Optical Society of America* 10: 137–148

Anderson, B. L., and Winawer, J. 2008. "Layered Image Representations and the Computation of Surface Lightness." *Journal of Vision* 8 (7): 1–22.

Battu, B., Kappers, A. M. L., and Koenderink, J. J. 2007. "Ambiguity in Pictorial Depth." *Perception* 36: 1290–1304.

Buckley, D., and Frisby, J. P. (1993). "Interaction of stereo, texture and outline cues in the shape perception of three-dimensional ridges." *Vision Research* 33: 919–933.

Bülthoff, H. H., and Mallot, H. A. 1988. *Journal of the Optical Society of America A* 5: 1749–1758.

Clark, J. J., and Yuille, A. L. 1990. *Data Fusion for Sensory Information Processing Systems*. Dordrecht: Kluwer.

Cutting, J. E. (2003). "Reconceiving Perceptual Space." In *Looking Into Pictures: An Interdisciplinary Approach to Pictorial Space*, edited by H. Hecht, R. Schwartz, and M. Atherton. Cambridge, MA: MIT Press. 215–238.

Cutting, J. E., and Vishton, P. M. 1995. "Perceiving Layout: The Integration, Relative Dominance, and Contextual Use of Different Information About Depth." In *Handbook of Perception and Cogni-

tion: Vol. 5: Perception of Space and Motion, edited by W. Epstein and S. Rogers. New York: Academic Press. 69–117.

Doorschot, P. C. A., Kappers, A. M. L., and Koenderink, J. J. 2001. "The Combined Influence of Binocular Disparity and Shading on Pictorial Shape." *Perception & Psychophysics* 63 (6): 1038–1047.

Ernst, M. 2005. "A Bayesian View on Multimodal Cue Integration." In *A Human Body Perception from the Inside Out*, edited by G. Knoblich, M. Grosjean, I. Thornton, and M. Shiffrar. New York: Oxford University Press. 105–131.

Glennerster, A., McKee, S. P., and Birch, M. D. 2002. "Evidence for Surface-Based Processing of Binocular Disparity." *Current Biology* 12: 825–828.

Glennerster, A., Rogers, B. J., and Bradshaw, M. F. 1996. "Stereoscopic Depth Constancy Depends on the Subject's Task." *Vision Research* 36: 3441–3456.

Hagen, M. A. 1980. *The Perception of Pictures I: Alberti's Window: The Projective Model of Pictures*. New York: Academic Press.

Hecht, H., Schwartz, R., and Atherton, M. 2003. *Looking Into Pictures: An Interdisciplinary Approach to Pictorial Space*. Cambridge, MA: MIT Press.

Hillis, J., Ernst, M., Banks, M., Landy, M. "Combining Sensory Information: Mandatory Fusion Within but not Between Senses. *Science* 298: 1627–1630.

Hillis, J. M., Watt, S. J., Landy, M. S., and Banks, M. S. 2004. "Slant From Texture and Disparity Cues: Optimal Cue Combination." *Journal of Vision* 4 (12): 967–992.

Hollins, M. 1976. "Does Accommodative Micropsia Exist?" *American Journal of Psychology* 89: 443–454.

Howard, I. P., and Rogers, J. B. 1995. *Binocular Vision and Stereopsis*. Oxford, UK: Oxford University Press.

Jepson, A. D., Richards, W., and Knill, D. 1996. "Modal Structure and Reliable Inference." In *Perception as Bayesian Inference*, edited by D. C. Knill and W. Richards. Cambridge, MA: Cambridge University Press. 93–122.

Judge, A. W. 1926. *Stereoscopic Photography*. London: Chapman & Hall.

Kanizsa, G. 1979. *Organization in Vision*. New York: Praeger.

Koenderink, J. J. 1998. "Pictorial Relief." *Philosophical Transactions of the Royal Society London A* 356: 1071–1086.

Koenderink, J. J., and van Doorn, A. J. 2003. "Pictorial Space." In *Looking Into Pictures: An Interdisciplinary Approach to Pictorial Space*, edited by H. Hecht, R. Schwartz, and M. Atherton. Cambridge, MA: MIT Press. 239–299.

Koenderink, J. J., van Doorn, A. J., and Kappers, A. M. L. 1992. "Surface Perception in Pictures." *Perception & Psychophysics* 52: 487–496.

Koenderink, J. J., van Doorn, A. J., and Kappers, A. M. L. 1994. "On So-Called Paradoxical Monocular Stereoscopy." *Perception* 23 (5): 583–594.

Koenderink, J. J., van Doorn, A. J., Kappers, A. M. L., and Todd, J. T. 2001. "Ambiguity and the 'Mental Eye' in Pictorial Relief." *Perception* 30: 431–448.

Kubovy, M. 1986. *The Psychology of Perspective and Renaissance Art.* New York: Cambridge University Press.

Landy, M. S., Maloney, L. T., Johnston, E. B., and Young, M. 1995. "Measurement and Modelling of Depth Cue Combination: In Defense of Weak Fusion." *Vision Research* 35: 389–412.

Leyton, M. 1992. *Symmetry, Causality, Mind.* Cambridge, MA: MIT Press.

Leyton, M. 2001. *A Generative Theory of Shape.* Heidelberg: Springer-Verlag.

Mamassian, P., and Landy, M. S. 2001. "Interaction of Visual Prior Constraints." *Vision Research* 41: 2653–2668.

Marr, D. 1982. *Vision: A Computational Investigation Into the Human Representation and Processing of Visual Information.* New York: W. H. Freeman.

Mausfeld, R. 2002. "The Physicalistic Trap in Perception." In *Perception and the Physical World*, edited by D. Heyer and R. Mausfeld. Chichester: Wiley.

Mausfeld, R. 2003. "Conjoint Representations and the Mental Capacity for Multiple Simultaneous Perspectives." In *Looking Into Pictures: An Interdisciplinary Approach to Pictorial Space*, edited by H. Hecht, R. Schwartz, and M. Atherton. Cambridge, MA: MIT Press.

McCready, D. 1965. "Size-Distance Perception and Accommodation-Convergence Micropsia: A Critique." *Vision Research* 5: 189–206.

Michotte, A. 1948. "The Psychological Enigma of Perspective in Outline Pictures" Translated in G. Thines, A. Costall & G. Butterworth (Eds.) (1991) *Michotte's Experimental Phenomenology of Perception.* Erlbaum: Hillsdale, New Jersey (manuscript originally published in 1948).

Nakayama, K., He, Z. J., and Shimojo, S. 1995. "Visual Surface Representation: A Critical Link Between Lower-Level and Higher-Level Vision." In *Frontiers in Cognitive Neuroscience*, edited by S. Kosslyn and D. N. Osherson. 2nd ed. Cambridge, MA: MIT Press.

Neri, P. 2005. "A Stereoscopic Look at Visual Cortex." *Journal of Neurophysiology* 93: 1823–1826.

Neri, P., Bridge, H., and Heeger, D. J. 2004. "Stereoscopic Processing of Absolute and Relative Disparity in Human Visual Cortex." *Journal of Neurophysiology* 92: 1880–1891.

Niederée, R., and Heyer, D. 2003. "The Dual Nature of Picture Perception: A Challenge to Current General Accounts of Visual Perception." In *Looking Into Pictures: An Interdisciplinary Approach to Pictorial Space*, edited by H. Hecht, R. Schwartz, and M. Atherton. Cambridge, MA: MIT Press. 77–98.

Norman, J. F., Todd, J. T., and Phillips, F. 1995. "The Perception of Surface Orientation from Multiple Sources of Optical Information." *Perception & Psychophysics*, 57: 629–636.

Pirenne, M. H. 1970. *Optics, Painting, and Photography*. Cambridge, UK: Cambridge University Press.

Predebon, J. 1993. "The Familiar-size Cue to Distance and Stereoscopic Depth Perception." *Perception* 22: 985–995.

Richards, W., and Jepson, A. 1991. "What Makes a Good Feature?" *Technical Report, MIT Artificial Intelligence Laboratory*, AIM-1356.

Richards, W., Jepson, A., and Feldman, J. 1996. "Priors, Preferences and Categorical Percepts." In *Perception as Bayesian Inference*, edited by D. C. Knill and W. Richards. Cambridge, MA: Cambridge University Press. 93–122.

Rogers, B. J., and Graham, M. E. 1982. "Similarities between Motion Parallax and Stereopsis in Human Depth Perception." *Vision Research* 22: 261–270.

Sacks, O. 2006. "Stereo Sue." *The New Yorker*, June 19, 2006, p. 64.

Schlosberg, H. 1941. "Stereoscopic Depth from Single Pictures." *The American Journal of Psychology* 54 (4): 601–605.

Stevens, K. A., and Brookes, A. 1988. "Integrating Stereopsis with Monocular Interpretations of Planar Surfaces." *Vision Research* 28: 371–386.

Stevens, K. A., Lees, M., and Brookes, A. 1991. "Combining Binocular and Monocular Curvature Features." *Perception*, 20: 425–440.

Tassinari, H., Domini, F., and Caudek, C. 2008. "The Intrinsic Constraint Model for Stereo-motion Integration." *Perception*, 37: 79–95.

Todd, J. T., Koenderink, J. J., van Doorn, A. J., and Kappers, A. M. L. 1996. "Effects of Changing Viewing Conditions on the Perceived Structure of Smoothly Curved Surfaces." *Journal of Experimental Psychology: Human Perception and Performance* 22: 695–706.

van Ee, R. L., van Dam, C. J., and Erkelens, C. J. 2003. "Bi-Stability in Perceived Slant When Binocular Disparity and Monocular Perspective Specify Different Slants." *Journal of Vision* 2 (9): 597–607.

Vishwanath, D. 2005. "The Epistemological Status of Vision and Its Implications for Design." *Axiomathes* 15: 399–486.

Vishwanath, D. 2006. "Coplanar Reflectance Change and the Ontology of Surface Perception." In *Visual Thought*, edited by L. Albertazzi. Amsterdam: Benjamins.

Vishwanath, D. 2007. "Is Focal Blur an Absolute Cue to Depth?" *Journal of Vision* 7 (9): 845, 845a. [Abstract]

Vishwanath, D. 2008. "The Focal Blur Gradient Affects Perceived Absolute Distance." *Perception* 37 (ECVP Abstract Supplement): 130.

Vishwanath, D., Girshick, A. R., and Banks, M. S. 2005. "Why Pictures Look Right When Viewed From the Wrong Place." *Nature Neuroscience* 8 (10): 1401–1410.

Wade, N. J., Ono, H., and Lillakas, L. 2001. "Leonardo da Vinci's Struggles with Representations of Reality." *Leonardo* 34: 231–235.

Yuille, A. L., and Bülthoff, H. H. 1996. "Bayesian Decision Theory and Psychophysics." In *Perception as Bayesian Inference*, edited by D. C. Knill and W. Richards. Cambridge: Cambridge University Press. 123–161.

Zimmerman, D. L., Legge, G. E., and Cavanagh, P. 1995. "Pictorial Depth Cues: A New Slant." *Journal of the Optical Society of America A* 12: 17–26.

8 Good Continuation in Layers: Shading Flows, Color Flows, Surfaces, and Shadows

Ohad Ben-Shahar and Steven W. Zucker

... space and color are not distinct elements but, rather, are interdependent aspects of a unitary process of perceptual organization.
—Gaetano Kanizsa (1979, p. 17)

Image segmentation is normally taken to be that process of partitioning the image into a complete cover of nonoverlapping regions, with the boundaries of these regions related to the (projected) boundaries of objects in the world. One source of complexity in this process is shadowing, by which image intensities vary as a function of both surface orientation (e.g., shading) and light sources (e.g., cast shadows). Land's *retinex theory* (Land and McCann, 1971) suggested one way to manage this complexity—by ascribing abrupt image changes to material (or reflectance) discontinuities and smooth gradient changes to lighting. This developed into the intrinsic image concept (Witkin and Tenenbaum, 1983), which emphasized that surface properties, geometry, and lighting all map into the image, and suggested representing them separately as images. Undoing this map clearly involves an inverse problem, which requires a model of some sort. One possibility is to try to learn the context of every possible measurement, a type of pseudoinverse (Tappen, Freeman, and Adelson, 2005). Here we extend the notion of context in a different way, by considering natural images such as those in figure 8.1. Notice how space, reflectance, and lighting conspire together. We seek to find a representation rich enough to support unwinding this.

The first requirement for such a representation is that it be rich enough to capture the previous phenomena. But unlike special-purpose algorithms applicable in one situation (e.g., Garg and Nayar, 2005; Horn and Brooks, 1989), our second requirement is that it be general purpose. That is, the information that it makes explicit must support computations for unraveling many such phenomena.

We do not yet have a formal solution to this problem that we can prove is complete. Instead, and consistent with the goals of this workshop, we develop an argument based

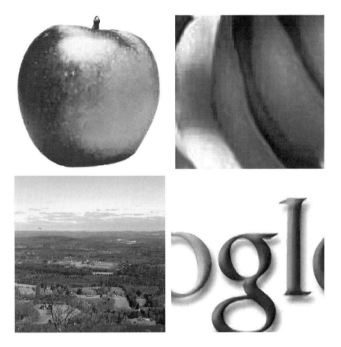

Figure 8.1
The rich interaction among surfaces, lighting, pigmentation, and atmosphere work together to provide a diversity of appearance phenomena in natural images. To simply claim that "apples are red," or "bananas are yellow," or "the sky is blue" amounts to an assumption that physical processes in the world are constant in a way that only artificial examples can really achieve.

on a neurobiological analogy, several steps of which have been formalized and are complete. The demonstrations in the final section of this chapter involve phenomena beyond the current capability of any single existing algorithm and provide counter-examples to many. Constructively, however, we submit that any final solution has an intermediate representation at least as rich as the one we describe. Thus we see the contribution of this workshop submission as consisting of (1) an enlargement of the framework for perceptual organization informed by (2) the rich foundation for perceptual organization in primate visual systems.

The core of our argument is that good continuation applies to several key domains: boundaries, intensity (shading), hue, texture, saturation, and so on, all of which enjoy a certain differential geometric structure. It is this structure that relates to the Gestalt notion of *good continuation*. Computationally we propose a layered representation— similar in spirit to intrinsic images (Witkin and Tenenbaum, 1983)—but different in that all share the property that they are flows in a technical sense. This is what we meant by layered flows implied in the title, and computations across these flows then reflect subtle lighting, surface, and space interactions.

Figure 8.1 illustrates this point in several different domains (see also Beck, 1972). Apples are not a single color; rather, fruits mature differentially, and this is reflected in their pigmentation. Attempts to remove these slow variations as lighting are one reason that lightness and color constancy algorithms have problems. Atmospheric depth effects impose a blue tint with distance because of increased scattering and despite surface reflection effects. Mutual illumination and color bleeding mix everything.

We approach the *lift* of these images into layered flows in two stages, both of which are mathematical but motivated by biology. We concentrate on one flow (from the color pathway) because, as becomes clear later, the others fit naturally into our framework and are more widely discussed in the literature. Specifically, we first consider the question of how to represent color information as a dimensionality-reduction problem, which leads formally to intensity-hue-saturation coordinates at each point. This is important for us because it suggests that there is more to color processing than simple detection tasks (e.g., locating a red fruit among green foliage; Sumner and Mollon, 2000), for which the standard cone pigments are tuned. We next consider (hue) interactions between points and adopt a technique previously used to denoise color patterns to articulate the flow of hue across image coordinates. The resultant computations are then run on the examples in figure 8.1.

Representation of Color at a Point

Take as data the Munsell patches considered as points in wavelength space. Although wavelength space is rather high-dimensional, our strategy is motivated by the observation that colors are not randomly distributed throughout wavelength space but rather occupy only a small portion of it. One possibility, suggested by the visual photopigments in primates, is that this structured space of colors is three-dimensional. Although this is a classical view of color, many of the classical algorithms have been modified in an ad hoc fashion to take account of nonlinearities among colors (e.g., multidimensional scaling). For this reason, we use a new algorithm (Coifman et al., 2005a,b) derived from the *geometric harmonics* (reviewed below) that can handle inherently non-linear data. It is in the class of spectral methods, and is related to the algorithm in Belkin and Niyogi (2003).

Geometric Harmonics

Let $X = \{x_1, x_2, \ldots, x_N\}$ be the set of data points, in this case Munsell patches, with each $x_i \in R^n$. We seek to find a projection of these data into much lower dimension, under the assumption that they are not randomly distributed throughout R^n, but rather that they lie on (or near) a lower-dimensional manifold embedded in R^n.

The structure of these data is revealed via a symmetric, positivity-preserving, and positive semidefinite *kernel* $k(x, y)$, which provides a measure of similarity between data points. The result is a graph, with edges between nearby (according to the similarity kernel) data points. (The similarity value can be truncated to 0 for all but very similiar points.)

From this we construct a diffusion kernel $a(x, y)$ on the data set using the weighted graph Laplacian normalized as follows:

$$a(x,y) = \frac{k(x,y)}{v(x)},$$

where $v = \sum_{y \in X} k(x, y)$. Note that, although symmetry is lost, we do have $\sum_{y \in X} a(x, y) = 1$ so the kernel $a(x, y)$ can be interpreted as the transition matrix of a Markov chain on the data X. The kernel $a^{(m)}$ of the mth power of this matrix then represents the probability of getting from x to y in m steps.

If we now define the averaging operator for a function f defined on the data:

$$Af(x) = \sum_{y \in X} a(x,y)f(y)$$

then A admits a spectral theory. To develop this we symmetrize a by:

$$\tilde{a}(x,y) = \frac{\sqrt{v(x)}}{\sqrt{v(y)}} a(x,y)$$

which makes $\tilde{a}$ symmetric and positive semidefinite (although no longer row-stochastic). The spectral decomposition is then given by $\tilde{a} = \sum_{i \geq 0} \lambda_i^2 \phi_i(x) \phi_i(y)$ with the important consequence

$$\widetilde{a^{(m)}(x,y)} = \sum_{i \geq 0} \lambda_i^{2m} \phi_i(x) \phi_i(y)$$

where $\lambda_0 = 1$.

Increasing powers of the operator A can be obtained by running the chain through the spectral decomposition. This gives rise to the family of *diffusion maps* $\{\Phi_m\}_{m \in N}$ given by

$$\Phi_m(x) = \begin{pmatrix} \lambda_0^m \phi_0(x) \\ \lambda_1^{2m} \phi_1(x) \\ \vdots \end{pmatrix}$$

Diffusion distances $D_m^2(x, y) = \tilde{a}^{(m)}(x, x) + \tilde{a}^{(m)}(y, y) - 2\tilde{a}^{(m)}(x, y)$ within the high-dimensional measurement space then approximate Euclidean distance in the diffusion map space.

The Munsell Color Space

The Munsell (1905) patches were chosen according to human psychophysics, with each step between patches perceptually equal, and they are now known to be physiologically relevant (Hanazawa, Komatsu, and Murakami, 2000; Wachtler, Sejnowski, and Albright, 2003; Xiao, Wang, and Felleman, 2003). Thus, they represent data spanning those portions of color space relevant to our interactions with the visible world. We now seek to understand whether these data lie on or near a well-defined structure in wavelength-space.

Two experiments were performed. We used $N = 1,269$ patches, each with $n = 421$ wavelengths (380 nm – 800 nm in 1 nm steps). The kernel is $\exp(-d_{ij}^2/\sigma)$, where d_{ij} is the Euclidian distance between patch i and patch j. Although the patch data are given in no particular order, the geometric harmonic map arranges them so that patches are close to one another provided the diffusion distance between them in wavelength space is small. The results are shown in figure 8.2. Note that the natural representation emerges—intensity, hue, saturation—even though the hue (color circle) is nonlinear. The diffusion maps recover the Munsell representation, thus demonstrating that the structure is in the wavelength data. In the second experiment, we first projected the wavelength data through the human cone photopigments, and again the color circle emerged (figure 8.2, bottom).

Spatiospectral Interactions

Now that we know there is a preferred representation for color at a point, we next consider the question of how colors interact between nearby points. We first observe that the primate visual system is well organized to address this problem. Although it is widely accepted that perceptual organization is first accomplished via the long-range horizontal connections in superficial V1, consideration of these connections has been limited to orientation good continuation for boundaries (Adini, Sagi, and Tsodyks, 1997; Beaudot and Mullen, 2003; Parent and Zucker, 1989) and textures (Ben-Shahar and Zucker, 2003). However, there exists a specialized structure for color (and contrast) information in the cytochrome oxidase blobs, within which neurons also enjoy long-range horizontal interactions (figure 8.3; Yabuta and Callaway, 1998). We submit that it is precisely these connections that implement a geometry for hue (and color) that is formally analagous to that for texture (Ben-Shahar and Zucker, 2003) and shading (Breton and Zucker, 1996; Lehky and Sejnowski, 1988) flows. A sketch of this geometry is developed next. The extension to include boundaries is found in Ben-Shahar, Huggins, and Zucker (2002).

Geometry of Hue Fields

Within the (intensity, hue, saturation) color space, the hue component across the image is a mapping $\mathcal{H}: \mathbb{R}^2 \to \mathcal{S}^1$ and thus can be represented as a unit length

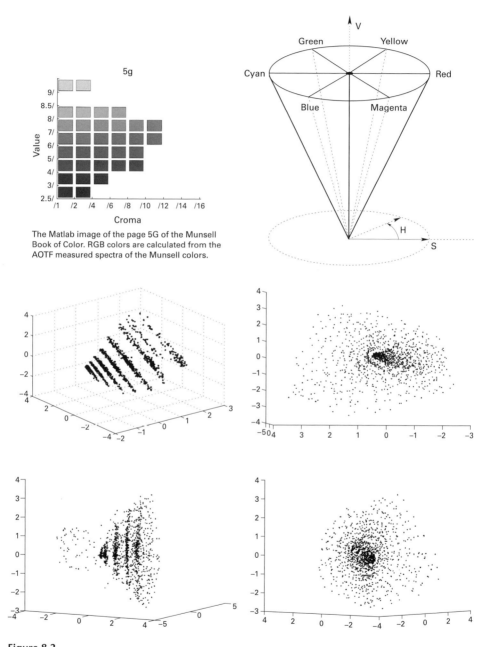

The Matlab image of the page 5G of the Munsell Book of Color. RGB colors are calculated from the AOTF measured spectra of the Munsell colors.

Figure 8.2

Geometric harmonics organize Munsell color patches. (Top row, left) Typical "page" of the patch data used in the experiment. Data from <http://spectral.joensuu.fi/databases/download/munsell _spec_matt.htm>. (Right) Classical intensity, hue, saturation color space. Note that hue is orga-

vector field over the image. In many images this hue field is piecewise smooth (figure 8.4) with singularities corresponding to significant scene events (e.g., occlusion boundaries or material changes).

The frame field (O'Neill, 1966) obtained by attaching a (tangent, normal) frame $\{E_T, E_N\}$ to each point in the image domain is the representation suggested by modern differential geometry. This provides a local coordinate system in which the hue vector and related structures can be represented. Most important among these are the covariant derivatives of E_T and E_N, which represent the initial rate of change of the frame when it is moved in a direction v expressed by the connection equation (O'Neill, 1966):

$$\begin{pmatrix} \nabla_V E_T \\ \nabla_V E_N \end{pmatrix} = \begin{bmatrix} 0 & w_{12}(V) \\ -w_{12}(V) & 0 \end{bmatrix} \begin{pmatrix} E_T \\ E_N \end{pmatrix}$$

The coefficient $w_{12}(V)$ is a function of the tangent vector V, which represents the fact that the local behavior of the flow depends on the direction along which it is measured. $w_{12}(V)$ is a linear 1-form, so it can be represented with two scalars at each point:

$$\kappa_T \triangleq w_{12}(E_T)$$

$$\kappa_N \triangleq w_{12}(E_N).$$

We call κ_T the hue's *tangential curvature* and κ_N the hue's *normal curvature*. They represent the rate of change of the hue in the tangential and normal directions, respectively.

Because the local behavior of the hue is characterized (up to Euclidean transformation) by a pair of curvatures, it is natural to conclude that nearby measurements of hue should relate to each other based on these curvatures. Put differently, measuring a particular curvature pair $(\kappa_T(q), \kappa_N(q))$ at a point q should induce a field of coherent measurements (i.e., a hue function $\widetilde{HUE}(x, y)$, in the neighborhood of q). Coherence of $HUE(q)$ to its spatial context $HUE(x, y)$ can then be determined by

nized around the circle. (Middle row) The geometric harmonic organization of the Munsell data. Each point represents a single patch, and the scatterplots show the distribution of points in the subspace spanned by the first three nontrivial eigenfunctions. Two views are shown, with (left) illustrating different clusters according to the Munsell chromaticity parameters and (right) a view showing the hue circle. That this noninear organization of the data is recovered by geometric harmonics is significant because it provides the foundation for the next, geometric stage of processing. (Bottom row) Organization of the Munsell data first projected through the three human cone photopigments. Since the two views are essentially the same as (middle), the Munsell representation is largely invariant to the order of projection.

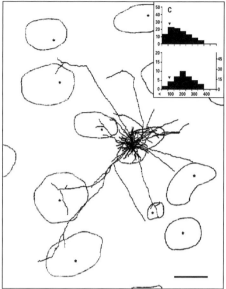

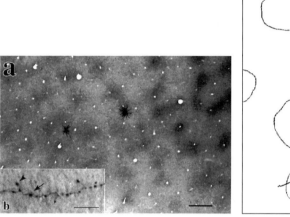

Figure 8.3
The cytochrome oxidase blobs in superficial primate visual cortex are specialized for the processing of color. The left figure shows the blobs selectively stained to highlight their locations regularly interspersed between orientation hypercolumns. (Right) When single cells are filled with dye, their long-range connections become clear. Note how axons tend to terminate within (or near) other cytochrome oxidase blobs (drawn in outline). We submit that it is these long-range connections that enforce "good continuation" between hues at nearby positions. Images courtesy of E. Callaway, Salk Insitute.

examining how well $HUE(x,y)$ fits $\widetilde{HUE}(x,y)$ around q. Clearly, this should be a function of the local hue curvatures $(\kappa_T(q), \kappa_N(q))$, it should agree with these curvatures at q, and it should extend around q according to some variation in both curvatures.

Although many local coherence models $\widetilde{HUE}(x,y)$ are possible, we exploit the fact that the hue field is a unit length vector field which suggests that it behaves similarly to oriented texture flows (Ben-Shahar and Zucker, 2001); Ben-Shahar and Zucker (2003) and adopt a similar curvature-tuned local model.

$$\widetilde{HUE}(x,y) = tan^{-1}\left(\frac{\kappa_T(q)x + \kappa_N(q)y}{1 + \kappa_N(q)x - \kappa_T(q)y}\right).$$

Unlike texture flows, however, the local model for the hue function is not a *double* helicoid because the hue function takes values in $[\pi, \pi)$, where texture flows are constrained to $[-\frac{\pi}{2}, \frac{\pi}{2})$.

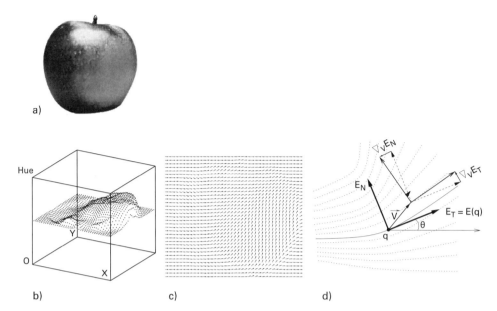

a)

Hue

O

Y

X

b)   c)   d)

Figure 8.4
Color images of natural objects are piecewise smooth and the hue flow captures this. (A) An apple with varying hue. (B) A representation of hue as a scalar field, with value corresponding to height. (C) The hue field, with each value represented as a vector pointing to location on the hue circle. (D) The geometry of the hue flow, illustrating that nearby values can be represented as a differentiable frame field that is tangent (and normal) to the streamlines of the flow. Interations between nearby hue values then correspond to an (infinitesimal) transport of the frame in direction V, which rotates it according to the connection form of the frame field. Since E_T, E_N are unit length, their covariant derivative lies in a normal direction, regardless of V. This diagram also suggests a relationship between hue and texture and shading flows.

This local model possesses many properties that suit good continuation, in particular, it is both a minimal surface in the $(x, y, \widetilde{HUE}(x,y))$ representation and a critical point of the p-harmonic energy for all p. It is also the only local model that does not bias the changes in one hue curvature relative to the other—that is, it satisfies

$$\frac{\kappa_T(x,y)}{\kappa_N(x,y)} = \text{const} = \frac{\kappa_T(q)}{\kappa_N(q)}.$$

Examples of the model for different curvature tuning is illustrated in figure 8.5. A detailed technical account of the model in the texture flow domain can be found in Ben-Shahar and Zucker (2003).

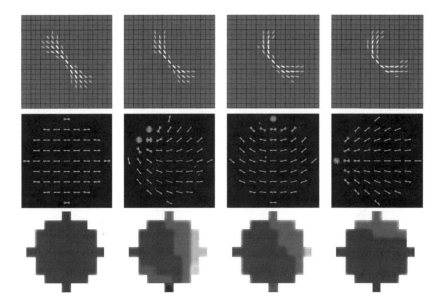

Figure 8.5
Illustration of the different types of compatibility fields that can be used for early forms of good continuation. In each case the central unit is supported by the contextual arrangement of surrounding units and can be used as the constraints within quadratic programming, relaxation labeling, and belief propagation engines. (Top) For boundary continuation, the orientation at a position is enhanced by consistent tangential (co-circular) boundary measurements at nearby positions (Geisler et al., 2001; Parent and Zucker, 1989). (Middle) For oriented texture measurements, both tangential and normal curvatures arise. Similar models can be used for shading flows, which are the tangent fields to the intensity level sets (Ben-Shahar and Zucker, 2004). (Bottom) For hue flows the orientations are replaced by colors. In the first column zero curvature continuations are shown. In the last column, a single large curvature is shown. For the texture and hue compatibilities, the tangential curvature is zero and the normal curvature is not. Note the emergence of singularities.

Examples of Flows

We now illustrate the prior computations on several examples. We begin with artificial ones to illustrate the points most clearly, and then we proceed to natural ones to illustrate the complexities that arise.

We stress that, for space reasons, some of these flows are not visible unless one zooms in to enlarge the manuscript.

In figure 8.6, we show one of the few examples from the psychophysical literature. In an important article, Kingdom (2003) created images consisting of superimposed

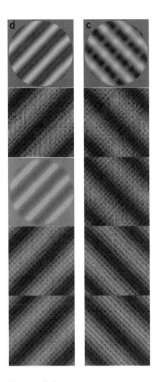

Figure 8.6
Results on the test Kingdom (2003) images. Note how both provide the impression of an undulating surface with color on it. The left column is Kingdom figure 2d; the right column is Kingdom figure 2c. From top to bottom are original images; initial estimate of shading flow (tangents to intensity level sets); final estimate of shading flow; initial estimate of hue flow; final estimate of hue flow. The shading flow corresponds to the undulations; the hue flows are smooth and do not interfere with them.

sinusoids, one in brightness and the other in color. He demonstrated that it is the intensity component that drives the impression of shape-from-shading, whereas the color information appears "painted" onto the undulating surface. We reproduced this separation with our flows, from which it follows that the shading flow is suffcent (for these examples) to derive the shape.

The shading flow is estimated by evaluating a gradient operator (an orientationally selective receptive field tuned to low spatial frequency) over the image. It demonstrates one role for the long-range interactions: correcting local artifacts in shading flow estimation.

Our next examples (figure 8.7) on artificial images confirm the classical view that color remains invariant across shadows while shading affects surface percepts (Ruzon

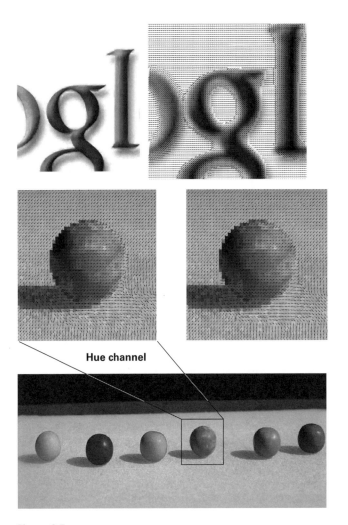

Hue channel

Figure 8.7
Shading and hue flows for artificial objects. Although the shading flow fields are not shown,
notice how the hue flows (superimposed on the original image) are constant over the "plastic" objects. This is the way such materials were designed. The case of the sphere also introduces two more complex lighting effects. First, note how the hue flow remains constant
through the shadow. This is a classical cue for separating shadow boundaries from surface
boundaries. (Surface boundaries are taken to involve different materials, and therefore a hue
discontinuity together with the intensity discontinuity.) Second, and less familiar, is the
mutual illumination between the sphere and the tabletop, which is captured by the hue flow
but not the shading flow. The left magnification shows the initial local measurements of hue;
the right magnification shows the converged hue flow. A boundary has been introduced
around the hue flow on the table top illustrating an elongation in the direction of the source.

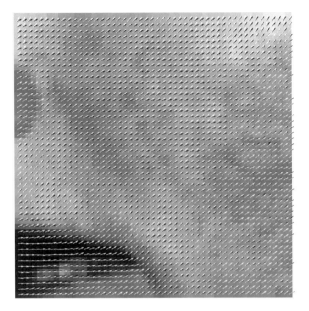

Figure 8.8
Hue flows vary for natural objects. This shows a portion of a woman's face (the lips are lower left) when she is blushing (gray vectors) and not blushing (black vectors). Note how hue varies both spatially and as a function of emotional and physical states.

and Tomasi, 1999). This is most clear in the plastic sphere, and the same effect is reproduced in the Google logo, which appears both three-dimensional and colored. However, unlike the plastic sphere, there are no mutual illumination effects.

The next examples show how hue can vary over a natural object. Figure 8.4 shows the hue flow for an apple, and figure 8.8 is a close-up of a woman's face in which a blush has been introduced. Note in particular how variant the "color" is, a point of some relevance to both face identification and emotional estimation. Hue can also vary systematically over a scene. Atmospheric depth scattering is shown in figure 8.9.

Our next two examples illustrate the beautiful complexity of shading, hue, and boundary interactions. The first shows an apple photographed on a highly reflective surface in bright sunlight (figure 8.10). The flows are varied with respect to one another and with respect to the boundaries (of both the apple and the shadow). In particular, the mutual illumination modulating the shadow (Langer, 1999) introduces a smooth shading flow not unlike the one for the plastic sphere or the Kingdom examples, but this time it is due to a lighting effect and not a surface normal effect. The mutual illumination effect is also strong on the bananas image (figure 8.11), which illustrates a shading flow effect due to a highly diffuse cast shadow. In this case, the

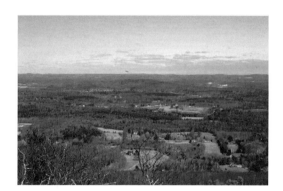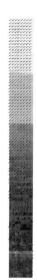

Figure 8.9
Hue flows and atmospheric depth effects. The flow is shown along a thin strip on the right side of the photograph. Note the dominant shift toward blue for the upper half.

cast shadow phenomenon is readily identified because the hue flow is constant across it.

Our final example (figure 8.12) illustrates the complement to shading and hue; notice how the hue remains invariant through the highlight, although it is a complex pattern for the pepper.

Summary and Conclusions

Perceptual organization was viewed within Gestalt psychology as pervasive in perception, but discussion of such issues in computer vision is significantly more limited. Our goal in this chapter was to take a step back and raise the profile of questions for which perceptual organization is relevant. Following a biological analogy, we introduced the construct of multiple (spatially) aligned flows within which Gestalt good continuation can be enforced geometrically but between which information can be inferred about the many complexities of lighting, space, and geometry. The computation of each flow was global based on local measurements and differential (covariant derivative) constraints between them. At the same time, the computation of each flow was local within an information (sometimes within a sensor) source, and logical relationships between flows provide a new foundation for many computer vision computations. Hue flows smoothly through shadows, whereas intensity often jumps. Shading flows

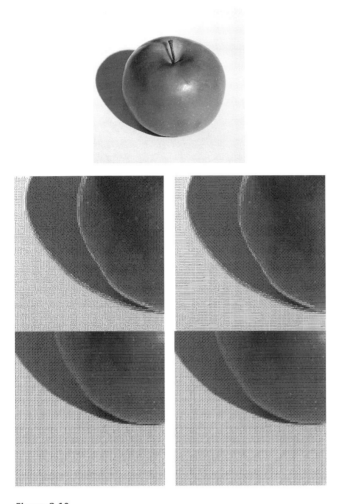

Figure 8.10

An image of an apple on colored cardboard in bright sunlight. It illustrates the complexities that can arise both for shading due to surface irregularities from packing and from mutual illumination. In particular, the shaded area now exhibits a shading flow derived from mutual illumination, in which the gradient decreases in magnitude away from the concavity between the apple and the table. At the same time, there is strong mutual illumination between the apple and the cardboard and the cardboard and the apple. The result are smooth shading and hue flows, with discontinuities at neither object nor shadow edges.

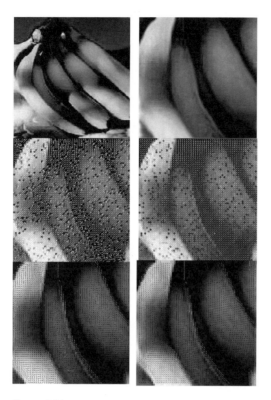

Figure 8.11

A photograph of bananas illustrates the richness of mutual illumination in a complex scene. The result is an essentially constant hue flow (middle row, left: initial measurement; right: consistent flow). The shading flow (bottom) illustrates a special interaction between boundaries and shading flows, in which multiple surfaces fold away from each other along them. Such situations are geometrically rare.

smoothly over many man-made objects, whereas hue is often constant. Natural objects often imply smooth shading and hue flows, although they are typically independent of one another. The involvement of boundaries is both necessary and complicated Elder and Zucker (1998).

Although the list of interactions must be extended (motion and stereo should at least be included), it is useful to conclude on an enlargement of the biological metaphor underlying this chapter. The centrality of long-range horizontal connections as defining each flow suggests that the flows be layered on top of one another, enabling "vertical" connections for their interactions. Recent breakthoughs in color processing demonstrate that hue and orientation are not independent, as was once thought, and

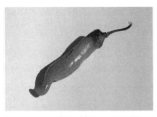
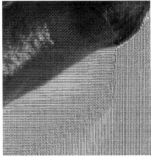

Figure 8.12
A photograph of a pepper illustrates how the hue flow remains constant through highlights, even when the hue is varying. The mutual illumination on the background is very interesting as well. (Top) Pepper image. (Bottom) Hue flow through a portion of the pepper image. The flow is superimposed on the image for identification purposes only.

that such vertical connections exist Shapley and Hawken (2002). Computationally, it remains an open question whether only two interaction "dimensions" suffice.

Acknowledgments

Research supported by AFOSR, DARPA, ONR and the Toman and Frankel Funds from Ben-Gurion University.

References

Adini, Y., Sagi, D., and Tsodyks, M., 1997. "Excitatory-inhibitory network in the visual cortex: Psychophysical evidence." *Proc. Natl. Acad. Sci. (USA)* 94: 10426–10431.

Beaudot, W., and Mullen, K., 2003. How long range is contour integration in human color vision. *Visual Neurosci.* 20: 51–64.

Beck, J., 1972. *Surface Color Perception.* Cornell University Press.

Belkin, M., and Niyogi, P., 2003. Laplacian eigenmaps for dimensionality reduction and data representation. *Neural Computation* 6(15): 1373–1396.

Ben-Shahar, O., Huggins, P., and Zucker, S., 2002. On computing visual flows with boundaries: The case of shading and edges. In *Workshop on Biologically Motivated Computer Vision*.

Ben-Shahar, O., and Zucker, S., 2001. On the perceptual organization of texture and shading flows: From a geometrical model to coherence computation. In *Proc. Computer Vision and Pattern Recognition*. 1048–1055.

Ben-Shahar, O., and Zucker, S., 2003. The perceptual organization of texture flows: A contextual inference approach. *IEEE Trans. Pattern Anal. Machine Intell.* 25(4): 401–417.

Ben-Shahar, O., and Zucker, S., 2004. Geometrical computations explain projection patterns of long range horizontal connections in visual cortex. *Neural Comput.* 16(3): 445–476.

Breton, P., and Zucker, S., 1996. Shadows and shading flow fields. In *Proc. Computer Vision and Pattern Recognition*. 782–789.

Coifman, R., Lafon, S., Lee, A., Maggioni, M., Nadler, B., Warner, F., and Zucker, S. 2005a. Geometric diffusions as a tool for harmonic analysis and structure definition of data: Diffusion maps. *Proc. Nat. Acad. Sci. (USA)* 102(21): 7426–7431.

Coifman, R., Lafon, S., Lee, A., Maggioni, M., Nadler, B., Warner, F., and Zucker, S. 2005b. Geometric diffusions as a tool for harmonic analysis and structure definition of data: Multiscale methods. *Proc. Nat. Acad. Sci. (USA)* 102(21): 7432–7437.

Elder, J., and Zucker, S., 1998. Evidence for boundary-specific grouping. *Vision Res.* 38(1): 143–152.

Garg, K., and Nayar, S., 2005. When does a camera see rain? *ICCV*.

Geisler, W., Perry, J., Super, B., and Gallogly, D., 2001. Edge co-occurrence in natural images predicts contour grouping performance. *Vision Res.* 41(6): 711–724.

Hanazawa, A., Komatsu, H., and Murakami, I., 2000. Neural selectivity for hue and saturation of colour in the primary visual cortex of the monkey. *Eur. J. Neurosci.* 12: 1753–1763.

Horn, B., and Brooks, M. (Eds.), 1989. *Shape from Shading*. Cambridge, MA: MIT Press.

Kanizsa, G., 1979. *Organization in Vision: Essays on Gestalt Perception*. Praeger Publishers.

Kingdom, F., 2003. Color brings relief to human vision. *Nature Neuroscience* 6(6): 641–644.

Land, E., and McCann, J., 1971. Lightness and retinex theory. *American Journal of Optical Society of America* 61: 1–11.

Langer, M., 1999. When shadows become interreflections. *Int. J. Comput. Vision* 34(2/3): 193–204.

Lehky, S., and Sejnowski, T., 1988. Network model of shape-from-shading: neural function arises from both receptive and projective fields. *Nature* 333: 452–454.

Munsell, A., 1905. *A Color Notation*. Boston: G.H.Ellis.

O'Neill, B., 1966. *Elementary Differential Geometry*. New York: Academic Press.

Parent, P., and Zucker, S., 1989. Trace inference, curvature consistency, and curve detection. *IEEE Trans. Pattern Anal. Machine Intell.* 11(8): 823–839.

Ruzon, M., and Tomasi, C., 1999. Color edge detection with the compass operator. In *Proc. Computer Vision and Pattern Recognition.* 160–166.

Shapley, R., and Hawken, M., 2002. Neural mechanisms for color perception in the primary visual cortex. *Curr. Opin. Neurobiol.* 12: 426–432.

Sumner, P., and Mollon, J., 2000. Chromaticity as a signal of ripeness in fruits taken by primates. *Journal of Experimental Biology* 203(13): 1987–2000.

Tappen, M., Freeman, W., and Adelson, E., 2005. Recovering intrinsic images from a single image. *IEEE Trans. Pattern Anal. Machine Intell.* 27(9): 1459–1472.

Wachtler, T., Sejnowski, T., and Albright, T., 2003. Representation of color stimuli in awake macaque primary visual cortex. *Neuron* 37: 681–691.

Witkin, A., and Tenenbaum, J., 1983. On the role of structure in vision. In J. Beck, B. Hope, and A. Rosenfeld (Eds.) *Human and Machine Vision.* New York: Academic Press. 481–542.

Xiao, Y., Wang, Y., and Felleman, D., 2003. A spatially organized representation a colour in macaque cortical area v2. *Nature* 421: 535–539.

Yabuta, N., and Callaway, E., 1998. Cytochrome oxidase blobs and intrinsic horizontal connections of layer 2/3 pyramidal neurons in primate v1. *Visual Neurosci.* 15: 1007–1027.

9 Illusory Contours and Neon Color Spreading Reconsidered in the Light of Petter's Rule

Baingio Pinna

The problem of perceptual organization is one of the basic problems of visual neuroscience. It concerns the how and why separated elements of the retinal image combine and group to create visual objects. Within the problem of organization, there are three well-known phenomena useful to understand how and why the visual system segregates objects with a particular shape, color, and depth stratification: illusory contours, neon color spreading, and Petter's figures.

Illusory Contours

Kanizsa's triangle (Kanizsa, 1955) is the most known example of illusory contour (Schumann 1900), where brightness enhancement and contours are perceived without a luminance or color change across the contour. In figure 9.1a, three black circular sectors and three black angles on a white background, arranged in alternated order on the vertexes and sides of a virtual triangle, are perceived as three black disks and an outline triangle placed behind an illusory triangle with clear boundary contours and brighter than the white background. Ehrenstein's illusion (1941), illustrated in figure 9.1b, is another well-known example of illusory contours, where a bright illusory disk appears superimposed on the radial lines that complete amodally behind the disk.

Neon Color Spreading

Varin (1971) studied a "chromatic spreading" effect induced when four sets of concentric black circumferences are arranged in a cross-like shape and partially composed of red arcs creating a virtual large central red circle (see figure 9.2a). The central virtual circle appears as a ghostly transparent veil or a chromatic translucent diffusion of reddish tint spreading among the red arcs. The illusory neon has a depth stratification appearing in front of the component elements. The appearance of the spreading color is diaphanous and glows like a smoggy neon upon the background or (mostly under achromatic conditions) like a shadowy, foggy, dirty, or filmy transparent veil. The

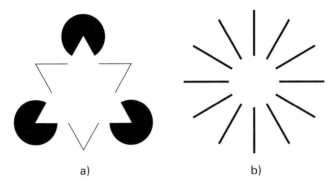

Figure 9.1
(a) Kanizsa's triangle, and (b) Ehrenstein's illusion.

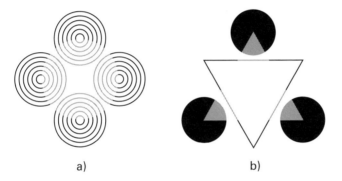

Figure 9.2
(a) Neon color spreading, and (b) neon-like version of Kanizsa's triangle.

chromatic spreading fills the whole illusory circle induced by the terminations of the black arcs and is strongly related to Ehrenstein's illusion. The neon effect was independently reported in 1975 by van Tuijl (see also van Tuijl and de Weert, 1979), who named it "neon-like color spreading." The neon-like version of Kanizsa's triangle is illustrated in figure 9.2b.

Petter's Figures

Petter's figures (Petter, 1956) concern all the conditions where a black irregular pattern can be seen as made up of independent surface components separated in depth and delineated by illusory contours in the area of apparent intersection and stratification. In figure 9.3a, the irregular black shape splits in two or three intersecting surfaces: one horizontal scalene triangle and two vertical scalene triangles. These surfaces intersect

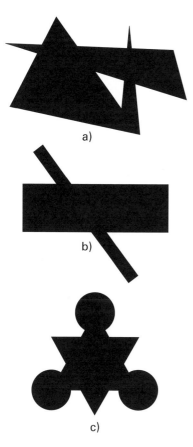

a)

b)

c)

Figure 9.3

Petter's figures. (a) These surfaces intersect and appear segregated in depth (i.e., the horizontal triangle is perceived in front of the narrow vertical triangle and behind the wide vertical one). (b) The irregular shape splits in two rectangles: The narrow one is seen behind the wide one. (c) Three disks placed in front of a triangle intersected by another triangle rotated of 180 degrees.

and appear segregated in depth: The horizontal triangle is perceived in front of the narrow vertical triangle and behind the wide vertical one. Illusory contours, clearly perceived in the intersecting portions of the stimulus, belong to the portion of the surface perceived closer to the observer. On the basis of the previous description, two kinds of boundaries can be seen: illusory modal contours of the occluding surface and amodal ones (Michotte, 1951; Michotte et al., 1964) belonging to the partially occluded surface completing behind the occluding one. In figure 9.3b, the irregular shape splits in two rectangles: The narrow one is seen behind the wide one. In figure 9.3c, Petter's version of Kanizsa's triangle shows the segregation of three disks placed in front of a triangle intersected by another triangle rotated by 180 degrees. The two triangles can reversibly appear one in front of the other.

Petter's Rule

Given the perceived stratification of two overlapping surfaces, depth information and, more specifically, relative size cues seem to be the only responsible factors of the previous results (i.e., the larger surface appears in front of the smaller one). However, by studying chromatically homogenous patterns like those illustrated in figure 9.3, Petter (1956) suggested that the perceived stratification occurs according to a general rule stating that the surface with the shorter contours, placed in the region where the surfaces look superimposed, has a greater probability of appearing in front of the other surface (see also Kanizsa, 1969, 1979; Metzger, 1975; Shipley and Kellman, 1992).

In figure 9.4, four examples test this rule. Conditions a–b and c–d show that by increasing the width of the annulus, it pops out in front of, respectively, the four squares and the radial lines. In fact, the intersecting border between the annuli and the other

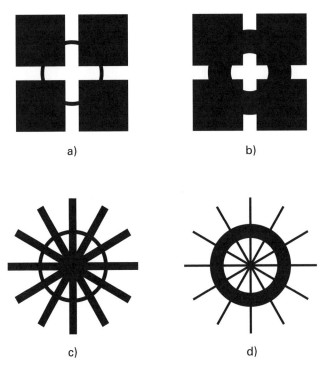

a)   b)

c)   d)

Figure 9.4
Four examples to test Petter's rule.

surfaces is a contour shorter (a–c) or longer (b–d) than the size of the continuation of the annuli within the other black surfaces. If the contour is shorter, it appears as a modal illusory contour belonging to the squares or radial lines. As a consequence, squares and radial lines appear in front of the annuli. If the contour is longer, it does not appear as such but becomes part of the annulus surfaces. Therefore, the annuli complete modally similarly to illusory figures in front of the other black surfaces.

Can Petter's Rule Explain Illusory Contours and Neon Color Spreading?

On the basis of the previous phenomenal results, the main question is whether Petter's rule may have a bearing on illusory contour formation or neon color spreading. More precisely, we suggest that Petter's rule can influence the presence/absence, strength, and depth perception of illusory contour formation and neon color spreading. As a consequence, this rule can be considered as a new basic factor for the formation of the two known illusions. If this is true, it should be possible to create competitions between known factors and Petter's rule eliciting unexpected effects. To better understand the theoretical extent and relevance of this hypothesis, let us consider some of the main explanations proposed to account for illusory contours and neon color spreading.

Some of the Main Explanations of Illusory Contours

Kanizsa (1955, 1979) proposed that the main factor for the formation of the illusory triangle is the presence of incompletenesses or open figures, which activates the amodal completion processes toward closure that in their turn induce complete elements partially occluded by an illusory triangle. Gregory (1972, 1987) suggested that illusory figures are similar to perceptual hypotheses (see Helmholtz's [1867] likelihood principle) postulated to explain the unlikely gaps within the stimulus. Therefore, a top-down cognitive hypothesis, namely, the illusory triangle, explains the gaps in the stimulus (i.e., the missing sectors of the disks and the missing parts of the outline triangle). Rock (1983, 1987) explained the illusory contours on the basis of fragments similar to familiar figures that elicit a cognitive hypothesis, similar to the one suggested by Gregory, according to which a surface is occluding missing parts of inducing elements. Other cues triggering the cognitive problem-solving process are: symmetry, incompleteness, interruptions, gaps, alignments among interruptions, expectations, and general knowledge. As a consequence, the alignment among gap terminations and the familiarity of the fragments (the circular sectors and the angles) should elicit a cognitive hypothesis of a triangle occluding three disks and an outline triangle. Also, Coren (1972) considered the incompleteness of the stimulus as a depth cue that generates the cognitive hypothesis of an occluding triangle.

Grossberg and Mingolla (1985a, 1985b) suggested that illusory contours can be explained by end-stopped cells in the primary visual cortex in conjunction with a grouping mechanism. End-stopped cells have elongated receptive fields with an excitatory region in the middle and inhibitory zones at their ends. Their role is to bridge the gap between two aligned inducers. Completion of illusory contours in a horizontal direction occurs between pairs of end-stopped cells that are tuned to vertically oriented edges or lines. This is related to the fact that spatial inhibition underlying end-stopped cells, interacting with the inhibition among cells tuned to different orientations, induces enhanced activity in cells whose orientational tuning had a peak in the orientation perpendicular to that of a thin line whose end fell into the cells' receptive fields (end cutting). Activity at spatially disjoint pairs of such end-stopped cells can activate a gating mechanism in V2 through a multiplicative interaction of activity triggered by those end-stopped cells called "cooperative bipole cells" (Grossberg and Mingolla, 1985a, 1985b). Peterhans and von der Heydt (1987) suggested that the output of the gating cell signals illusory contours. This output is then combined with the output of cells signaling real contours, thus forming an integrated perceptual representation of illusory contours.

Some of the Main Explanations of Neon Color Spreading

The explanations of the neon color spreading are based on the main effects involved, mainly illusory contours and color spreading (see Bressan et al., 1997, for a review). The illusory contours formation in the neon color spreading can be explained through the same hypotheses described in the previous section. The distinction between figural and coloration effects in the neon color spreading suggests that different mechanisms give rise to these properties. The FAÇADE model (Grossberg, 1994, 1997) proposes how parallel boundary grouping and surface filling-in processes are carried out, respectively, by a Boundary Contour System (BCS) and a Feature Contour System (FCS) (Cohen and Grossberg, 1984; Grossberg and Mingolla, 1985a, 1985b; Grossberg and Todorovic, 1988). These two processes are predicted to be realized by the cortical interblob and blob streams, respectively, within cortical areas V1 through V4.

The boundary and surface processes exhibit *complementary* properties (Grossberg, 2000). Boundaries form *inwardly* between similarly *oriented* contrasts and are *insensitive* to contrast polarity or pool contrast information at each position from opposite contrast polarities. Boundaries pool opposite contrasts so that they can form around objects on textured backgrounds. In particular, a boundary can continuously surround an object even if its contrast relative to the background reverses multiple times as the object boundary is traversed. Because of this contrast-pooling property, all boundaries are predicted to be *amodal* within the interblob cortical stream where they form. (The previous explanation suggested to account for illusory contours is included within the FAÇADE model.) Visible colors and brightnesses, including neon color spreading, are predicted to be a property of the surface formation stream. Surfaces fill in *outwardly* from individual lightness or color inducers in an *unoriented* way using a process that is *sensitive* to contrast polarity. Surface filling in is contained by boundaries, which act as barriers or gates that restrict the spread of color or brightness. This hypothesis implies that, whenever surface colors are seen at locations far from their inducers, they must have spread there via surface filling in. Moreover, if surface color does manage to spread to positions beyond which they occur in a scene or image the boundaries, which might otherwise have contained their spread, must be broken or otherwise weakened to permit the leakage of color beyond them (see Pinna and Grossberg, 2005).

The Role of Petter's Rule within Illusory Contours and Neon Color Spreading

The previous explanation pointed out some properties of the stimulus considered as basic to explain both illusory contours and neon color spreading. They are: incompleteness, gap, missing region, interruption, alignment, and past experience. These properties are related to a correlated mechanism involving end-stopped cells in conjunction with grouping and boundary contour processes.

In figure 9.5a, Petter's rule can influence the presence/absence of illusory contours even if, under these conditions, the general illusory contours conditions are satisfied given the presence of line ends, interruptions, gaps, and so on. They should produce a strong illusory annulus partially occluding the radial lines. However, unexpectedly the annulus is perceived only virtually (i.e., as a result of the circular connection [not illusory] among the gaps). In fact, the gaps appear as disjoint bright spots overlapped on each radial line without any illusory contours bridging and completing them (Pinna and Grossberg, 2006). The bright spots do not spread but remain localized in the region of the gaps. These phenomenal observations imply that there is a brightness induction only in the region close to the line terminations, but it does not complete modally in the region in between each radial line neither as brightness enhancement nor as illusory contours. The white among the lines is the same as the background.

The previous unexpected results are strongly related to Petter's rule. In fact, under illusory contours conditions, this rule can be expressed as follows: The region with the shortest contour appears surrounded by modal illusory contours. Because the length of each gap is shorter than the distance between each radial line, the illusory contours tend to be formed along the boundaries of the gaps and not on the boundaries of the region connecting the gaps thus creating *ipso facto* a virtual (but not illusory) annulus.

By increasing the size of the gaps of figure 9.5a (see figure 9.5b), the ratio between the gap size and the distance among the lines tends to 1 but still remains in favor of the gap size. As a consequence, the illusory contours and the brightness enhancement among the radial lines start to be perceived even if the bright spots appear as the strongest effects. This result is supported by the clear difference of the perceived brightness present in each gap and in the regions among the radial lines. The brightness among the lines is stronger than the one of the background but less strong than the one within the gaps. This induces a brighter and darker alternation in the annulus that

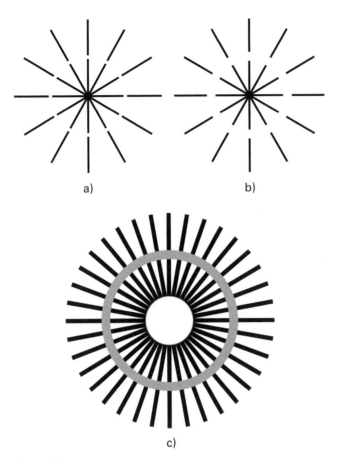

Figure 9.5
Petter's rule can influence the presence/absence of illusory contours (a–b and d–f). In (c) a new illusion is illustrated: By keeping the gaze on the center of the figure, the brightness and darkness inductions clearly deform the shape of the annulus that appears as full of bulges.

appears like a whole illusory shape with wavy contours. This shape effect is much stronger in figure 9.5c, where, by keeping the gaze on the center of the figure, the brightness and darkness inductions clearly deform the shape of the annulus that appears as full of bulges.

By further increasing the gap sizes so that Petter's rule is now slightly in favor of the distance among radial lines (figure 9.5d), the illusory annulus is perceived more easily than the bright spots on the gaps. However, being the ratio near the equilibrium, the strength of both illusory contours and brightness enhancement is not as strong as those conditions where the ratio is more definitively in favor of one or the other size

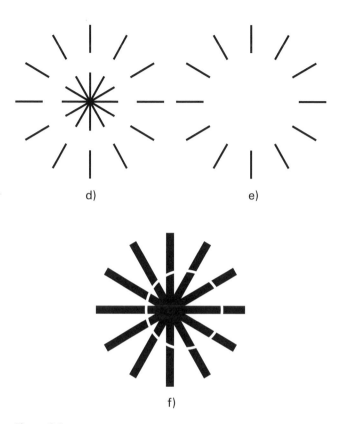

d)   e)

f)

Figure 9.5
(continued)

of Petter's ratio. Figure 9.5e corroborates this hypothesis. Under these conditions, only the distance among lines is present, and then both the illusory contours and the brightness enhancement are stronger than those perceived in figure 9.5d.

In figure 9.5f, variations in Petter's ratio are illustrated within the same condition. On the left side, where the ratio is about 1, a portion of an illusory annulus can be perceived more strongly than on the right side, where bright curved rectangles within each black stripe can be seen instead. It is worthwhile noticing that on the left side the illusory shape appears like a perfect arc of a circle, whereas on the right side, although the bright inset rectangular shapes are real arcs of a circle whose alignment should elicit portions of an annulus, they appear more rectilinear. This happens because in between the radial stripes no illusory contours can be perceived.

The right side of figure 9.5f can also be perceived in another way (i.e., black rectangular windows or holes on a black background through which portions of a white annulus are seen). This result is stronger in figure 9.6a, where the inducers are not radial

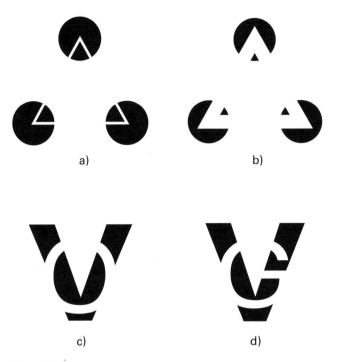

Figure 9.6
Other examples testing Petter's rule with illusory contours.

lines but surfaces like the circular sectors of Kanizsa's triangle. This change from a line to a surface reveals more clearly the role of Petter's rule.

The three corners are not grouped to produce an illusory triangular contour across the white space in between the disks partially occluding them. But they become a white triangle partially perceived through three circular windows or holes in a white surface on a black background. The boundaries of the holes belong to the white surface. The black achromatic color, seen through the windows, completes amodally becoming a homogenous black background. The white space becomes a punched surface partially occluding a white triangle (see also Pinna and Grossberg, 2006). Like figure 9.5a, this figure clearly demonstrates that, given incompletenesses, gaps, missing regions, interruptions, and alignments, favored by gestalt principles of good continuation, closure, proximity, and Prägnanz working synergistically, the perceived result depends on Petter's rule, which creates illusory contours closing the circles instead of connecting the corners to form an illusory triangle. By increasing the width of the corners and changing Petter's ratio (figure 9.6b), an illusory triangle is more easily perceivable.

Figure 9.6c–d investigates the role of past experience when pitted against Petter's rule. Two black Vs appear partially occluded by an illusory O and G. In the outside edges of the Vs, the O and the G do not appear in front of the Vs but rather behind the white region that now appears as a figure and that is the background of the Vs. In other words, the perceived results are two holes having V shapes partially showing a black background and a white O and G partially perceived through them (see also Pinna and Grossberg, 2006). If the global observation of these stimuli reveals immediately the alphabetical letters, the local perception across the intersecting regions change the global result on the basis of Petter's rule. This implies that past experience plays only a partial and temporary role.

The role of Petter's rule within neon color spreading is similar to the one played within illusory contours. Figure 9.7 shows some examples similar to those illustrated in figure 9.5. By varying Petter's ratio, four conditions can be obtained: one in favor of neon color spreading (a–d), one against it (c), and a reversible condition where both blue stripes and neon color spreading can be perceived (b–e). The phenomenal results on the left and right side of figure 9.7e are the same as those described for figure 9.5f.

A Synoptic Phenomenal Comparison among Illusory Contours, Neon Color Spreading, and Petter's Figures

To demonstrate a clear role of Petter's rule in the formation of illusory contours and neon color spreading, some conditions should be fulfilled: (1) The rule should work properly and consistently with the predictions (i.e., by creating at least three possible results) in favor of one size of the ratio, in favor of the other and, when the two sizes are about the same, reversibly in favor of both; (2) it should influence the presence/absence, the strength, and the depth organization of the component parts of illusory contours and neon color spreading; and (3) Petter's rule should predict similar results (presence/absence, strength, and depth organization) in the three effects: Petter's figures, illusory contours, and neon color spreading.

In figure 9.8, three conditions of Petter's figures are illustrated where Petter's rule works consistently with predicted depth organizations and different perceived strengths: In (a) the horizontal bar is strongly perceived behind the vertical ones, in (b) it appears reversibly in front of the vertical bars or behind them (i.e., the strength of the two possible depth segregations is about the same [50%]), and in (c) the horizontal bar is clearly perceived in front of the vertical ones.

The same results should be expected under illusory contours and neon color spreading conditions. In figure 9.9, the same examples of Petter's figures are illustrated as illusory contours. The main argument is: If Petter's horizontal bar (figure 9.8a) is perceived behind the vertical black bars, then in figure 9.9a no illusory horizontal bar is expected to be perceived; instead, the gaps should appear like bright dashes in front of the black bars. Another possible result, consistent with Petter's rule is: a horizontal

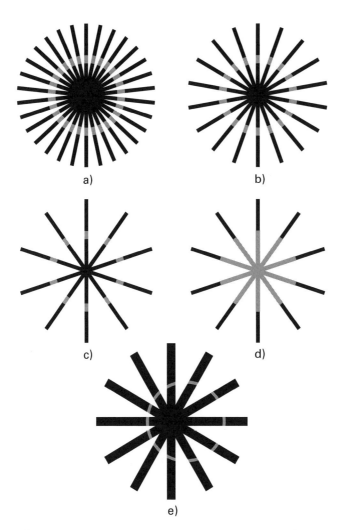

Figure 9.7
Petter's rule can influence the presence/absence of neon color spreading.

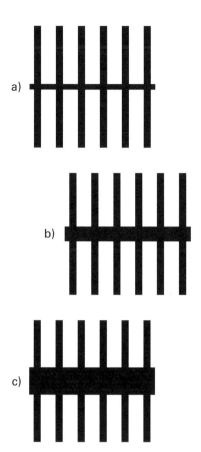

Figure 9.8
Three conditions of Petter's figures, where Petter's rule works consistently with predicted depth organizations and different perceived strengths.

bright bar partially perceived through rectangular holes showing a black background and completing amodally behind the white surface on which the holes are cut. These are indeed the two strongest results perceived in figure 9.9a. They clearly depend on Petter's rule and on the illusory contour formation along the vertical side of the white gaps and in the continuation of the black bars across the gaps. Very weak or no illusory contours are perceived in between the bars because the interspaces are much longer than the vertical heights of the gaps. These results disagree with the previous explanations of illusory contours, which take into account only the gaps but not the role of Petter's ratio. Therefore, they predict an illusory horizontal stripe partially occluding black vertical bars.

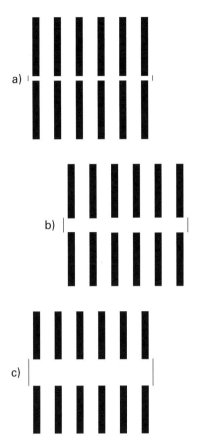

Figure 9.9
The same examples of Petter's figures, illustrated as illusory contours, elicit result consistent with Petter's rule.

In figure 9.9b, the ratio between the height of the gaps and distance in between bars is approximately 1. Under these conditions, a reversible shift between the two previous possible results is expected on the basis of Petter's rule as it really happens (i.e., bright dash/amodal bar vs. illusory white stripe partially occluding black bars). The perceived strength of the two kinds of results (~50%) is also consistent with Petter's rule. The complement of figure 9.9a is illustrated in figure 9.9c. The expected and perceived result is a large illusory rectangle partially occluding the vertical bars while the dash/amodal bar effect is hardly perceived.

The change of the results perceived in figure 9.9 cannot be predicted from any of the main explanations of illusory contours described earlier.

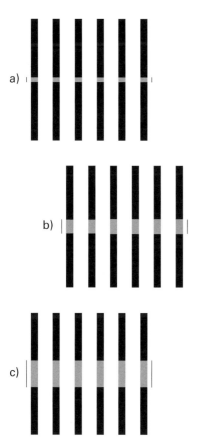

Figure 9.10
Under neon color-spreading conditions, Petter's rule predicts results similar to those obtained with illusory contours and Petter's figures.

Under neon color spreading conditions, Petter's rule predicts results similar to those obtained with illusory contours. In figure 9.10, the neon-like counterparts of the three previous cases are illustrated.

The color spreading is not expected and perceived in figure 9.10a. This is due to the formation of vertical illusory contours on the continuation of the boundaries of the vertical bars that prevents the spread of color. In figure 9.10b, the color spreading is weak but is clearly perceived in figure 9.10c, where it is favored by the formation of horizontal illusory contours in between the vertical bars.

By changing Petter's ratio more and more in favor of the height of the gaps or the distance among vertical bars, the previous results are expected to become stronger and stronger. This can be done, for example, by changing the distance among the vertical bars. The aim of the next experiment is to obtain a quantitative study of the role of Petter's rule on the three phenomena: Petter's figures, illusory contours, and neon color spreading.

Methods

Subjects

Three independent groups of fourteen (male and female) undergraduate students participated in the experiment. Subjects were naive as to the purpose of the experiment, and all had normal or corrected-to-normal acuity.

Stimuli

Three sets of nine stimuli were, respectively, created for the three illusions: Petter's figures, illusory contours, and neon color spreading. The stimuli were composed of figures like those illustrated in figures 9.8 to 9.10: one horizontal component placed at the center of several vertical bars. According to Petter's ratio, two sizes of the stimulus were systematically varied: the height of the horizontal component (0.5, 1.44, 2.75 degrees of visual angle) and the distance among the vertical black bars (1.15, 2.3, 3.8 degrees).

All the other properties of the stimulus were kept constant. The length of the horizontal component was 12.9 degrees. The sizes of the vertical bars were 0.7 × 12.15 degrees. The luminance of the white background was 88.5 cd/m2. The CIE chromaticity coordinates for the red chromatic color were 0.62, 0.34. Stimuli were presented on a computer screen with ambient illumination from an Osram Daylight fluorescent light (250 lux, 5600° K) in a frontoparallel plane. Subjects viewed the stimuli positioned at 50 cm with freely moving eyes using a chin-and-forehead rest.

Procedure

The tasks of the subjects were: (1) *Phenomenological task*—to describe freely what they perceived and, more particularly, to give an exhaustive description of the depth organization of the perceived components of the stimulus, and (2) *Rating task*—to scale the relative strength or salience (in percent) of the perceived results.

Each independent group evaluated only one of the three illusions. The stimuli were presented consecutively to each observer in a random order. Observation time was unlimited, but responses were prompt.

Results and Discussion

Phenomenological Task   The results of this task are described separately for the three illusions. Three qualitatively different descriptions were reported for all the illusions relatively to the three main values of Petter's ratio: The size of the height of the horizontal bar is smaller than the distance size in between the vertical bars (we call this condition "small bar"), the difference between the two sizes is small or about the same (we call this "size equilibrium"), and, finally, the distance size in between the vertical bars is smaller than the size of the width of the horizontal bar (we call this "small distance").

Petter's figures   In small bar, the horizontal bar appears clearly behind the vertical ones. In size equilibrium, the horizontal bar appears alternately and reversibly in front of the vertical bars or behind them. In small distance, the horizontal bar appears strongly in front of the vertical ones.

Illusory contours   In small bar, the gaps are perceived like bright dashes in front of the black bars or like an amodal horizontal bar partially perceived through black holes and completing behind a large white surface. In size equilibrium, the results of small bar are alternated with the results of small distance. In small distance, an illusory horizontal bar appears strongly in front of the vertical ones.

Neon color spreading   In small bar, the red dashes are perceived as red dashes in front of the black bars or like an amodal red horizontal bar partially perceived through black holes and completing behind a large white surface. In size equilibrium, the results of small bar are alternated with the results of small distance. In small distance, a neon-like horizontal bar appears strongly in front of the vertical ones.

Rating Task   In figure 9.11, mean ratings of the strength of the horizontal component perceived like (1) a figure of Petter's placed in front of the vertical bars (figure 9.11a), (2) an illusory surface partially occluding the vertical bars (figure 9.11b), and (3) a neon-like transparent bar (figure 9.11c) are plotted as a function of the height (size width) of the horizontal bar for the three variations of the distance in between the vertical bars.

The results of Petter's figure condition showed that, by increasing the size of the height of the horizontal bar, it appears more and more in front of the vertical bars in all the distance sizes (figure 9.11a). The three components of Petter's ratio emerge clearly from the results. The descriptions of the phenomenological task coincide with the three groups of mean ratings: closest to 0%, ~50%, and closest to 100%. These results are also supported by the fact that each mean rating is related to the strength of the horizontal component perceived in front of the vertical bars but at the same time to the complementary result (i.e., the horizontal component seen behind the vertical bars). If one rating suggested by a subject is closest to 0 (e.g., 5%), then its complement is closest to 100 (95%).

A two-way analysis of variance (ANOVA) (size of the height of the horizontal bar x distance in between the vertical bars) yielded an overall effect of variation in the size of the height of the horizontal bar ($F_{2,26} = 18.7$, $p < 0.001$) and in the distance in

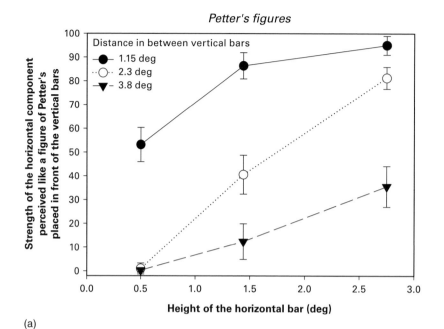

(a)

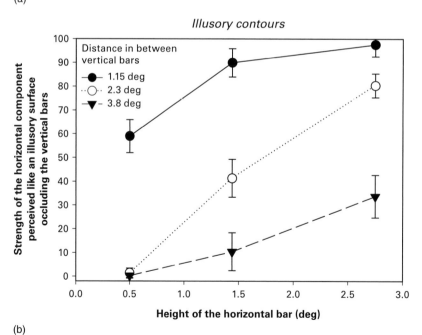

(b)

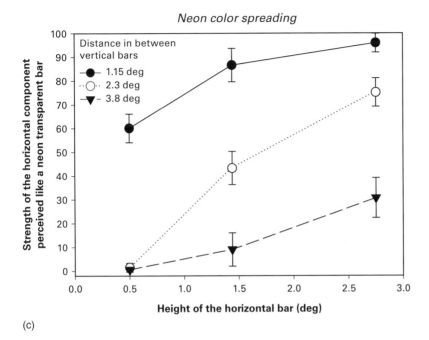

(c)

Figure 9.11

Mean ratings of the strength of the horizontal component perceived like (a) a Petter's figure placed in front of the vertical bars, (b) an illusory surface partially occluding the vertical bars, and (c) a neon-like transparent bar.

between the vertical bars ($F_{2,26} = 19.7$, $p < 0.001$). The interaction between these two factors was also significant ($F_{4,26} = 15.5$, $p < 0.001$).

The results of illusory contours and neon color spreading conditions showed results similar to those obtained with Petter's figures but related to the three main effects of these two illusions.

A two-way ANOVA yielded an overall effect of variation in the height of the horizontal bar (illusory contours: $F_{2,26} = 18.5$, $p < 0.001$; neon color spreading: $F_{2,26} = 15.8$, $p < 0.001$) and in the distance in between the vertical bars (illusory contours: $F_{2,26} = 13.2$, $p < 0.001$; neon color spreading: $F_{2,26} = 17.5$, $p < 0.001$). The interaction between these two factors was also significant (illusory contours: $F_{4,52} = 13.2$, $p < 0.001$; neon color spreading: $F_{4,52} = 18.7$, $p < 0.001$).

Discussion

In summary, the results of the two experimental tasks clearly demonstrated a basic role played by Petter's ratio in influencing presence/absence, strength, and depth

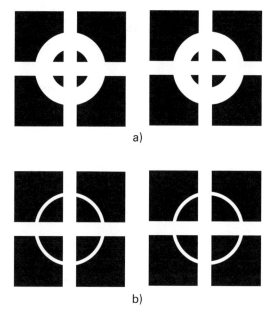

a)

b)

Figure 9.12
Petter's rule pitted against stereopsis.

organization of the component parts of Petter's figures, illusory contours, and neon color spreading. Therefore, Petter's rule is a valid principle not only for chromatically homogenous patterns (Singh et al., 1999) but also for inhomogenous ones.

These results suggest that Petter's rule is a contour formation rule due to global boundary contours interactions determining the depth organization of the visual components. This rule derives from the formation of two different kinds of contours, modal and amodal, linked together by the dynamics of filling in of contour gaps.

The strength of Petter's rule in determining depth perception and therefore illusory contours and neon color spreading can be carried to extremes by pitting this rule against the strongest way to obtain depth perception: the stereopsis (Julesz, 1971). In figure 9.12a, the stereogram was created by introducing small horizontal disparities in the position of the annulus. The square shapes were at zero disparity in relation to the annulus. By viewing this pattern stereoscopically, a white illusory annulus appears standing out clearly in front of the four squares, seen at the same depth plane. The annulus appears opaque with a surface color similar to the illusory figure that can be observed monocularly.

The stereogram of figure 9.12a is the control of the next one illustrated in figure 9.12b, where Petter's rule is pitted against the stereoscopic depth organization. When the two eye patterns are fused, the unity and integrity of the annulus expected from the stereoscopic viewing is broken due to Petter's rule: The annulus is split in four arcs standing out in stereoscopic depth and separated by empty spaces right by the intersecting regions with the crossed empty space among the squares. Another possible description is a stereoscopic annulus with four gaps. The same results can be obtained under Petter's figures and neon color spreading conditions (not illustrated). These results demonstrate that Petter's rule wins against stereopsis.

The effectiveness and strength of this rule induce a reassessment of all the theories of illusory contours previously considered, but they also suggest new researches in terms of neural correlate. Von der Heydt et al. (1984) and Peterhans and von der Heydt (1987) demonstrated that neurons in area V2 of the monkey cortex respond to both real and illusory contours. Sasaki and Watanabe (2004) reported distinct functional magnetic resonance imaging (fMRI) signatures in the human visual cortex for illusory contours and for color spreading processes, including color spreading in V1. Zhou et al. (2000) found a substantial fraction of cells that are sensitive to border ownership in area V2. fMRI studies of Kanizsa squares by Hirsch et al. (1995) revealed that there was activation of the occipital cortex lateral to V1 where signals related to segmentation were present. Mendola et al. (1999) found that signals related to illusory contours were observed in cortical area V3 and also in LO, the lateral occipital area (Malach et al., 1995). These studies deserve to be reconsidered in the light of Petter's rule.

How can Petter's rule be explained? Petter (1956; see also Kanizsa 1979) suggested that the generation of modal illusory contours in the intersecting regions where the surfaces appear overlapped require an extra amount of "energy" and that the visual system has a tendency to save this (never defined) energy. To save energy, the visual system generates only the shortest possible modal illusory contours. As a consequence, the surface with the shorter contours in the intersecting region would more probably appear to be in front.

Grossberg's FAÇADE model can explain Petter's rule in reductionist terms of neural circuitry. The bipole grouping cells (Grossberg and Mingolla, 1985a, 1985b; Raizada and Grossberg, 2003) form real and illusory boundaries via long-range excitatory connections and short-range inhibitory connections. Some of the short-range inhibitory connections ensure that the groupings form inwardly between pairs or greater numbers of (quasi) collinear contours. Other inhibitory connections suppress weaker boundary groupings at nearby positions and at different orientations and depths.

Another key step in this explanation is based on the fact that (Grossberg, 1987, 1994, 1997) the stronger boundary can break the weaker boundary where it abuts the stronger boundary, thereby creating a gap in the weaker boundary. This step triggers depth figure-ground percepts through a feedback interaction between boundary and surface representations. This hypothesis is useful to explain how the visual cortex generates illusory contours and neon color-spreading percepts.

Acknowledgments

Supported by Finanziamento della Regione Autonoma della Sardegna, ai sensi della L.R. 7 agosto 2007, n. 7, Fondo d'Ateneo (ex 60%), Fondazione Banco di Sardegna, and Alexander von Humboldt Foundation. Special thanks to Maria Tanca for assistance in testing the subjects.

References

Bressan, P., Mingolla, E., Spillmann, L., and Watanabe, T. 1997. "Neon Colour Spreading: A Review." *Perception* 26: 1353–1366.

Cohen, M., and Grossberg, S. 1984. "Neural Dynamics of Brightness Perception: Features, Boundaries, Diffusion, and Resonance." *Perception & Psychophysics* 36: 428–456.

Coren, S. 1972. "Subjective Contours and Apparent Depth." *Psychological Review* 79: 359–367.

Ehrenstein, W. 1941. "Über Abwandlungen der L. Hermannschen Helligkeitserscheinung" (On the Variations of the Hermann Grid). *Zeitschrift für Psychologie* 150: 83–91.

Gregory, R. 1972. "Cognitive Contours." *Nature* 238: 51–52.

Gregory, R. L. 1987. "Illusory Contours and Occluding Surfaces." In *The Perception of Illusory Contours*, edited by S. Petry and G. E. Meyer. New York, Berlin, Heidelberg: Springer-Verlag. 81–89.

Grossberg, S. 1987. "Cortical Dynamics of Three-Dimensional Form, Color, and Brightness Perception: II. Binocular Theory." *Perception & Psychophysics* 41: 117–158.

Grossberg, S. 1994. "3-D Vision and Figure-Ground Separation by Visual Cortex." *Perception & Psychophysics* 55: 48–120.

Grossberg, S. 1997. "Cortical Dynamics of Three-Dimensional Figure-Ground Perception of Two-Dimensional Pictures." *Psychological Review* 104: 618–658.

Grossberg, S. 2000. "The Complementary Brain: Unifying Brain Dynamics and Modularity." *Trends in Cognitive Sciences* 4: 233–245.

Grossberg, S., and Mingolla, E. 1985a. "Neural Dynamics of Form Perception: Boundary Completion, Illusory Figures and Neon Color Spreading." *Psychological Review* 92: 173–211.

Grossberg, S., and Mingolla, E. 1985b. "Neural Dynamics of Perceptual Grouping: Textures, Boundaries, and Emergent Segmentations." *Perception & Psychophysics* 38: 141–171.

Grossberg, S., and Todorovic, D. 1988. "Neural Dynamics of 1-D and 2-D Brightness Perception: A Unified Model of Classical and Recent Phenomena." *Perception & Psychophysics* 43: 241–277.

Helmholtz, H. L. F. von. 1867. *Handbuch der physiologischen Optik* (Handbook of Physiological Optics). Leipzig: Voss.

Hirsch, J., DeLaPaz, R. L., Relkin, N. L., Victor, J., Kim, K., Li, T., Borden, P., Nava, R., and Shapley, R. 1995. "Illusory Contours Activate Specific Regions in Human Visual Cortex: Evidence From Functional Magnetic Resonance Imaging." *Proceedings of the National Academy of Science* 92: 6469–6473.

Julesz, B. 1971. *Foundations of Cyclopean Perception*. Chicago: University of Chicago Press.

Kanizsa, G. 1955. "Margini quasi-percettivi in campi con stimolazione omogenea" (Quasi-perceptual margins in homogenously stimulated fields). *Rivista di Psicologia* 49: 7–30.

Kanizsa, G. 1969. "Perception, Past Experience and the Impossible Experiment." *Acta Psychologica* 31: 66–96.

Kanizsa, G. 1979. *Organization in Vision*. New York: Praeger.

Malach, R., Reppas, J. B., Benson, R. R., Kwong, K. K., Jiang, H., Kennedy, W. A., Ledden, P. J., Brady, T. J., Rosen, B. R., and Tootell, R. B. 1995. "Object-Related Activity Revealed by Functional Magnetic Resonance Imaging in Human Occipital Cortex." *Proceedings of the National Academy of Science* 92: 8135–8139.

Mendola, J. D., Dale, A. M., Fischl, B., Liu, A. K., and Tootell, R. B. 1999. "The Representation of Illusory and Real Contours in Human Cortical Visual Areas Revealed by Functional Magnetic Resonance Imaging." *Journal of Neuroscience* 19: 8560–8572.

Metzger, W. 1975. *Gesetze des Sehens* (Laws of Seeing). Frankfurt am Main: Kramer.

Michotte, A. 1951. "Une nouvelle énigme de la psychologie de la perception: le 'donné amodal' dans l'expérience" (A New Enigma of the Psychology of Perception: The 'Amodal Datum' in the Experience). *Stockholm: Actes du Congrés Internationale de Psychologie*, pp. 179–180.

Michotte, A., Thinès, G., and Crabbé, G. 1964. "Les compléments amodaux des structures perceptives" (Amodal Completion of Perceptual Structures). In *Michotte's Experimental Phenomenology of Perception*, edited by G. Thinès, A. Costall, and G. Hillsdale, NJ: Lawrence Erlbaum Associates, 1991.

Peterhans, E., and von der Heydt, R. 1987. "The Role of End-Stopped Receptive Fields in Contour Perception." In *New Frontiers in Brain Research: Proceedings of the 15th Göttingen Neurobiology Conference*, edited by N. Elsner and O. Creutzfeldt. Stuttgart: Thieme. 29.

Petter, G. 1956. "Nuove ricerche sperimentali sulla totalizzazione percettiva" (New Experimental Researches on Perceptual Totalization). *Rivista di Psicologia* 50: 213–227.

Pinna, B., and Grossberg, S. 2005. "The Watercolor Illusion and Neon Color Spreading: A Unified Analysis of New Cases and Neural Mechanisms." *Journal of the Optical Society of America A* 22: 1–15.

Pinna, B., and Grossberg, S. 2006. "Logic and Phenomenology of Incompleteness in Illusory Figures: New Cases and Hypotheses." *Psychofenia* 9: 93–135.

Raizada, R. D. S., and Grossberg, S. 2003. "Towards a Theory of the Laminar Architecture of Cerebral Cortex: Computational Clues From the Visual System." *Cerebral Cortex* 13: 100–113.

Rock, I. 1983. *The Logic of Perception*. Cambridge, MA: MIT Press.

Rock, I. 1987. "A Problem-Solving Approach to Illusory Contours." In *The Perception of Illusory Contours*, edited by S. Petry and G. E. Meyer. New York: Springer. 62–70.

Sasaki, Y., and Watanabe, T. 2004. "The Primary Visual Cortex Fills in Color." *Proceedings of the National Academy of Sciences* 101: 18251–18256.

Schumann, F. 1900. "Beiträge zur Analyse der Gesichtswahrnehmungen. Zur Schätzung räumlicher Größen" (Contributions to the Analysis of Visual Perception. On the Estimate of Size). *Zeitschrift für Psychologie und Physiologie der Sinnesorgane* 24: 1–33.

Shipley, T. F., and Kellman, P. J. 1992. "Perception of Partly Occluded Objects and Illusory Figures: Evidences for an Identity Hypothesis." *Journal of Experimental Psychology: Human Perception and Performance* 18: 106–120.

Singh, M., Hoffman, D. D., and Albert, M. K. 1999. "Contour Completion and Relative Depth: Petter's Rule and Support Ratio." *Psychological Science* 10: 423–428.

van Tuijl, H. F. J. M. 1975. "A New Visual Illusion: Neon-Like Color Spreading and Complementary Color Induction Between Subjective Contours." *Acta Psychologica* 39: 441–445.

van Tuijl, H. F. J. M., and de Weert, C. M. M. 1979. "Sensory Conditions for the Occurrence of the Neon Spreading Illusion." *Perception* 8: 211–215.

Varin, D. 1971. "Fenomeni di contrasto e diffusione cromatica nell'organizzazione spaziale del campo percettivo" (Contrast Phenomena and Color Spreading within the Spatial Organization of the Perceptual Field). *Rivista di Psicologia* 65: 101–128.

von der Heydt, R., Peterhans, E., and Baumgartner, G. 1984. "Illusory Contours and Cortical Neuron Responses." *Science* 224: 1260–1262.

Zhou, H., Friedman, H. S., and von der Heydt, R. 2000. "Coding of Border Ownership in Monkey Visual Cortex." *Journal of Neuroscience* 20: 6594–6611.

III Language and Perception

10   From Grouping to Visual Meanings: A New Theory of Perceptual Organization

Baingio Pinna and Liliana Albertazzi

This chapter proposes a foundation of meaning on a perceptual basis, providing experimental evidence to the thesis that the contents and structures of the phenomenal world are transposed into language as nuclei bearing semantic and syntactic features. The arguments presented are in favor of a universalist position in language, however, not in the sense of the analytic approach to semantics (logical syntax and model theory applied to natural language).

More generally, we follow the hypothesis that semantic contents and syntactic structures of natural language can be broken down into meaningful (i.e., not purely formal) traits, parts, or aspects rooted in perception. Accordingly, in the analysis of the structure of language, we make use of phenomenological concepts and principles drawn from Gestalt psychology.

Antecedents to this line of research are to be sought in the Brentanian tradition, specifically in Anton Marty and his idea of *figurative internal form* (Albertazzi, 1996; Marty, 1893, 1908, 1910). To the internal form belong those presentations that accompany the act of signifying. Because these presentations are figurative, they are often constituted of images or imaginative contents drawn from the field of visual perception, and they enable the interlocutor to make associations in the spoken language. As a first approximation, we may say that internal form comprises those expressions to which the intuitive presentation of a nameable object corresponds. Internal form, however, is not merely a matter of names. It also involves propositions, verbs, and adjectives (as the Brentano, Marty, and Twardowski [Twardowski, 1977] theory of modification would show), and it therefore more generally involves the phenomena of grammar (see Husserl 1910).

For several reasons, however, the Brentano–Marty approach to language has never had an experimental development. This chapter is one of the first attempts to shed light on the grammar of the figural internal form starting from the perceptual organization.

The problem of perceptual organization represents one of the basic topics of vision science. It concerns the reason that we perceive a world articulated in objects such as people, cities, houses, cars, and trees, and not scattered differences of luminances, edges, and bars. It was traditionally studied by Gestalt psychologists in terms of group-ing (Wertheimer, 1912a, 1912b, 1922, 1923) (i.e., how individual elements group into parts of a whole that in their turn group into larger wholes) and figure-ground segrega-tion (Rubin, 1921) (i.e., what appears as a figure and what appears as a background). However the complexity process of perceptual organization does not end with group-ing and figure-ground segregation. Recently, Pinna and Reeves (2006) introduced some principles of figurality, defining the phenomenal appearance of what is perceived as a figure within the three-dimensional space and under a perceived illumination: the figurality being due to the color and volume of the appearance with light and shaded regions and the direction and color of the light reflected by it.

Human perception goes beyond the perception of appearances and figures versus backgrounds. It is mostly perception of shapes and meanings that are at the basis of the construction of perceptual "objects." Strictly speaking, in Gestalt psychology, given their intrinsic dynamics, perceptual objects are considered to be events. From this point of view, with regard to the visual objects, we will use the category event instead of the category object and precisely, according to Metzger's definition, those of (1) stationary events (relative to the perception of stationary things), (2) nonstationary events (relative to the perception of movement or change), (3) quasi-stationary events (relative to variable stimulation in space), and (4) quasi-continuous events (relative to islands of stability in an event perceived overall in evolution in phases) (Albertazzi, 1998, 2004, 2005; Metzger, 1941; Musatti, 1928; Vicario, 2005).

Each perceptual event has a precise shape related to other shapes that conveys and signifies one or more meanings related to other meanings, thus creating a net of what the complex world we perceive in everyday life is.

Some of the basic questions concerning the complexity of such a net are: What is the connection in terms of perceptual organization between grouping and shape? Can grouping and shape be reduced to the same perceptual item? Then, what is the percep-tual connection between shape and meaning? Can both be considered as parts of the perceptual organization process? If so, what are the main phenomenal rules governing their formation? Specifically, what is a perceptual meaning? Finally, is it possible to speak of a "visual language" arising from the rules of perceptual organization, whose conceptualizations are embedded in the grammar and lexicon of natural languages?

The aims of this chapter are to suggest that perception is perceiving appearances of grouping, shapes, and meanings, and to propose a new theory of perceptual organiza-tion based on three different forms of organization: grouping, shape, and meaning. This tripartite distinction can widen the domain of vision science up to the item of meanings, usually considered as a specific issue of the cognitive science domain and usually considered to be top down. More specific purposes are to (1) suggest a link among perceptual grouping, shape perception, and visual meaning; (2) trace the visual meanings back to organizational processes eliciting objects and shapes while going beyond the principles studied by Gestalt psychologists; (3) define the phenomenal underlying structure and principles ruling the formation of meanings; and, finally, (4) define the main properties common to the three forms of perceptual organization.

Furthermore, our purpose is to show how the "invariants" of the structures of phenomenal appearances are transposed and expressed in natural language organization.

As to the last point, this work assumes a cognitive approach to semantics. The issue of cognition in semantics centers on an old Aristotelian issue regarding the natural origin (*physei*) of language (Aristotle, 1984). The question raised by cognitive semantics—by cognitive linguistics in particular (Evans and Green, 2006; Langacker, 1988; Rudzka-Ostyn, 1988)—is whether there exist contents and structures of the phenomenal world that are transposed into language as nuclei bearing semantic and syntactic features (Albertazzi, 1998a). If this were demonstrable, then it would be a strong argument in favor of the nonconventionality—at least in principle—of language (Albertazzi, 2002a).

To answer the question, philosophical and experimental analyses of the prelinguistic and precategorical structures are required, as well as an explanation of how the successive levels of predication develop on this basis (Husserl, 1973). In other words, it must be shown whether and how perception gives rise to the semantic categories of substantive, verb, and adjective (Husserl, 1975, Second Logical Investigation), to the linguistic modes (declarative, hypothetical, etc.), and especially whether and how the expressive modes of language are based on specific types of qualities of visual percepts (Albertazzi, 1997; Massironi and Bonaiuto, 1966). These questions have been entirely neglected by the formal analyses of a great part of the last century, and especially by analytic philosophy, because of the separation between syntax (a set of symbols) and semantics (the formal connection between symbols and the universe of discourse) (Albertazzi, 2000; Tarski, 1944).

Such a cognitive approach to semantics has a lot of aspects in common with experimental phenomenology. Experimental phenomenology, in fact, takes the point of departure of conceptual analysis to be the nature, structure, and organizing laws of perceptual phenomena and of the schemes embedded within them. From this point of view, therefore, meaning is not mentalist and/or propositional in character; on the contrary, it is an immediate datum of perception (the so-called experienced [*erlebt*] as opposed to represented) closely dependent on the spatiotemporal structure of events and their interconnections (see Husserl, 1973; Michotte, 1963). On the system used by language to schematize and structure space-time with properties of visual perception, see Talmy (1988).

At the ontological level, phenomenology takes a view that is both nonreductionist (the phenomenal level of experience does not coincide with that of physics or neurophysiology) and dynamic (perception is eminently temporal, and a phase of action) (Albertazzi, 2005, 2006).

An example of the contribution of experimental research to phenomenological analysis consists in singling out the "perceptual invariants" in a situation that—on the basis of the existence of particular structural characteristics—renders phenomenal events meaningful and ensures that "physically" distinct events are "perceived" as unitary. Experimental phenomenology therefore not only supports an anti-reductionist and anti-physicalist conception of meaning but also analyzes the origin and characteristics of the conceptual domain of representation and meaning in relation to perception.

From a semantic point of view, in particular, the analysis of the perceptual invariants reveals the connection between the forms of categorization that regulate the meaning of perceptual situations, on the one hand, and the linguistic product of those perceptions in their various construal expressions, on the other hand (Albertazzi, 1998a, 1998b; Langacker, 2000). The results of experimental research, in fact, show that the classic epistemological categories (e.g., that of "causality") are also in large part those that we use in language because they comprise conceptualization schemes, which are active in both (Albertazzi, 2002a; Schlottman, 2000; Schlottman and Shanks, 1992; Scholl and Tremoulet, 2000; Talmy, 1988).

Consequently, specification of the categorical structure at the perceptual level provides important insights into linguistic categorization, and it confirms the main tenets of cognitive linguistics.

Finally, an analysis of this type shows that the linguistic categorization does not simply come about through the metaphorical extension of semantic concepts because it is perception that accounts for different conceptualizations at the mental level (Barsalou, 1992).

In the specific cases examined here, as we see, the instruments of experimental phenomenology are able to demonstrate that the structural characteristics of certain phenomenal events involving, for example, the perception of events of causation constitute the origin of conceptual categories expressed linguistically by causatives of the type "melting," "cutting," "deforming," "mutilate," "eject," "crash," "pull," and so on, also in passive forms ("being melted," "being cut," "being deformed," "being mutilated," "being ejected," "being crashed," and "being pulled"). Thus, experimental analysis provides support for the force dynamics scheme of cognitive linguistics, which analyzes the structure of "causing into finer primitives" (Talmy, 1988). In particular, the analysis that follows shows how certain conceptual categories of perceptual causation and certain conceptual categories of psychological causation are strictly connected and expressed in natural language.

Unlike cognitive linguistics, however, we argue that the concept of causation is not simply a linguistic extension of the concept of physical domain to the conceptual domain that expresses the psychic relations. Rather, it is based on specific categorical perceptual structures.

In short, language is essentially "by nature," and even syntax is semantically interpreted as the case of spatial prepositions (along, into, around, over, etc.) show (Vandeloise, 1991).

The Form of Grouping

In 1923, Wertheimer studied one of the basic problems of vision: perceptual grouping. The questions he answered were: How do the elements in the visual field "go together" to form a holistic percept (Gestalt)? How do individual elements group into wholes separated from others?

A general mereological problem concerning the nature of Gestalten is that they are not static products but rather processes and parts of processes (Albertazzi, 2006; Wertheimer, 1922). A specific mereological problem, instead, concerns the characteristics of the parts of a whole, which can be considered per se (red) or as dependent on others (red ball) or even as nondetachable (color and extension). In principle, a mereological theory of parts is not independent from a more general theory of relations. There are different ways to be part of a whole, in fact: There is the relation of having parts, which concerns the action of the whole on its parts and vice versa (e.g., having four angles named as different items/having a quadrangular form), and the relation of similarity between the whole and its parts, where it can be similar under several aspects and dissimilar under others (square/diamond, square/incomplete square) (see below).

Through phenomenological experiments, Wertheimer suggested some basic "grouping principles."

In figure 10.1, there are "small squares groups in columns (a) and rows (b)" (see Methods section). The form of grouping, columns or rows, depends on the similarity of achromatic color (black and white) among squares. Figure 10.1 illustrates one of

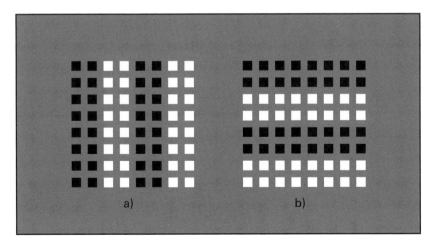

Figure 10.1
Small squares group in columns (a) and rows (b). *The local/global square/rectangle effect.* Both small and large squares appear similar to vertical (a) and horizontal (b) rectangles.

Wertheimer's grouping principles, stating that, all else being equal, the most similar elements (in color, size, orientation, etc.) tend to be grouped together.

Wertheimer identified other grouping principles in analogy with the similarity one and representing principles defining what determines the emerging whole when all else is equal. In addition to similarity, Wertheimer (1923) and other Gestalt psychologists discovered other basic "grouping principles": proximity, good continuation, closure, symmetry, convexity, *Prägnanz*, past experience, common fate, and parallelism. Furthermore, a number of new principles have been more recently discovered: common region (Palmer, 1992), synchrony (Palmer, 1999), and element connectedness (Palmer, 1999; Palmer and Rock, 1994). However, despite their novel appearance, these principles can be traced back to the classical ones because they likely represent special cases of at least one of the classical principles. Through the following figures (figures 10.2–10.5), the similarity principle is mostly considered and deepened.

Methods

Subjects   Independent groups of 14 undergraduate students participated in the phenomenological experiments described in the next sections. Subjects were naïve as to the purpose of these experiments, and all had normal or corrected-to-normal acuity.

Stimuli   The stimuli were composed of the figures illustrated and described in the next sections. Stimuli were presented on a computer screen with ambient illumination from an Osram Daylight fluorescent light (250 lux, 5600° K). The mean overall size of the stimuli was about 10×10 degrees of visual angle. The luminance of the white background was 88.3 cd/m^2. Black contours had a luminance contrast of 0.97 (luminance value of 2.6 cd/m^2). The stroke width was approximately 6 arc/min.

Stimuli, for all experimental conditions, were viewed binocularly and presented in a frontoparallel plane at a distance of 50 cm from the observer. The head position of the observer was stabilized by a chin rest.

Procedure   The subjects' task was to report freely what they perceived by giving, as much as possible, an exhaustive description of the main visual properties. Unless otherwise stated, different groups of 14 naïve observers each described only one stimulus. This was done to avoid interactions and contaminations among stimuli. The descriptions reported in angle quotes (guillemets) through the paper used similar phrases and words as those provided by the spontaneous descriptions of no less than 11 out of 14 subjects but edited for brevity and representativeness. Some individual differences were found, but we report only those descriptions generated by at least 11 of the 14 subjects in each group. We report all of these descriptions unless otherwise noted. The edited descriptions were judged by five graduate students of linguistics, who were naïve as to the hypotheses of the present research, to provide a fair representation of those provided by the observers. The descriptions are incorporated within the text to aid the reader in the stream of argumentations.

From the Form of Grouping to the Form of Shape

The Local/Global Square/Rectangle Effect

The descriptions of figure 10.1 continued spontaneously as follows: "columns (a) and rows (b) group creating a large square. Both small and large squares appear similar to vertical (a) and horizontal (b) rectangles" (i.e., the components group and also orient and elongate the shape of each inner small square and of the whole squares in the same direction as the perceptual organization). The shapes of small and large squares do not appear isotropic (directional invariant) but with a clear directional symmetry (see also Pinna, 2010).

This effect is likely related to Oppel-Kundt group of illusions, where an empty (unfilled) space looks wider than a space filled by some objects (Da Pos and Zambianchi, 1996; Kristof, 1961; Oppel, 1854–1855), and to Helmholtz's (1866) square illusion, where a square appears wider when it is filled with vertical lines and higher when filled with horizontal lines. Nevertheless, there are several important differences: (1) in our stimuli, the whole shape distortion is induced by grouping and not by filled versus unfilled space; (2) the direction of the illusory distortion is the opposite of the one perceived in both Oppel-Kundt's and Helmholtz's square illusions; and (3) the shape distortion involves both the small squares and the whole square shape.

The previous descriptions suggest that the form of grouping influences the form of the shape: Squares appear as rectangles. These results might depend on the directional symmetry derived from the grouping by similarity. It is necessary to reassert that the role of the Gestalt principles is to define the rules of "what is or stays with what" and, therefore, the grouping and not the shape. There is nothing within these principles that suggests that they can describe the form of shape beyond the form of grouping. Under our condition (see the next figures), it is necessary to introduce the notion of form of shape as a complementary evolution of the form of grouping. This is not a literal or fictitious distinction but a phenomenal necessity that can have consequences in terms of neural circuitry. The phenomenal nature of this distinction is deepened through the next figures that prelude to a further necessary distinction: the form of visual meaning.

The Local/Global Square/Diamond Effect

In figure 10.2, the inner organization of elements forms the shape of both the elements and the whole.

In figure 10.2a, both the small and the whole composite squares are rotated by 35 degrees, and the similarity principle groups the components in columns along the

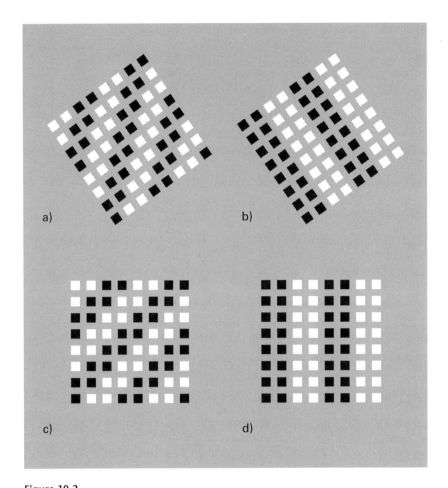

Figure 10.2

The local/global square/diamond effect. The inner and the whole squares appear as having a diamond shape (a). Small squares organized in columns and creating a rotated large square and both appear elongated in the same direction as the columns (b). The small and the large squares are perceived as having diamond shapes (c). Control—squares forming a large square and both appearing elongated (d).

diagonal of the whole square. As a consequence, "the inner and the whole squares appear as having a diamond shape." This result is strongly related to the square-diamond illusion (Schumann, 1900), according to which a square rotated by 45 degrees is perceived larger and like a diamond-shaped or rhombic figure. This effect is clearly enhanced by the grouping of the components along the diagonal of the whole diamond.

In figure 10.2b, the same components of figure 10.2a are perceived like "small squares organized in columns and creating a rotated large square and both appear elongated in the same direction as the columns." This result demonstrates the strength of the grouping due to similarity in forming the shape on the basis of the directional symmetry independently from or against the square-diamond illusion. It is worthwhile noticing that, by comparing figures 10.2a and 10.2b, the rotation with respect to the vertical-horizontal axis of both small and large squares appears different: The elements and the whole square are perceived as rotated and oriented in the same direction as the grouping, then in figure 10.2a more vertical than in figure 10.2b. This means that the directional symmetry also forms the orientation that is a perceptual component of the shape. In the next sections, other similar cases are considered. Another interesting effect likely depends on the directional symmetry: The inner structure of figure 10.2a, due to the alternation between black and white components, appears sinusoid or wave-like compared with the one perceived in figure 10.2b, where the waved alternation appears as having a square shape.

In figure 10.2c, the grouping forms similarly to figure 10.2a the shapes of the local and global components: "The small and the large squares are perceived as having diamond shapes." All the previous results emerge more clearly through the comparison with the control illustrated in figure 10.2d, where "squares forming a large square and both appearing elongated" are clearly perceived. The similarity principle induces a directional symmetry that determines the shape of the small and the whole components (see also Pinna, 2010).

Differently from figure 10.1, in figures 10.2a and 10.2c the similarity principle operates either against the main orientation of the small squares or against the one of the whole square. This implies that there are at least two grouping principles working at the same time. As a consequence, the similarity of the achromatic color is pitted against one of the local or global orientations. By comparing figures 10.2a and c, the role of the similarity of the main local and global orientations is clearer and stronger in figure 10.2c. Under these conditions, and all else being equal, one principle (similarity of achromatic color) wins over the other. More precisely, one principle defines what determines the emerging whole when all else is equal. Therefore, the strength of what emerges by virtue of the winner principle is weakened by the strength of the alternative grouping resulting from the loser principle.

This important point is useful to understand the role of the directional symmetry due to the grouping by similarity. Although the previous two similarities (achromatic and local/global orientation) are placed on the same phenomenal plane competing against each other, under our conditions, the similarity and directional symmetry are placed in different consequential planes or perceptual levels. In fact, they do not compete and do not cooperate but create different kinds of perceptual outcomes placed at different levels. They are also perceived phenomenally as different forms that can be considered as the result of different kinds of perceptual organization: form of grouping and form of shape. With regard to figure 10.1, this distinction can be expressed as follows: The achromatic similarity groups elements in rows and columns that in their turn form the whole shape on the basis of the directional symmetry. The latter principle is some kind of meta-principle that operates at another organization level after (or at the same time as) the result due to the former. More precisely, the similarity is a part-whole grouping principle that puts together elements (the small squares) that are perceived as parts of a whole grouping (the rows). By contrast, the directional symmetry is like a part-whole shape principle, where the elements (the rows) are perceived as parts (small rectangular shapes) of a whole shape (a large square) that appears similar to a horizontal rectangle. This distinction between principles and meta-principles or between grouping principles and shape principles is not trivial or merely linguistic but mostly phenomenological. It can be further perceived in the following figures, where the role of the form of shape emerges more clearly as an organizational process independent from the form of grouping.

The Tilt Grouping/Shape Effect
In figure 10.3, the similarity of the relative rotation of the elements groups the squares, respectively, in "alternated columns (a) and rows (b)."

The directional symmetry, due to the grouping, forms the shape of each column and row and of the whole configuration that "appears globally tilted in opposite directions and alternately converging and diverging." "The whole shape appears as an isosceles trapezium with the smallest side at the base (a) or on the right-hand side (b)." A circular arrangement of this tilt illusion is illustrated in figure 10.4, where "the concentric circles appear intertwined and forming a double spiral (a) or a spiral (b)." "In figure 10.4a the two spirals rotate in opposite directions." In this description both the form of grouping and the form of shape are clearly distinct. They are, respectively, the circular arrangement, due to the good continuation, and the spiral form of the shape.

These results are likely related to the Fraser (1908) illusion and to its special case, called "obliquity integration effect," suggested by Ehrenstein (1925), where a linear arrangement of slightly tilted segments, twisted like in a cord, appears globally tilted in the same direction as one of its components. However, unlike these well-known effects, under our conditions, the directional symmetry creates not only the simple or double spiral shapes but also the shape of the single elements. "The square elements in the double spiral of figure 10.4a appear more like diamonds than those of figure 10.4b."

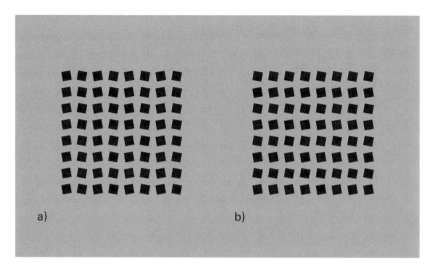

Figure 10.3
The tilt grouping/shape effect. Alternated columns (a) and rows (b). The whole shape appears as an isosceles trapezium with the smallest side at the base (a) or on the right-hand side (b).

This depends on the intertwining of the two spirals and their rotation in opposite ways that determines their directional symmetry along the square diagonal. In figure 10.4b, in contrast, the directional symmetry is oriented along the side of each square. Another difference with the Fraser illusion is that the components are not twisted like in a cord but are clearly perceived as separated individual elements. They can then be grouped in different ways when the similarity of achromatic color is introduced (see figure 10.5).

If the two similarities (tilt and achromatic color) are pitted one against or in favor of the other, the illusory tilt can be weakened (figures 10.5a, b, e, and f) or enhanced (figures 10.5c and d). They also create two directional symmetries that can change the whole shape (figures 10.5c, d, and f). In figure 10.5c, the synergistic separation among alternated columns and the consequent grouping by achromatic color induce "a 3-D segregation of the black components from the white ones creating some sort of X-shape in depth." In figure 10.5d, the grouping of differently tilted columns on the basis of similarity creates "a flat alternation of columns that, when going from the bottom to the top, appear diverging." The form of shape is the flat arrangement. Furthermore, depending on the kind of grouping and directional symmetry, "the small geometrical squares appear like squares or diamonds." In figures 10.5a, e, and f, "they appear more like diamonds than those of all the other conditions (figures 10.5b, c, and d)."

Again, these figures demonstrate that grouping can induce directional symmetries that form both local and global shapes. But these shapes are formed differently from

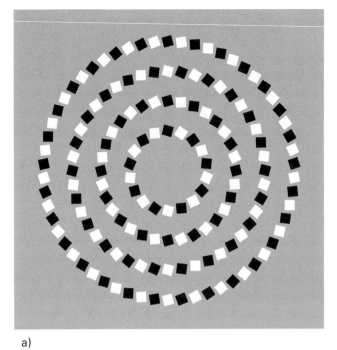

a)

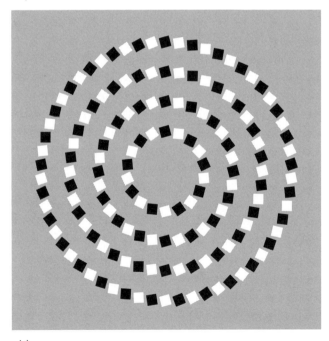

b)

Figure 10.4

The tilt grouping/shape effect. The concentric circles appear intertwined and forming a double intertwined spiral (a) or a spiral (b).

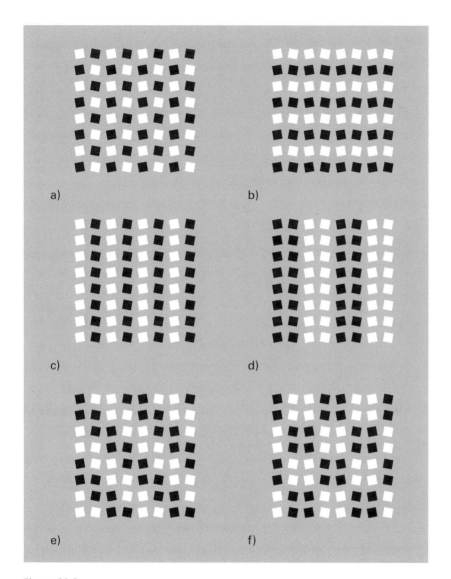

Figure 10.5

If the two similarity principles (tilt and achromatic color) are pitted one against or in favor of the other, the illusory tilt can be weakened (a, b, e, and f) or enhanced (c and d). They also create two directional symmetries that can change the whole shape (c, d, and f).

the one of the Fraser illusion and of its variants (i.e., not only in the tilt or in the converging/diverging effect). This is a more direct shape deformation that, even if it cannot be easily perceived in figures 10.4 and 10.5, is much stronger in the next figures.

The Trapezoidal Effect

In figure 10.6 (see also Pinna, 1990), the rotation of columns of squares in opposite directions induces: "a shape deformation of the vertically/horizontally oriented squares, placed in between the two columns, that both locally and globally appear as having a trapezoidal shape" (a, b, d, e); "a whole anticlockwise tilt of the large square which contains the empty tilted small squares" (c); and "a convex/concave deformation of the large square where the empty small square are included" (f; see also figure 10.7).

The shape deformation can involve the whole perimeter surrounded by the tilted squares (e) or the perimeter surrounding them (c, d, f). By pitting the similarity of tilt against the one induced by the achromatic color, the previous deformation effects are not reduced (not illustrated). This trapezoidal effect clearly demonstrates the role of the form of shape as a level of organization independent from the form of grouping. This effect depends on interactions between different directional symmetries (see next sections).

The Concave/Convex Effect

Similarly to figure 10.6f, the straight sides of the large inset squares of figure 10.7 appear to be illusory deformed: In (a) "the vertical sides appear convex, while the horizontal ones concave," and in (b) "the opposite of (a)" is perceived. This effect is reminiscent of the Zöllner, Wundt-Hering, Orbison, and Tilt illusions (Hering, 1861; Orbison, 1939; Schilder and Wechsler, 1936; Wundt, 1898; Zöllner, 1860), but it differs from them because it does not contain crossing lines or segments. Our conditions are more complex and also include other kinds of effects.

The trapezoidal shape distortions of figure 10.6, and more particularly of figure 10.6a, reveal a possible connection with the Ponzo (1912) illusion, where two parallel and identical segments, like the sides of our small squares, appear to be of different lengths when they are placed along the axis of two oblique lines forming an acute angle. The segment, placed in the smaller region of the converging oblique lines, appears longer than the one placed in the larger region. This illusion has been considered (Ponzo, 1912) as a consequence of the convergence of lines similar to the linear perspective where parallel lines converge by receding in depth. Despite the structural similarities of our conditions with the Ponzo illusion, in figures 10.6a, b, and e or in figure 10.7, there are juxtaposed squares with different orientations and not parallel lines converging by receding in depth as in the Ponzo illusion. A further difference is that these figures are strongly related to figures 10.6c, d, and f, where another known

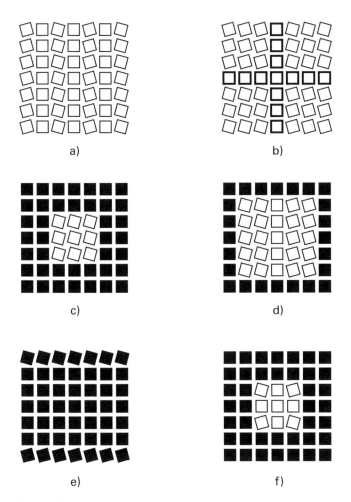

Figure 10.6
The trapezoidal effect. Shape deformations.

illusion can be involved. It is the rod and frame illusion (Kopfermann, 1930), where the orientation of a surrounding frame tilts, apparently in the opposite direction, the orientation of an inset element, a segment, or a rectangle. However, under our conditions, the effect proceeds in the opposite direction (i.e., the orientation of the inset elements affects the orientation of the surrounding frame).

The Frame/Rod Effect
The frame/rod effect is clearly demonstrated in figure 10.8, where "the white rectangles, inset within the squares, tilt them in a direction opposite to the smaller angle

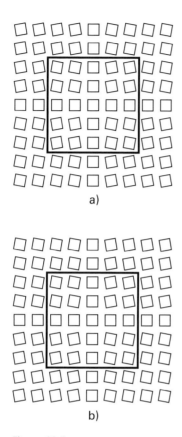

a)

b)

Figure 10.7
The concave/convex effect. The sides appear convex and concave.

created by the rectangle and the square, thus apparently increasing the acute angle."
The whole effect resulting from the organization of the local tilts is "a large square with
concave vertical and convex horizontal sides in figure 10.8a and, conversely, a large
square with convex vertical and concave horizontal sides in figure 10.8b." If each inset
rectangle is 45 degrees tilted with respect to the square, then by creating two equal
angles, the illusory effect is annulled (not illustrated).

By rotating the squares of figure 10.8a, as illustrated in figure 10.9, "the concave/
convex effect is enhanced when the inset rectangles follow the diagonal of each square
and weakened or annulled when they are parallel to the side orientation." Therefore,
the perceived result is switched from the diamond to the square illusion when the directional symmetry of the inset rectangles is synergistic with those of the shapes that now
appear as tilted squares. If, alternately, the squares or rectangles are removed by leaving
only the rectangles or squares of figure 10.9, thus annulling the square-diamond illu-

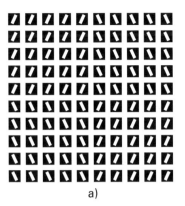

a)

b)

Figure 10.8
The frame/rod effect. The white rectangles, inset within the squares, tilt them in a direction oppo-site to the smaller angle created by the rectangle and the square, thus apparently increasing the acute angle.

sion due to the inset rectangles, the concave/convex effect is restored (not illustrated). This result demonstrates the role played by the inverse rod and frame illusion that can be called the "frame/rod illusion."

In figures 10.10a and b, some effects similar to figures 10.8 and 10.9 but elicited by simpler inducers are illustrated. Under these conditions, the position of the small white squares—along the diagonal or parallel to one side of the squares—polarizes the directional symmetry of each shape like a diamond (a, b) or a square (c) but less strongly than in figures 10.8 and 10.9b. The results are whole deformed squares similar to those illustrated in figure 10.8. In figure 10.10c (control), the position of the small inset squares placed parallel to the sides annuls the concave/convex effect. It is worthwhile noticing that the same effects are perceived when the contrast of the small and large

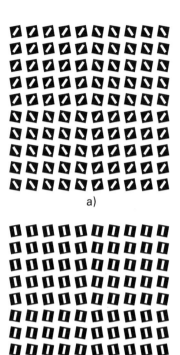

a)

b)

Figure 10.9
The concave/convex effect is enhanced when the inset rectangles follow the diagonal of each square and weakened or annulled when they are parallel to the side orientation.

squares is reversed (not illustrated) and when the small inner white squares are more distant from the large square boundaries (not illustrated).

The role of the directional symmetry in forming the shape of a square is clearly shown in figures 10.11a–d, where "the shapes within the four rows appear as diamonds (a and d) or tilted squares (b and c)," respectively, by virtue of the orientation of the inner rectangle (a and b) or the position of the circle (c and d). To be more precise, "the square shapes appear slightly elongated as a rectangle in the same direction as the inner small rectangle and the circle." By changing the directional symmetry, the shape and the apparent tilt of the shapes change: The shapes perceived as squares are perceived more clearly rotated anticlockwise than the diamond shapes. It is important to notice that in figures 10.11b–d, there are two different orientations of the directional symmetry: The strongest and local one is due to the orientation of the rectangles and

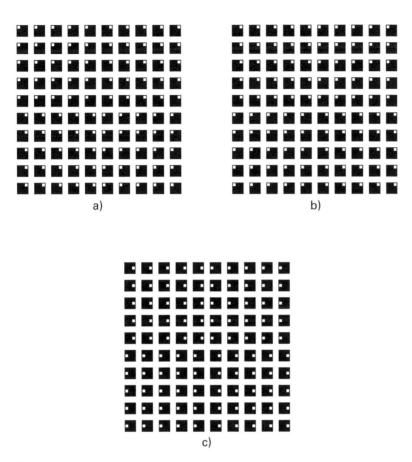

Figure 10.10
Similar to figures 10.8 and 10.9 but elicited by simpler inducers.

the position of the circles; the weakest and global one is due to the alignment of shapes that is in favor of a vertex and hence in favor of the diamond shape. This entails that in figures 10.11b and c, the two directional symmetries are not synergistic, like in the other two figures, but pitted one against the other. The grouping principles cannot explain the form of shapes in any of these cases and especially the one of figures 10.11c and d. Under our conditions, the notion of directional symmetry cannot be assimilated or considered like a grouping principle. In fact, it does not form the grouping but rather the shape of the elements (see also Pinna, 2010).

In figures 10.11e and f, the grouping and position of the white components define the directional symmetry that forms the orientation and shape of the small and whole elements (diamonds in figure 10.11e and squares in figure 10.11f).

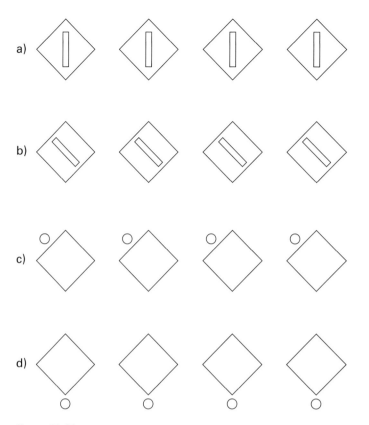

Figure 10.11
The shapes within the four rows appear as diamonds (a and d) or tilted squares (b and c), respectively, by virtue of the orientation of the inner rectangle (a and b) or the position of the circle (c and d). The grouping and position of the white components define the shape: diamonds (e) and squares (f).

The Pointing Effect
Because of the alignment of the equilateral triangles (see figure 10.12a), directional symmetry makes them "point in the right direction," even though as equilateral triangles they should in theory point toward the other two vertexes. Under these conditions, the directional symmetry corresponds to the "configural orientation effect" studied by Attneave (1968), Palmer (1980, 1989), and Palmer and Bucher (1981). These authors used stimuli similar to those illustrated in figure 10.12a to investigate the pointing of equilateral triangles aligned along their axes of symmetry or along one of their sides. They showed that the perception of local spatial orientation (the pointing of each triangle) is determined by the overall spatial orientational structure.

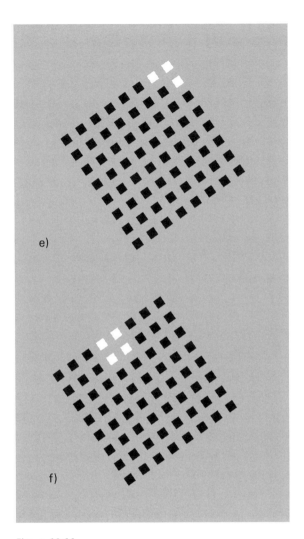

Figure 10.11
(continued)

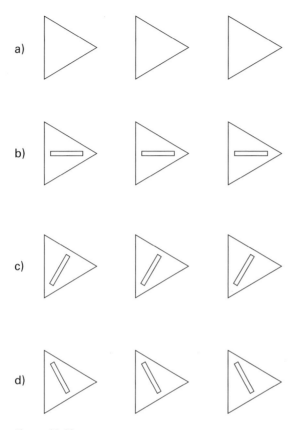

Figure 10.12

The pointing effect. Small squares group in columns (a) and rows (b). Both small and large squares appear similar to vertical (a) and horizontal (b) rectangles.

In figure 10.12b, the orientations of the directional symmetries, the alignment of the triangles and of the rectangles, and the orientation of the rectangle are synergistic. Here, the triangles apparently point more strongly rightward than they do in figure 10.12a. But in figures 10.12c and d, the two directional symmetries are oriented differently from each other. The rectangles are oriented, respectively, toward the bottom-left and top-left corners of the triangles, whereas, owing to the configural orientation effect, the triangles are all oriented in the same rightward direction. In this case, the configural orientation effect does not operate, and each triangle's pointing is due to the directional symmetry induced by the rectangles. The type of shape entails not only the pointing but also the shape of the equilateral rectangles, which now appear as "isosceles triangles with the two longer sides converging towards the apparent pointing direction." Hence, the tilt of each triangle in figure 10.12b is also perceived

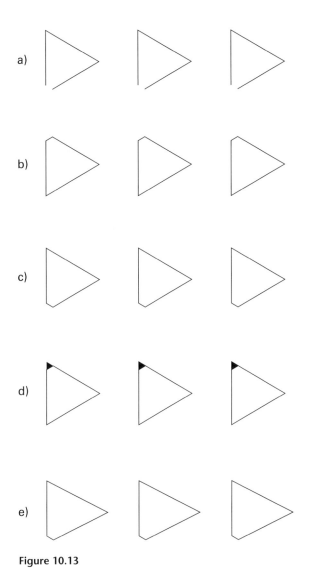

Figure 10.13
The pointing effect. Other ways to create a strong directional symmetry that form the shape and its components like the apparent tilt and the pointing.

differently from those in figures 10.12c and d: "The perceived orientation appears more clearly tilted in the direction of the pointing."

There are other ways to create a strong directional symmetry, which forms the shape and its components, such as the apparent tilt and the pointing (see figure 10.13). In figure 10.13a, the missing or cut vertexes of the triangles define the directional symmetry and, consequently, "their pointing (bottom-left) and their shape (as an equilateral triangle now appearing as slightly isosceles)." Similar effects are apparent in figures 10.13b–d, where, respectively, "beveled triangles (b, c) or triangles with one blackened point" are the phenomenal inducers of the directional symmetry. In figure 10.13e, isosceles triangles with their longest sides converging rightward are beveled at their bottom-left vertexes (see also Pinna and Reeves, 2009). The resulting effects are "three scalene triangles pointing towards the bottom-left corner." The directional symmetry determines the shape (scalene triangle) and its attributes (pointing and orientation) (see also Pinna, 2010).

The Loss of Collinearity Effect

There is another shape attribute deriving from the orientation and determined by the directional symmetry: perceived collinearity. In figure 10.14a, "circles and concentric dots appear to be collinear" as they are in actual fact. Giovannelli (1966) discovered a deformation in dot collinearity by changing the arrangement of the surrounding circles, as illustrated in figure 10.14b. In this case, "the dots do not appear as collinear but as slightly misaligned or slightly zig-zagged." Giovannelli attributed this effect (see also Kanizsa, 1972) to the conflict between the position of the wider scheme of reference (the circles) and the components (the dots) and hence to the predominance of the former over the latter.

We suggest that the factor mainly responsible for the loss of collinearity in figure 10.14b is the interaction between the two directional symmetries due to the circles and the dots, rather than the effect induced by the wider scheme of reference. Indeed, the apparent misalignment in figure 10.14c concerns the circles and then the wider scheme of reference. Put otherwise: The wider scheme of reference is now misaligned by the components so that the opposite of the Giovannelli illusion comes about: "The circles surrounding the dots appear to be slightly misaligned and alternately shifted upwards and downwards according to the direction and position of the dots." In figure 10.14d, rotation of the lines within the circles induces their "slight misalignment and loss of collinearity" (compare this result with the control illustrated in figure 10.14e). A similar loss of collinearity is apparent in figure 10.14f, where it is induced by the position of the missing part within each circle. Changing the distance among the dots apparently alters not only the collinearity among the circles but also their distance. In figure 10.14g, "the circles are not perceived as equidistant." The form of grouping is entirely irrelevant to eliciting these effects.

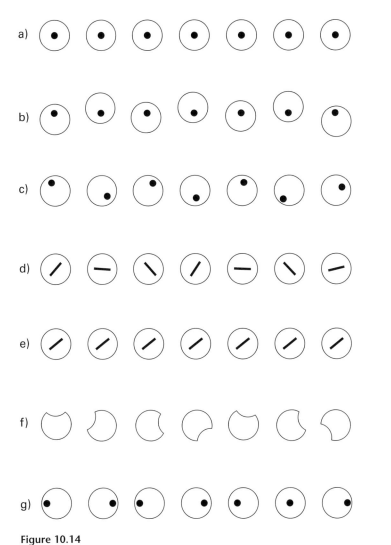

Figure 10.14
The loss of collinearity effect and the Giovannelli illusion.

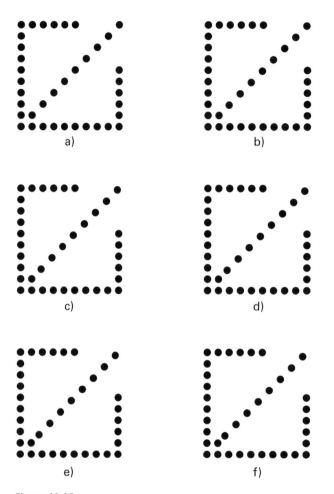

Figure 10.15

The illusion of the diagonal. Which is the true diagonal of the square: the one that reaches perfectly the virtual vertex where the two incomplete sides should meet?

The Illusion of the Diagonal

By using the principle of directional symmetry, another effect can be obtained. This is the illusion of the diagonal (figure 10.15). In figure 10.15, six squares, made up of dots, incomplete in the top right-hand corner and crossed by a dotted oblique line, are illustrated. The dotted oblique line stops before it reaches or goes beyond the virtual vertex, where the two incomplete sides should meet to complete the square. The question is: Which is the true diagonal of the square: the one that reaches perfectly the virtual vertex where the two incomplete sides should meet? The subjects chose the diagonal illustrated in figures 10.15c (3 out of 14), 10.15d (7 out of 14), and 10.15e

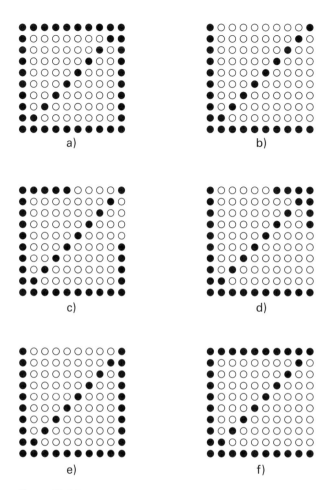

Figure 10.16
The illusion of the diagonal is perceived even within perfect arrays of filled and empty dots.

(4 out of 14). The true geometrical diagonal of the virtual square is the one illustrated in figure 10.15a, even if it appears clearly going much beyond the corner. In all other cases (figures 10.15b–f), each point is gradually pulled down about 0.35 × 0.353 mm for each figure toward the bottom left-hand corner.

In figure 10.16, the directional symmetry creates similar size and shape distortions even when the directionality of the elements emerges from perfect arrays of filled and empty dots. In figure 10.16a, a control without any open directional symmetry that elicits the illusion of the diagonal is illustrated. It is worth noticing that the filled dotted diagonal induces a diamond shape effect in the whole configuration that can be enhanced if this figure is used similarly to the elements illustrated (e.g., in figure 10.11).

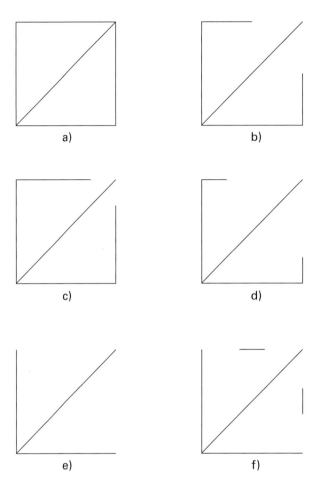

Figure 10.17
The illusion of the diagonal is elicited similarly by continuous lines.

In figure 10.16a, the whole array appears like a virtual "regular square and the filled dotted diagonal is perceived as the true one." In figure 10.16b, where the two top and right sides of the array are now made of empty dots, the whole array appears "tilted like a diamond or distorted toward the top right-hand direction and following the directionality of the diagonal that pushes and distorts the shape of the array and appears longer than it would be if it were the true diagonal of a square array." A similar result is illustrated in figure 10.16c, where "the diagonal is perceived longer than the true diagonal of a square array and the empty dots appear eructating, thus distorting or protruding the square shape in the direction of the diagonal." In figure 10.16d, the empty dots are those close to the vertical and horizontal sides of the array that now "do not end when the square array ends but appear to continue and then to be perceived longer than the top right-hand corner where the diagonal ends like an arrow." This result suggests that, within the directional symmetry, there is some kind of virtual or apparent continuation of lines (dotted or continuous, as can be seen in figure 10.17) that, even if they modally end, perceptually they seem to virtually or amodally continue when they are not interrupted by perpendicular lines. A demonstration of this underlying tendency is illustrated in figures 10.16e and f, where by emptying the dots at the top or on the right sides of the square array of figure 10.16a, "the size of the arrays appear elongated or enlarged making them similar to narrower (higher) or wider container of small circles." This result is related to the one illustrated in figure 10.1.

In figure 10.17, by replacing the dots with lines, the illusion of the diagonal is perceived similarly to those illustrated in figure 10.15. (Compare the results of figures 10.17b–e with the control illustrated in figure 10.17a). In figure 10.17f, "the two dashes appear indented with respect to the sides and diagonal ends," even if they are physically aligned. These effects are likely related to the illusion of unbounded figures (Lipps, 1897; Müller-Lyer, 1889), where a square, whose upper side is missing, appears higher than the one with the right side missing, which appears wider. Nevertheless, the conditions illustrated in figures 10.1, 10.15a, and 10.16e and f demonstrated that these effects cannot be considered as a subset of the illusion of unbounded figures, but likely the opposite is true (i.e., this classical illusion can be interpreted as due to the directional symmetry and the underlying amodal or virtual continuation that in terms of form of grouping is based on the similarity principle).

The Empty Misalignment Effect

The directional symmetry plays a basic role in the variation of the Poggendorff illusion (Zöllner, 1860) illustrated in figure 10.18a, where although all the empty and filled dots belong to a regular square array, "the oblique filled dotted lines lose their continuation and appear broken and misaligned: the right oblique line is perceived moved upward with respect to the true continuation of the left oblique line." In figure 10.18b, an adjusted or a corrected version of the illusion is illustrated: "The two oblique lines are perceived aligned" even if they are geometrically misaligned. The perception of the regular array and the continuation of the oblique lines is ineffective in correcting the misalignment effect. This is due to the interaction among the directional symmetries of each segregated component (vertical rectangle made up of filled dots, oblique dotted lines crossing or completing amodally behind the rectangle, and empty dots that induce a vertical direction or become the background) on the basis of filled/empty and orientation similarity.

In figure 10.19a, by removing the filled dots of figure 10.18, the perceived absence of dots elicits the same kind of illusion of figure 10.18. It is worth noticing that the

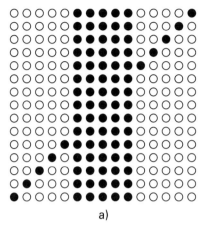

a)

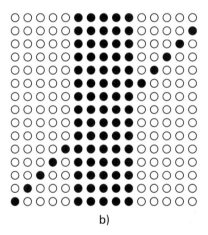

b)

Figure 10.18
The misalignment effect. The oblique-filled dotted lines lose their continuation and appear broken and misaligned: The right oblique line is perceived moved upward with respect to the true continuation of the left oblique line.

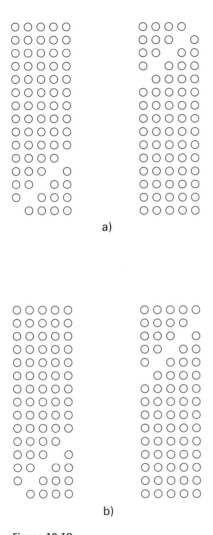

Figure 10.19

The empty misalignment effect. By removing the filled dots of figure 10.18, the perceived absence of dots elicits the same kind of misalignment effect.

absences and not their boundaries are perceived to be misaligned. Figure 10.19b is corresponding to figure 10.18b with removed filled dots. Under these conditions, the role of amodal completion, angles, and intersecting lines is annulled. What remains are the directional symmetries and their interaction.

If the directional symmetries interact by revealing, for example, the misalignment of the modified Poggendorff illusion illustrated in figure 10.19, then by introducing an oblique line of empty dots, it can influence the strength of the misalignment. This is the case of figure 10.20, where the apparent misalignment of figure 10.19a is now perceived as "aligned" and the apparent alignment of figure 10.19b is now perceived as "misaligned." In other words, the variation of the Poggendorff illusion is now corrected by virtue of new interactions among directional symmetries.

Beyond the Form of Grouping and the Form of Shape: Toward the Form of Meaning

The previous results demonstrated that many classical illusions, like those previously quoted, can be reduced to the more general problem of formation of shape, where the directional symmetry plays a basic role in creating both the local and the whole shapes and their attributes. Through experimental phenomenology, we also traced a distinction between the form of grouping, as described by the Gestalt principles, and the form of shape that complements the form of grouping in a more holistic shape organization. The form of grouping puts together the elements, while the form of shape draws the perceptual structure and spatial attributes of the figure both locally and globally. The form of grouping cannot explain the form of shape and vice versa, but the form of both grouping and shape cannot explain another kind of form that we have already encountered in the previous figures and can be observed in the following variation of figure 10.11 (see figure 10.21).

In figure 10.21, the form of grouping puts together the black elements parallel to the sides of the large figures on the basis of the proximity principle. Given the empty space in the top corner (figure 10.21a) or on the top left-hand side (figure 10.21b) of the whole figures, the directional asymmetry creates "diamonds" in figure 10.21a and "squares" in figure 10.21b, "both locally (in each element) and globally (in the whole figure)."

It is worthwhile noticing that under these conditions the directional symmetry is different from the Gestalt principle of symmetry that defines uniquely the grouping arrangement of the elements but not the shape of the elements and of the whole figure. In other words, the Gestalt grouping symmetry does not polarize the shape. The previous results of the form of shape are independent and parallel to the results of the form of grouping. This means that both forms live together one independently from or varying in line with the other. The form of grouping persists within the form of shape, and the form of shape does not influence the form of grouping.

The whole shapes of figure 10.21 are not only "a diamond" and "a square," but also "a diamond with the top corner missing or cut with the absence having a diamond

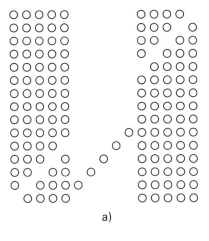

a)

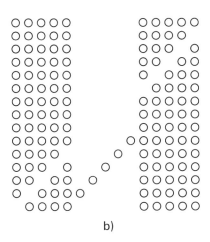

b)

Figure 10.20
The apparent misalignment of figure 10.19a is now perceived aligned, and the apparent alignment of figure 10.19b is now perceived misaligned.

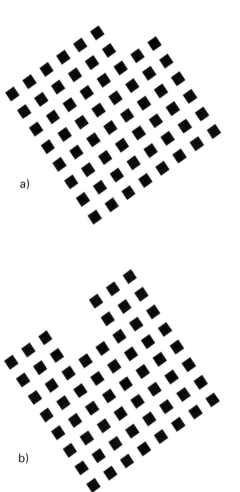

Figure 10.21

A diamond with the top corner missing or cut with the absence having a diamond shape (a) and a square with a missing or cut piece in the region of the top left-hand side with the absence having a square shape (b).

shape" and "a square with a missing or cut piece in the region of the top left-hand side with the absence having a square shape." This kind of form is far beyond both the form of grouping and the form of shape. It contains more "things" or couples of things—diamond/square and missing/cut pieces—that cannot be explained by the form of grouping and the form of shape. Both things do not exist in themselves. In fact, there are not a diamond and a square but, respectively, an irregular shape with six sides having the same size in pairs (figure 10.21a) and an irregular shape with eight sides, five and three of which have the same size. These are two descriptions derived from the form of grouping based on the principles of proximity, similarity, good continuation, and *Prägnanz*. Furthermore, the form of shape, through the directional symmetry, can only draw the shape of the whole irregular shapes, but it cannot say anything about the complex phenomenal description previously reported. Diamonds and squares can be shaped only locally but not globally due to the missing pieces.

Antinomic Properties of "Absences"

The same argument can be used for the "something" that is at the same time "nothing" (i.e., the missing or cut pieces). These "absences" are part of the organization process, together with phenomena of totalization, completion, integration, and gap-filling (Kanizsa, 1991; Metzger, 1941; see Albertazzi, 2003). These "absences" are not like the surrounding background but manifest figural properties. Conversely, they are not figures, but, like the background, they are nothing. Briefly, they are nothing and something at the same time, backgrounds and figures. The boundaries of the absences belong to them. This is demonstrated by the fact that the absences manifest figural attributes and like the figures are subjected to the same kind of illusions (diamond or square like in figure 10.21; see also the absence misalignment effect illustrated in figure 10.19). Nevertheless, the boundaries also belong to the complementary irregular figure, making the absences appear as a piece of background, a nothing, or an empty space. Even if under the form of grouping and figure-ground segregation, the emptiness is opposite to the figureness that is a solid-filled object property (Rubin, 1921). In the case of the absences, the dichotomous complementation is much more complex and can be understood only in the light of a new kind of form of organization. This is the form of meaning.

The Form of Meaning

Ideal and Contingent Levels within the Form of Meaning

In figure 10.21, the antinomic properties of both the figures and the absences are isomorphic with two levels of perceptual organizations that can be phenomenally observed and can be called "ideal" and "contingent" levels. The absence (missing or cut) is some kind of contingent and specific result of an action that happened to the figure ("happening"), making it appear incomplete and irregular. Without this happening and at an ideal perceptual level, it would have been complete, creating a full diamond or square. Both the figures and the absences have as ideal and contingent levels, respectively, the diamond/square (ideal) versus irregular shapes (contingent) and the filling-in and completeness of the absence (ideal) and its presence (contingent).

One level is related to the other (i.e., one is perceived only if the other is also perceived). Furthermore, they are directly and immediately perceived without any cognitive mediation but as a result of some kind of early part-whole organization eliciting perceptual meanings. The emerging meanings are the specific forms of the happenings that in figure 10.21 can be "missing, absence or cut." Other possible meanings can be invoked, but the phenomenal split in two levels does not change. Also the incompleteness versus completeness of the whole figure represents a specific meaning that can be formed or named in different ways: diamond, square, irregular figure, and so on.

One of the problems, therefore, is to understand: (1) how many potential meanings can be related to the same specific shape; (2) whether they are synonyms, and, specifically, (3) which aspect of the shape is the bearer of the one or the other resulting meaning.

In other words, which are boundaries of the subjective construal of a certain visual appearance or scene? After all, interpretation (Langacker, 1991) is not without limits (Eco, 2003).

The Amodal Wholeness

The two levels are not perceived in the same way, but the ideal level is perceived amodally, whereas the contingent one is perceived modally. The completed whole (diamond/square shape) is perceived amodally (amodal completeness), whereas the uncompleted whole (irregular shape) is perceived modally (modal incompleteness). The completed part (the absence that at the ideal level is filled with what is missing) is perceived amodally, whereas the uncompleted part (the absence as it is perceived) is perceived modally. Both ways coexist and reinforce each other. The term "amodal" refers to the fact that, although the complete figure and its contour are not actually seen, it appears with a vivid sense of completeness and object unity. Briefly, the diamond/square shape appears as the amodal whole object and the absence as the modal part of it. The diamond/square is the result of the amodal wholeness completion of something perceived as its visible modal portion. Like the absence, the diamond/square is perceived and not perceived at the same time, and its amodal whole completion occurs beyond (ideal perceptual level) the absence. It is the absence that makes the diamond/square appear as such and to complete amodally beyond it. In other words, the diamond/square shape cannot be perceived with this meaning if the absence is not perceived. Otherwise, the diamond/square shape would be perceived like an irregular shape. Vice versa, it is the perceptual meaning of the diamond/square that makes the empty space appear like an absence. None of these meanings can exist without the others.

Toward a Perceptual Language

The kind of organization illustrated in figure 10.21 can be regarded as a process of meaning assignment that reveals a sort of primitive perceptual language. One emergent object/meaning is the diamond/square shape. In phenomenal terms, this can be considered the subject of the description/proposition (i.e., it is the "noun" that refers to a thing and denotes what is described by the "predicate" or the term of the perceptual "sentence" with which something is affirmed or denied). The diamond/square shape appears to complete itself notwithstanding the absence that "occludes" its wholeness, thus eliciting its amodal completion. This absence is like a "doing" word or a "happening" (i.e., something that occurs to the diamond/square shape so that without it the diamond/square shape would have been complete). Hence, it follows that the happening is a visual "predicate" or a perceptual "verb" of the sentence expressing the subject's properties, existence, action, or occurrence.

These phenomenal properties belong to all the other figures previously shown. For example, figure 10.11 was fully described as: "a black diamond/square shape, made up of black small diamond/square shapes, with four white components." The free descriptions of the subjects play a fundamental role in understanding the nature of the perceptual meanings. In fact, it follows that the amodal wholeness creates complete diamond/square shapes, and the happenings are represented by the fact that some components are white instead of black as they should be. Also, figure 10.1, which can be considered the closest to the forms of grouping and shape, can be seen and therefore expressed in terms of perceptual meanings: "Two large squares/rectangles made up of alternated black and white columns and rows." The term "made up" reveals the happening occurred to the perceptual subject (i.e., the square/rectangle). The perceptual meanings are also reported by the spontaneous descriptions of figures 1 and 2b, where small and large squares appear elongated in the same direction as the perceptual organization. More precisely, they are "squares" that appear or "become" "elongated." The elongation represents the happening of the visual language. The square is the subject, and the elongated rectangular shape is the complement. In fact, the information pertaining to the act or process of elongation is not given by the static image but by a series or succession of implicit images (snapshots of evolution), of which the given image is a *nonindependent* part and to which it implicitly refers.

Every visual content (and auditory or tactile-kinetic as well) displays a *synthetic internal structure* that is manifest in its persistence, even if "illusory."

Once again, some key questions still remain. How do we recognize the implicit *deployment* of events in a stationary visual appearance? The same holds in daily life with warning signs—for example, "emergency exit." This sign usually consists of a figure represented in a *static* act of running indicated by the directionality of the legs, which evoke the perception of movement. The same applies to the sign "children," although in this case the movement is less evident.

Also at issue in this case is the role of the visual phenomena as *schemes* of experience that function as *props* for the development of thought. In favor of the hypothesis of an essentially temporal scheme operating in visual perception, there are plenty of other examples (Albertazzi, 2004, 2005).

From the Illusion of Shape to the Illusion of Meaning

More generally, we suggest that *the three forms of organization*—grouping, shape, and meaning—*are potentially and simultaneously present*. There is no perception without these three forms, even if there are several conditions where one of these forms can be seen more easily than the others. This is the case of the following figures, where the form of meaning emerges more clearly and where the forms of grouping and shape are unable to explain the emerging percepts. We will proceed from the simplest cases to the most complex ones, where the form of meaning becomes more and more important.

In figure 10.22a, alternating filled (black) and empty (white) squares are perceived as "a checkerboard." This is not a shape in the sense of the form of a shape kind of organization. Furthermore, although it is due to grouping, it is beyond grouping. The alternation creates some kind of homogenous structure with a precise meaning. This meaning is not due to its being a checkerboard because we know and use it as a checkerboard; rather, we know and use it as a checkerboard because it has that meaning. In figure 10.22b, "the checkerboard appears to be mutilated: a large piece of it has been removed from the top right corner" (see also Pinna, 2010).

This description is interesting for both its complexity and simplicity at the same time and because it contains several emerging "things" (from here onward, the term "thing" has been left in the text because it is expressly used in the naïve subjects' description of the relative appearances). The complexity is revealed by the emergence of terms/meanings apparently beyond what is represented and beyond the system constituent parts. These terms are: mutilation, removal, and piece of checkerboard (missing). The missing checkerboard has the form of a checkerboard. This apparent tautology suggests a general rule of the form of meanings: Every missing component has the shape of the whole object to which that component belongs. The amodal result is therefore very close to what is illustrated in figure 10.22c, where "a piece of checkerboard comes away from the main checkerboard and tumbles down." By comparing figures 10.22b and c, it seems that the piece illustrated in figure 10.22c is the one missing from figure 10.22b. However, this result emerges only through the comparison between the two figures. In fact, the amodal wholeness of figure 10.22b, when it is shown alone without any comparison, is the complete checkerboard illustrated in figure 10.22a and not the one in figure 10.22c.

The presentation of such simple appearances immediately raises again some questions: What are the signs, the discontinuities that enable us to perceive the temporal continuity of an apparently static perception? How can an essentially static presentation like figures 10.22d, e, and f immediately communicate the idea of movement and even act as a signal of danger ("falling squares")? How are the apparent perceived movement and velocity woven together in those static shapes? Moreover, why can we read the presentation of figures 10.22a, b, and c and following as connected by a story of possible events occurring to a certain shape?

First of all, if the presentation of the item of the phenomenal world were a substantially static representation enacted by an eye constructed to passively record events in a sequence of unconnected snapshots, we would never recognize these events as belonging to a continuing duration and, therefore, as signs of some events.

However, it is not sufficient to acknowledge that a duration is necessary to elaborate perceptual outcomes into meaningful events of experience. Other problems still remain: For instance, is the temporality of events due to our judgment of them or is it a characteristic of the modes of the perceptual presentation of events? In other words, does what I see have an immediate temporal connotation, or is the intervention of some form of top-down recognition subsequent to its presentation required?

One of the principal problems to solve, therefore, is the relationship between the continuity of a sequence of different perceptions and the unitary nature of these perceptions taken individually. A second problem is explaining the relationship between the actuality of the perceptions that we experience as directly present and the presence in the same situations of indices of directionality addressed to the past or the future (i.e., to absent states) (Benussi, 1913; Kanizsa, 1991; Meinong, 1899).

The temporal structure of the presentation, therefore, has to be considered as a constitutive component of the field structure of perceptual phenomena because it is in the extension of an act of seeing that we apprehend the being-before or being-after of phenomena, or simply their permanence (Husserl, 1991; Michotte et al., 1962). Every phenomenal spatial ordering into above-below, to the right-to the left, in front-behind, before-after, and so on presupposes a simultaneous flow of discretely ordered impressions, the temporal traces of which are also retained by the visual appearance and frozen in indices of direction that relate to the dynamics of the actual presentation of the event (Leyton, 1993, 2003). In other words, the reference system usually exemplified in terms of spatial ordering can only be understood within a temporal subjective completion of the scene, of which the absence is a constitutive component.

The checkerboard shape of the missing piece of figure 10.22b cannot be taken for granted. In fact, as illustrated in figure 10.22d, the missing part can be formed of "small scattered squares which seem to fly." In figure 10.22e, the small square components are instead perceived "as ejected or poured out from the checkerboard." From figures 10.22d and e, it follows that the large piece of checkerboard and the separated squares manifest different phenomenal properties. In fact, the checkerboard cannot be

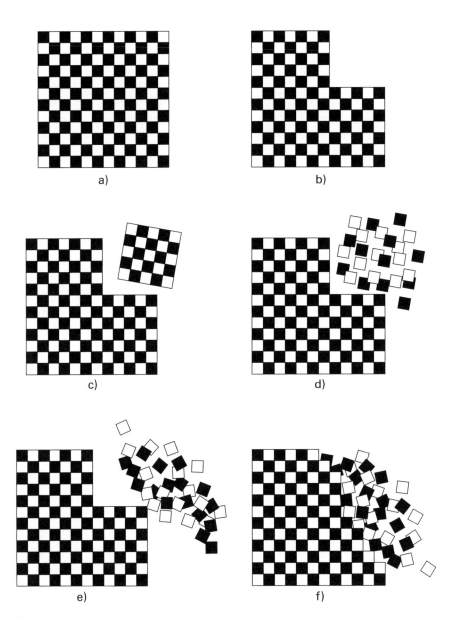

Figure 10.22

A checkerboard (a). A mutilated checkerboard (b). A piece of checkerboard comes away from the main checkerboard and tumbles down (c). Small scattered squares seem to fly (d). The small squares are perceived as ejected or poured out from the checkerboard (e). The checkerboard crashes, and its components made up of filled and empty squares come down rolling one over the other (f). While the squares are coming down and rolling, they are transformed in star-like shapes (g). A circle that after having hit the checkerboard and having caused the crash and the fall of its square components bounces on the left-hand side of the checkerboard following a curved trajectory (h). A rain of circles that destroys the arrangement of the squares making up the checkerboard (i). The direction of the rain of (i) changes from right to left (j).

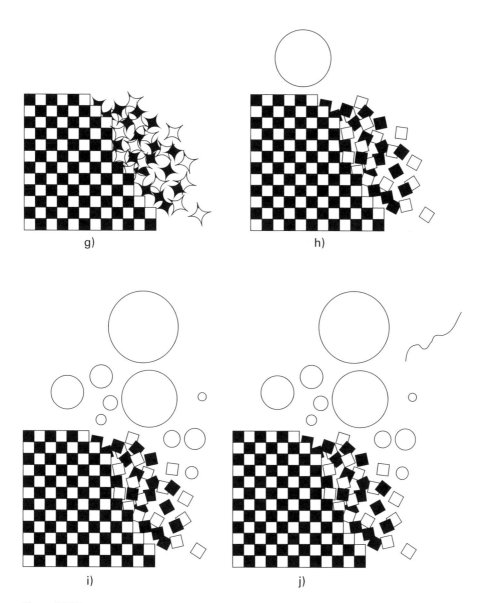

g)　　　　　　　h)

i)　　　　　　　j)

Figure 10.22
(continued)

phenomenally reduced to juxtaposed black and white squares. In terms of the form of grouping and of shape, they are segregated into at least two groups on the basis of similarity. Nevertheless, in the form of meaning, even different elements like these are put together and assume a meaningful kind of organization (see previous descriptions). In the form of meaning, anything can stay with anything else and become meaningful, provided that the invariants are maintained.

A second consequence of assuming a potential and temporal viewpoint in visual perception is that every distinguishable event endowed with certain characteristics of symmetry is virtually derivable from a principle of asymmetry and vice versa (see Leyton, 1993; Massironi, 2002).

Besides the complexity, the description of figure 10.22b also reveals a great simplicity. In fact, many kinds of variations in the checkerboard and many kinds of mutilations can be included in the same meaning organization, thus reducing the information load and the algorithmic information content.

In figure 10.22f, the checkerboard form of meaning is "weakened while it crashes and its components made up of filled and empty squares come down rolling one over the other." In figure 10.22g, falling squares are deformed, thus appearing more segregated from the checkerboard on the basis of the form of grouping. The form of grouping puts together both the checkerboard and the deformed squares that, "while coming down and rolling, they are transformed in star-like shapes." The power of the form of meaning to put together elements is much stronger than the other two kinds of forms. In figure 10.22h, the circle added to figure 10.22f becomes part of the whole meaning: "A circle that after having hit the checkerboard and having caused the crash and the fall of its square components bounces on the left hand side of the checkerboard following a curved trajectory." By adding other circles (figure 10.22i), they become "a rain of circles that destroys the arrangement of the squares making up the checkerboard." It is sufficient to add an undulated line that "the direction of the rain changes from right to left" (figure 10.22j). The line becomes an attribute of the perceived motion of the circles. In figures 10.22h–j, the perceived motion of the circles changes. It depends on the meaning assignment. The circles are perceived like the cause complement of the visual language that completes the predicate/happening. By causing the crash, they become subjects of a dependent clause with its own happening and so on. The circles with their happenings "explain" the crash of the checkerboard and the crash, being a more primary happening, and "explain" the checkerboard that can no longer be amodally perceived as a piece. In other words, the checkerboard can amodally complete its wholeness beyond the crush that in its turn can amodally complete its wholeness beyond the impact with the circle. Everything assumes a meaning within a context of other meanings. Everything is perceptually put together in a meaningful way. These are basic general principles of the form of meaning.

The Illusion of Meaning: Folding, Stretching, Deformation, and Transformation

The form of meaning is a process of amodal wholeness that corresponds to the directional symmetry of the form of shape and to the Gestalt principles in the form of grouping. One of the simplest and limiting cases of the amodal wholeness is the partial occlusion phenomenon that activates a process of amodal completion (Michotte, and Burke, 1951; Michotte, Thinès, and Crabbé, 1964). Therefore the object perceived as occluded is perceived as a unitary object with boundary contours that amodally complete behind the overlapped modal object. The "overlapping" is the happening that induces the amodal wholeness of the subject, which can now appear unitary at an ideal and amodal level. The amodal completion may be considered as an instance of the amodal wholeness: It phenomenally includes the completion or wholeness behind and beyond all the possible perceptible happenings.

The happenings do not necessarily amodally complete something that is modally perceived as a piece or portion of an entire or unitary object, but can also complete attributes of something that is already a unitary object. This is also true in the following conditions (figure 10.23), where the checkerboards are perceived deformed: folded, stretched, pulled, pushed, extended, and so on.

All of these happenings behave similarly to the amodal completion of partially occluded objects. They complete and amodally homogenize its subject. However, although in the case of occlusion the cause of the modal incompletion is modally perceived (i.e., the overlapped object), in figure 10.23, the happening is modally perceived as "occluding" the unity, integrity, and homogeneity of the checkerboard, but the cause is invisible although amodally it can be perceived. The cause of the deformations is the complement of the perceptual sentence and can be amodally completed on the basis of the specific meaning of the happening. Each happening, in describing a specific action occurred to the subject, also describes the shape and properties of the complement that causes that happening. It can be a sphere moving in a certain direction and at a specific speed that hit the checkerboard thus causing the deformation (see also figure 10.24). This example suggests that the form of meaning is not only a process of meaning assignment but also a process of meaning creation. Meanings create other meanings that create other meanings and so on, according to rules.

The meanings do not necessarily have a name and are not always identifiable. In figure 10.25, the happenings and checkerboards are clearly perceived, but it is extremely difficult to perceive and say what is "happening" and what is causing that "happening."

From the previous figures, it follows that the form of meaning and its processes of meaning assignment obey apparent antinomic rules. On the one hand, they put together everything so that everything can stay with everything else in a meaningful way. This imparts unity, integrity, and homogeneity among all the components. On the other hand, they divide, segregate, or discount everything that appears as the

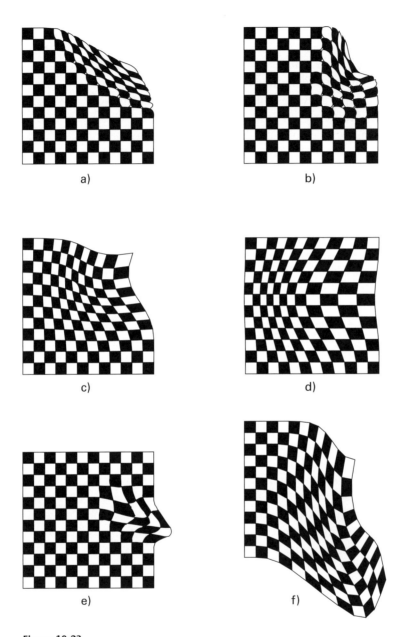

Figure 10.23
The checkerboards are perceived deformed: folded, stretched, pulled, pushed, extended, and so on.

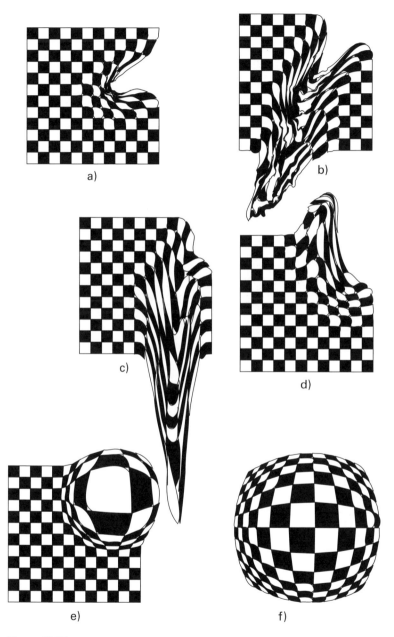

Figure 10.24
Other deformations of a checkerboard.

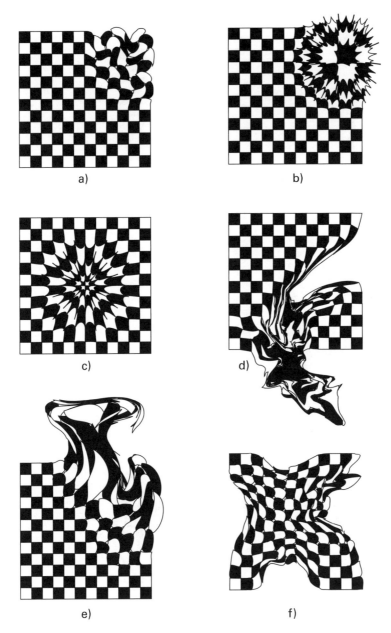

Figure 10.25
Deformations difficult to describe.

opposite of unity, integrity, and homogeneity. This process is not equivalent to the grouping/segregation formed by the Gestalt principle of similarity, but it does much more in terms of form of meaning. These two antinomic dynamics do not annul or weaken but strengthen each other in a very simple way (i.e., by creating the two perceptual levels [ideal and contingent] we previously mentioned). Then, what is segregated becomes the happening (i.e., something different from the main meaning [subject]). It is discounted, but at the same time it becomes part of the subject by qualifying it and explaining in terms of action the reason of the loss of homogeneity, integrity, and unity of the subject. In this way, the subject can assume, establish, or restore its homogeneity that is like a basic assumption within the process of meaning formation. In other words, differences, variations, and lack of homogeneity become the special emerging meanings that we called "happenings," whose aim is to create homogeneity and therefore unity. The paradox of meaning is avoided by creating and organizing the resulting meanings in two perceptual levels: amodal/ideal and modal/contingent.

The Perceptual Meanings

Complexity of the Form of Meaning

In summary, the complexity of emerging meanings has the following properties (see also Pinna, 2010):

1. Unpredictability   Unlike the forms of grouping and shape, the complex form of meaning can produce unexpected and unpredictable meanings. Moreover, as shown, some perceptual meanings cannot be easily seen and described despite being clearly perceived as happenings.
2. High connectedness   The form of meaning may involve a large number of components with numerous feedback loops enabling the system to restructure itself promptly. On comparing one figure with another, the emerging form of meaning may change according to whether it is perceived on its own or compared with a new figure. This is because the new figure becomes a new component and therefore part of the meaning as a whole.
3. Emergence   There are no perceived meanings in any of the individual subcomponents taken individually; rather, they emerge from composite interactions (e.g., the checkerboard form of the cut piece).
4. Non-decomposability   The emerging meanings are irreducible. The complex form of meaning cannot be resolved into isolated subcomponents without an uncoverable loss of meaning. Usually, if any part of the meaning assignment process is ignored, or if any of its connections are severed, essential aspects of the meaning structure are destroyed.

5. Hierarchical organization and centralized control   The complex form of meaning exhibits a hierarchical control structured in a manner similar to a perceptual language. But the power is distributed across a decentralized structure involving all the components. A number of units combine to generate the actual system of meanings so that the meaning of one component depends on the meanings of the others.

6. Invariability   The form of meaning is highly resistant and adaptable to changes. Because it introduces variations, changes, and happenings, the meaning as a whole tends to be modally invariant. This creates marked stability even in the presence of major disturbances.

7. Variability   Happenings manifest chaotic behavior, in the sense that minuscule variations in happenings may induce huge variations in their meanings. This gives rise to a high level of instability, which engenders mutations and hence the creativity of meanings. This is the source of the creativity of vision.

These properties suggest that the perception of a meaning is not the same as the perception of a shape or grouping, as it has been described in the previous sections. In general, a shape is the starting point of a meaning, and a meaning is the meaning of a shape. Yet the same shape may have different meanings. We assume that there is a continuum between shape and meaning perception: Phenomenally, a meaning represents what is expressed, indicated, or conveyed by a shape. The "checkerboard with a cut piece" is a shape expressing or indicating an entire meaning made up of meaning components, and the cut piece is organized so that one meaning component appears as such within the context of the other meaning (part/whole organization). Hence, the meaning is more than a shape, and it can be used to convey, represent, and denote something beyond its shape.

Propositions and Definitions of the Form of Meaning
The following general propositions and definitions can be put forward on the basis of the phenomenal observations described (see also Pinna, 2010):

Proposition 10.1   *There is no perception without the three forms of organization: grouping, shape, and meaning. To perceive is not just to perceive groups and shapes; it is also to perceive meanings. What we perceive always has a meaning. Vision is the perception of meanings.*

Proposition 10.2   *The form of shape extends beyond the form of grouping, and the form of meaning extends beyond the form of shape. The three kinds of forms are not mutually exclusive but reinforce one another by organizing the visual field at different perceptual levels.*

Proposition 10.3   *In the form of meaning, anything can stand with anything else, thus becoming meaningful.*

Proposition 10.4   *In the form of meaning, anything can stand with anything else, thus becoming meaningful and creating sentences of a visual language.*

Definition 10.1   *"Perceptual meaning" is what is expressed, indicated, or conveyed by a shape through "amodal wholeness" and "modal partialness" (see the following definitions).*

Definition 10.2   *"Amodal wholeness" is the vivid percept of object unity and wholeness that occurs even though the observer does not actually see a contour in regions where completion of the whole object takes place at a level above the "happening"* (see also Pinna and Reeves, 2009).

Definition 10.3   *"Modal partialness" is the clear modal emergence of a specific happening that occludes the completion of one part of the complementary region: for example, a square form that appears as the whole* (see also Pinna and Reeves, 2009).

Proposition 10.5   *Amodal wholeness and modal partialness are interrelated: Variations in the meaning of one component entail variations in the other. Because each happening partially "conceals" or "occludes" the whole, it determines the amodal wholeness. Conversely and simultaneously, each whole makes the discontinuities appear as they are and as its happenings or actions with that specific meaning* (see also Pinna and Reeves, 2009).

Proposition 10.6   *Stimulus variations split phenomenally into at least two independent and opposite phenomenal components: One component ("homogenous and invariant") is perceived not directly but amodally, whereas the other ("heterogeneous and variant") is perceived directly and modally. One component acts to discount or annul the variations, and thus it creates an amodal wholeness. The other subsumes all the variations attributing them to a different "thing or happening" of the whole, thus becoming the modal partialness. The two components reinforce each other, so that a certain variation in one component is counterbalanced by a contrary variation in the other component.*

Pinna and Reeves (2006) used this principle to explain the figurality consisting of the phenomenal appearance of what is perceived as a figure within the three-dimensional space and under a perceived illumination.

Unfortunately, there is nothing within the Gestalt grouping principles and the form of shape about the components that at one level are grouped and ungrouped at a different level. Although these levels were never envisaged by Gestalt psychologists, it is necessary to keep track of them because they are visual results.

The forms of meaning not only keep track of these levels but also combine phenomenal similarities and dissimilarities, homogeneities and heterogeneities, and continuity and discontinuity in a meaningful manner. They do not annul or weaken each other.

Instead, they are synergistically complementary, and they contribute to creating a whole meaning as described in proposition 6. By becoming meanings, the homogenous versus heterogeneous, continuous versus discontinuous components are made simpler and more economical because the level of complexity is shifted to a higher one. A mutilated checkerboard is much more economical than the irregular shape consisting of juxtaposed alternating black and white squares.

What Is a Perceptual Meaning?

The following list of properties (see also Pinna, 2010; Pinna and Reeves, 2009) can be used to define the properties subsumed by the form of meaning and necessary to furnish a more complete definition of perceptual meaning.

Property 1 *Many become few.*

Many elements are reduced to a few integrated meanings through the form of meaning. All the shapes illustrated in figures 10.22–10.25 are reduced to a checkerboard with a specific happening. Without this kind of organization, they would have been perceived as different irregular shapes.

Property 2 *What is segregated is integrated.*

Elements segregated by grouping principles or even disparate objects are integrated through the form of meaning.

Property 3 *Multiplicity and divergence become homogeneity and unity.*

Discontinuities, divergences, contrasts, and paradoxes are solved and "explained" within a whole meaning. The components are restructured in a meaningful manner: The discontinuity becomes the predicate (happening) of the subject (amodal meaning).

Property 4 *Homogenous and heterogeneous, continuous and discontinuous conditions, similarities and dissimilarities among elements within the form of meaning do not weaken or annul but strengthen one another.*

Property 5 *The form of meaning creates different perceptual levels of complexity (ideal and contingent).*

Property 6 *From one meaning to another: The form of meaning not only reduces the number of perceived elements that become meanings but also creates other meanings placed at higher perceptual levels connected in some kind of "perceptual net."*

Property 7 *From the grouped elements to the meaning formation to the perceptual language: The meanings organize themselves like the components of a language. The main components are the subject, the predicate (happening), and the complements.*

Property 8 *Every perceptual element communicates a meaning within a context of other meanings. Even the most senseless pattern creates and communicates a meaning.*

Conclusions

The theory of perceptual organization presented here suggests a three-level hierarchy given by the forms of grouping, shape, and meaning. The organization of the three forms becomes progressively more and more complex with the increasing complexity of the perceptual experience.

Why have we introduced multiple organizations rather than just one? The answer to this question is provided by the previous phenomenal results showing that all these organizations are simultaneously present when a figure is perceived, but they are located at different perceptual levels and produce different perceptual outcomes. Moreover, the results of one level do not influence the results of the others, although each of them is needed to trigger the other. This is the case of the similarity that triggers directional symmetry.

What is the advantage of introducing them? The apparent issue is the reduction of simplicity. However, the opposite is true. The final result emerging from each level is in fact much simpler than the number of its members. The algorithmic information content (Kolmogorov complexity) derived from each form is much reduced and simpler. The increase in complexity from one level to another is accompanied by a marked reduction in the number of contents and by increasing simplicity. Moreover, moving from one level to another eliminates the need to specify the initial condition of the previous level. The basic elements or atoms of one level are different from those of the other levels. Thus, the results of one level are the atoms of the next level. In fact, the result of each level is an emergent form comprising the grouping of components, the shape of the grouping, and the meanings of the shapes.

These hypotheses are consistent with the key feature of a knowledge-acquiring system such as the human brain. The latter has the capacity to abstract from the experience of many particulars or to minimize the number of elements. However, this capacity is accompanied by its complement (i.e., the capacity to maximize information and then create other meanings in a highly creative manner).

The drawback to introducing perceptual meanings is that they may also depend on cognitive processes operating at a higher level and involving past experience. Separating perceptual meanings from cognitive meanings may thus become impossible. We nevertheless suggest that perceptual meanings are the foundation of cognitive meanings and not necessarily in contrast with them, although a distinction between seeing and thinking is certainly necessary (Kanizsa, 1985, 1991). We propose that cognitive meanings can be reduced to perceptual ones. As Arnheim (1969) pointed out, abstraction already resides in the object. Perceptual meanings can be considered the components of some kind of primitive language prior to speech and therefore prior to cognitive meanings. They are the raw materials used by cognitive processes. Therefore, the advantages of proposing perceptual meanings are the following: (1) they pertain to perceptual processes primary with respect to cognitive ones; (2) the form of meaning and the underlying phenomenal processes described here are reduced to the problem of perceptual organization; (3) the form of meaning is closely linked to the form of shape and grouping; (4) perceptual meanings have a strong phenomenal status; (5) their inner structure can help explain how the brain creates meanings; (6) compared with other more complex explanations involving higher cognitive processes, they better fit the *lex parsimoniae* of Occam's razor.

The notion of "happening" may be related to that of "affordance" proposed by Gibson (1977, 1979). Put briefly, "affordances" are action possibilities latent in the environment, measurable and independent from the individual ability to recognize them. Happenings and affordances do not coincide, but they are not mutually exclusive. A happening is something that occurs to an object even beyond ecological possibilities: strange, paradoxical, nonsensical, unnatural meanings may occur beyond affordances. In this sense, happenings include affordances. The realm of happenings is accordingly broader and comprises affordances as a specific type.

Moreover, happenings are a specific class of perceptual meanings. The other meaning components are the subject and complement of the perceptual language without which happenings cannot be perceived as meanings. Subjects and complements lie beyond affordances.

There is another important difference. Happenings are not necessarily affordances. They are also meanings able to perform the role of subjects. In figure 10.26, the word ARTE (Italian for Art) is represented in different ways. Each way can be perceived or not as a happening. Even if it is perceived as a happening, the true subject is not the word but the happening itself if the question is: "Which is the most artistic word?" (The answer is left to the reader.) This means that, according to what we are seeking perceptually, how we see, how we organize meanings, and which visual "sentence" we "read," happenings may change in their meanings and become something other than affordances within perceptual language. This meaning variation of the happenings is fundamental for understanding art and its evolution (see also Pinna and Reeves, 2006).

The opposite of the previous argument is also true. A subject is also a happening, but as such it cannot be an affordance. A checkerboard is not only the subject of the form of meaning but also a happening, in the sense that it is the resulting action of combining in a whole object its elementary components.

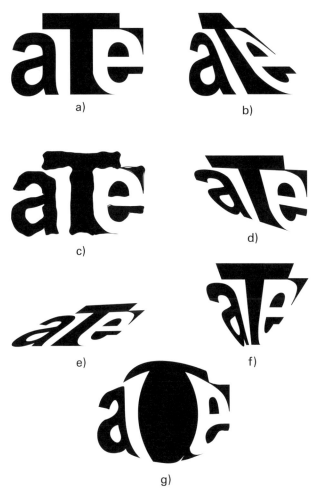

Figure 10.26
Which is the most artistic word?

In conclusion, the form of meaning explained in terms of perceptual organization related to the form of grouping and shape can help understand how the brain creates meanings. A possible neural scenario (see Pinna and Reeves, 2006) for the perceptual meanings is beyond the purpose of this chapter.

Acknowledgments

This chapter was supported by Finanziamento della Regione Autonoma della Sardegna, ai sensi della L.R. 7 agosto 2007, n. 7, Fondo d'Ateneo (ex 60%), Fondazione Banco di

Sardegna, and Alexander von Humboldt Foundation (to BP), and by CRS project on "Language and Perception," University of Trento (to LA). Special thanks to Maria Tanca for assistance in testing the subjects.

References

Albertazzi, L. 1996. "Anton Marty." In *The School of Franz Brentano*, edited by L. Albertazzi, M. Libardi, and R. Poli. Dordrecht: Kluwer. 83–109.

Albertazzi, L. 1997. "Continua, Adjectives and Tertiary Qualities." *Axiomathes* 8: 7–30.

Albertazzi, L. 1998a. "Perceptual Saliences and Nuclei of Meaning." In *The Brentano Puzzle*, edited by R. Poli. Aldershot: Ashgate. 113–138.

Albertazzi, L. 1998b. "Form Metaphysics." In *Shapes of Forms: From Gestalt Psychology to Phenomenology to Ontology and Mathematics*, edited by L. Albertazzi. Amsterdam: Kluwer. 261–310.

Albertazzi, L. 2000. "Which Semantics?" In *Meaning and Cognition: A Multidisciplinary Approach*, edited by L. Albertazzi. Amsterdam: Benjamins Publishing Company. 1–23.

Albertazzi, L. 2002a. "Causatives and Kinetic Structures." *Axiomathes* 1: 1–37.

Albertazzi, L. 2003. "From Kanizsa Back to Benussi: Varieties of Intentional Existence." *Axiomathes* 13: 239–259. [Special issue]

Albertazzi, L. 2004. "Stereokinetic Shapes and Their Shadows." *Perception* 33: 1437–1452.

Albertazzi, L. 2005. "Retrieving Intentionality. A Legacy From the Brentano School." In *The Lvov-Warsaw School: New Generation*, edited by J. Jadacki and J. Paśniczeck. Amsterdam: Rodopi. 291–314.

Albertazzi, L. 2006. "Das rein Figurale" (The Pure Figuration). *Gestalt Theory* 28 (1/2): 123–151.

Aristotle. 1984. *On Rhetoric*. Translated and edited by G. A. Kennedy, Oxford: Oxford University Press.

Arnheim, R. 1969. *Visual Thinking*. Berkeley: The Regents of the University of California.

Attneave, F. 1968. "Triangles as Ambiguous Figures." *American Journal of Psychology* 81: 447–453.

Barsalou, L. W. 1992. "Frames, Concepts, and Conceptual Fields." In *Frames, Fields, and Contrasts: New Essays in Semantics and Lexical Organization*, edited by A. Lehrer and E. Feder Kittay. Hillsdale: Hillsdale, NJ: Erlbaum Associates Publishers. 21–73.

Benussi, V. 1913. *Psychologie der Zeitauffassung* (Psychology of Time Apprehension). Leipzig: Hölder Publishing House.

Da Pos, O., and Zambianchi, E. 1996. *Visual Illusions and Effects*. Milan: Guerini.

Da Pos, O., and Albertazzi, L. 2010. "It Is in the Nature of Color . . ." *Seeing and Perceiving* 23: 39–73.

Eco, U. 2003. *Dire quasi la stessa cosa* (To Say almost the Same Thing). Milan: Bompiani.

Ehrenstein, W. 1925. "Versuche über die Beziehungen zwischen Bewegungs und Gestalt-Wahrnehmung" (Trials on the Relationship Between the Perception of Movement and of Gestalt). *Zeitschrift für Psychologie und Physiologie der Sinnesorgane* 96: 305–325.

Evans, V., and Green, M. 2006. *Cognitive Linguistics: An Introduction*. London: Routledge.

Fraser, J. 1908. "A New Visual Illusion of Direction." *British Journal of Psychology* 2: 307–320.

Gibson, J. J. 1977. "The Theory of Affordances." In *Perceiving, Acting, and Knowing: Toward an Ecological Psychology*, edited by R. Shaw and J. D. Bransford. Hillsdale, NJ: Erlbaum. 67–82.

Gibson, J. J. 1979. *The Ecological Approach to Visual Perception*. Boston: Houghton-Mifflin.

Giovannelli, G. 1966. "Stati di tensione e di equilibrio nel campo percettivo" (States of Tension and Equilibrium in the Perceptual Field). *Rivista di Psicologia* 60: 327–335.

Helmholtz, H. L. F. von. 1866. *Handbuch der Physiologischen Optik* (Part III) (Handbook of Physiological Optics). Leipzig: Voss.

Hering, E. 1861. *Beiträge zur Physiologie, I. Zur Lehre vom Ortsinne der Netzhaut* (Contributions to Physiology, I. On Gauging Localisation Through the Retina). Leipzig: Engelman.

Husserl, E. 1910. "Review of A. Marty, 'Recherches sur les fondements de la grammaire générale et de la philosophie du langage, 1908'" (Researches on the Foundations of the Universal Grammar and of the Philosophy of Language). *Deutsche Literaturzeitung* 31: 1106–1110.

Husserl, E. 1973. *Experience and Judgment*, translated by J. D. Churchill and K. Ameriks. Evanston, IL: Northwestern University Press.

Husserl, E. 1991. *On the Phenomenology of the Consciousness of Internal Time (1893–1917)*. Translated by J. B. Brough. Dordecht: Kluwer.

Husserl, E. 1975. *Logical Investigations*, translated by John N. Findlay. London: Routledge & Kegan Paul.

Kanizsa, G. 1972. "Errore del gestaltista e altri errori da aspettativa" (The Gestaltist Error and Expectation Errors). *Rivista di Psicologia* 66: 3–18.

Kanizsa, G. 1985. "Seeing and Thinking." *Acta Psychologica* 59: 23–33.

Kanizsa, G. 1991. *Vedere e pensare* (Seeing and Thinking). Bologna: Il Mulino.

Kopfermann, H. 1930. "Psychologische Untersuchungen über die Wirkung zweidimensionaler Darstellungen körperliche Gebilde" (Psychological Investigations on the Effects of Two-dimensional Representation of Corporeal Objects). *Psychologische Forschung* 13: 293–364.

Kristof, W. 1961. "Versuche mit der Waagrechten Strecke-Punkt-Figur" (Trials with the Horizontal Line-Point Figure). *Acta Psychologica* 18: 17–28.

Langacker, R. 1988. "An Overview of Cognitive Grammar." In *Topics in Cognitive Linguistics*, edited by B. Rudzka-Ostyn. Amsterdam: Benjamins Publishing Company. 3–48.

Langacker, R. 1991. *Concept, Image, and Symbol: The Cognitive Basis of Grammar*. Berlin, New York: De Gruyter.

Langacker, R. 2000. "Why a Mind is Necessary: Conceptualization, Grammar and Linguistic Semantics." In *Meaning and Cognition*, edited by L. Albertazzi. Amsterdam/Philadelphia: Benjamins Publishing Company. 25–38.

Leyton, M. 1993. *Symmetry, Causality, Mind*. Boston: MIT Press.

Leyton, M. 2003. *A Generative Theory of Shape*. Berlin/Heidelberg: Springer.

Lipps, Th. 1897. *Raumästhetik und geometrisch-optische Täuschungen* (Aesthetics of Space and Geometrical-Optical Illusions). Leipzig: Barth.

Marty, A. 1893. "*Über das Verhaltnis von Grammatik und Logik*" (On the Relationship between Grammar and Logic). Symbolae Pragenses, Festgabe der Deutschen Gesellschaft für Altertumskunde in Prag zur 42. Versammlung deutscher Philologen und Schulmänner in Wien. Vienna/Prague: Tempsky; Leipzig: Freytag. 99–126.

Marty, A. 1908. *Untersuchungen zur Grundlegung der allgemeinen Grammatik und Sprachphilosophie* (Researches on the Foundations of Universal Grammar and Philosophy of Language). Halle: Niemeyer. Repr. 1976, Hildesheim/New York: Olms.

Marty, A. 1910. *Gesammelte Schriften* (Collected Works). Edited by J. Eisenmeyer, A. Kastil, and O. Kraus, I. Bd., 1. Abt. mit einem Lebensabriss und einem Bildnis (und Bibliographie); I. Bd., 2. Abt., Schriften zur genetischen Sprachphilosophie. Halle: Niemeyer.

Massironi, M. 2002. *The Psychology of Graphic Images*. London: Elsevier.

Massironi, M., and Bonaiuto, P. 1966. "Ricerche sull'espressività. Qualità funzionali, intenzionali e relazione di causalità in assenza di 'movimento reale'" (Researches on Expressiveness. Functional and Intentional Qualities and Relation of Causality in Absence of "Real Motion"). *Rassegna di psicologia sperimentale e clinica* 8: 3–42.

Metzger, W. 1941. *Psychologie: die Entwicklung ihrer Grundannahmen seit der Einführung des Experiments* (Psychology: The Development of its Fundamental Assumptions since the Introduction of the Experiments). Dresden: Steinkopff.

Meinong, A. 1899. "Über Gegenstände höherer Ordnung und deren Verhältnis zur inneren Wahrnehmung" (On Higher Order Objects and Their Relation to Inner Perception). *Zeitschrift für Psychologie und Physiologie der Sinnesorgane* 21, 182–272. Repr. in *Alexius Meinong Gesamtausgabe* VII, edited by R. Haller. Graz: Akademische Druck- und Verlagsanstalt, II. 377–471.

Michotte, A. E., and Burke, L. 1951. "Une nouvelle énigme de la psychologie de la perception: le 'donné amodal' dans l'expérience" (A New Enigma of the Psychology of Perception. The 'Amodal Datum' in Experience). *Actes du Congrés Internationale de Psychologie*: 179–180.

Michotte, A. and collaborators. 1962. *Causalité, permanence et réalité phénoménales* (Causality, Permanence and Phenomenal Reality). Louvain: Studia Psychologica, Publications Universitaires.

Michotte, A. 1963. *The Perception of Causality*. London: Methuen.

Michotte, A., Thinès, G., and Crabbé, G. 1964. "Les compléments amodaux des structures percep-tuals" (Amodal Completion of Perceptual Structures). Louvain: Studia Psychologica, Publications Universitaires. Repr. 1991 in *Michotte's Experimental Phenomenology of Perception*, edited by G. Thinès, A. Costall, and G. Butterworth. Hillsdale, NJ: Lawrence Erlbaum.

Musatti, C. L. 1928. "Sui movimenti apparenti dovuti a identità di figura" (On Apparent Move-ments Due to Figure Identity). *Archivio Italiano di Psicologia* 6: 205–219.

Müller-Lyer, F. C. 1889. "Optische Urtheilstäuschungen" (Optical Illusions of Judgment). *Archiv für Anatomie und Physiologie, Physiologische Abteilung* 2: 263–270.

Oppel, J. J. 1854–1855. "Über Geometrisch-optische Täuschungen" (On Geometrical-Optical Illu-sions). *Jahresbericht des Physikalischen Vereins zu Frankfurt am Main*: 37–47.

Orbison, W. D. 1939. "Shape as Function of the Vector-Field." *American Journal of Psychology* 52: 31–54.

Palmer, S. E. 1980. "What Makes Triangles Point: Local and Global Effects in Configurations of Ambiguous Triangles." *Cognitive Psychology* 12: 285–305.

Palmer, S. E. 1989. "Reference Frames in the Perception of Shape and Orientation." In *Object Per-ception: Structure and Process*, edited by B. E. Shepp, and S. Ballesteros. Hillsdale, NJ: Lawrence Erl-baum. 121–163.

Palmer, S. E. 1992. "Common Region: A New Principle of Perceptual Grouping." *Cognitive Psychol-ogy* 24: 436–447.

Palmer, S. E. 1999. *Vision Science: Photons to Phenomenology*. Cambridge, MA, London, England: MIT Press.

Palmer, S. E., and Bucher, N. M. 1981. "Textural Effect in Perceiving Pointing of Ambiguous Tri-angles." *Journal of Experimental Psychology: Human Perception & Performance* 8 (5): 693–708.

Palmer, S. E., and Rock, I. 1994. "Rethinking Perceptual Organization: The Role of Uniform Con-nectedness." *Psychonomic Bulletin & Review* 1: 29–55.

Pinna, B. 1990. *Il dubbio sull'apparire* (The Doubt on the Appearance). Padova: Upsel Editore.

Pinna, B. 2010. "New Gestalt Principles of Perceptual Organization: An Extension from Grouping to Shape and Meaning." *Gestalt Theory* 32: 1–67.

Pinna, B., and Reeves, A. 2006. "Lighting, Backlighting and Watercolor Illusions and the Laws of Figurality." *Spatial Vision* 19: 341–373.

Pinna, B., and Reeves, A. 2009. "From Perception to Art: How the Brain Creates Meanings." *Spatial Vision* 22: 225–272.

Ponzo, M. 1912. "Rapports de contraste angulaire et l'appréciation de grandeur des asters à l'horizon" (The Relationship between Angular Contrast and Gauging the Size of the Stars on the Horizon). *Archives Italiennes de Biologie* 58: 327–329.

Rubin, E. 1921. *Visuell wahrgenommene Figuren* (Visual Perceived Figures). Kobenhavn: Gyldendal-ske Boghandel.

Rudzka-Ostyn, B. 1988. *Topics in Cognitive Linguistics*. Amsterdam: Benjamins Publishing Company.

Schilder, P., and Wechsler, D. 1936. "The Illusion of the Oblique Intercept." *Journal of Experimental Psychology* 19: 747–757.

Schlottman, A. 2000. "Is Perception of Causality Modular?" *Trends in Cognitive Sciences* 4: 441–442.

Schlottman, A., and Shanks, D. R. 1992. "Evidence for a Distinction Between Judged and Perceived Causality." *Quarterly Journal of Experimental Psychology: Human Experimental Psychology* 44 (2): 321–342.

Scholl, B. J., and Tremoulet, P. D. 2000. "Perceptual Causality and Animacy." *Trends in Cognitive Science* 4: 299–309.

Schumann, F. 1900. "Beiträge zur Analyse der Gesichtswahrnehmungen. Zur Schätzung räumlicher Grössen" (Contributions to the Analysis of Facial Recognition and Gauging Spatial Dimensions). *Zeitschrift für Psychologie und Physiologie der Sinnersorgane* 24: 1–33.

Talmy, L. 1988. "Force Dynamics in Language and Cognition." *Cognitive Science* 12: 49–100.

Tarski, A. 1944. "The Semantic Conception of Truth and the Foundations of Semantics." *Philosophy and Phenomenological Research* 4: 341–375.

Twardowski, K. 1977. *On Content and Object of Presentations*, edited by R. Grossman. The Hague: Nijhoff (1st German ed. 1894, Wien: Hölder Publishing House).

Vandeloise, C. 1991. *Spatial Prepositions: A Case Study From French*. Chicago/London: University of Chicago Press.

Vicario, G. B. 2005. *Il tempo* (Time). Bologna: Il Mulino.

Wertheimer, M. 1912a. "Über das Denken der Naturvölker" (On the Thought Patterns of Native People). *Zeitschrift für Psychologie* 60: 321–378.

Wertheimer, M. 1912b. "Untersuchungen über das Sehen von Bewegung" (Investigations on Visual Perception of Movement). *Zeitschrift für Psychologie* 61: 161–265.

Wertheimer, M. 1922. "Untersuchungen zur Lehre von der Gestalt. I" (Investigations on Gestalt Theory. I) *Psychologische Forschung* 1: 47–58.

Wertheimer, M. 1923. "Untersuchungen zur Lehre von der Gestalt. II" (Investigations on Gestalt Theory. II) *Psychologische Forschung* 4: 301–350.

Wundt, W. M. 1898. "Die geometrisch-optischen Täuschungen" (Geometrical-Optical Illusions) *Abhandlungen der Mathematisch-Physischen Classen der Königl. Sächsischen Gesellschaft der Wissenschaften*, Leipzig 24: 53–178.

Zöllner, J. K. Fr. 1860. "Über eine neue Art von Pseudoskopie und ihre Beziehungen zu den von Plateau und Oppel beschriebenen Bewegungsphänomenen" (On a New Kind of Pseudoskopics and its Relationship to the Motion Phenomena Described by Plateau and Oppel). *Annalen der Physik und Chemie* 110: 500–523.

11   The Perceptual Roots of Metaphor

Liliana Albertazzi

The garden in the brain
—Emily Dickinson

"Metaphor. What would that be?" In a memorable dialogue with delicate overtones between the postman of a remote Mediterranean island and Pablo Neruda, in a film of some years ago, the poet answered the question as follows: "Better than any explanation is the direct experience of the emotions, which can explain metaphor to a mind willing to understand it." It is probably thus for a poet, who does not set out to *explain* contents but rather to *express* them perfectly.

After all, the absolute taxonomic and dictionarial nonsense of poems like Ungaretti's: (Ungaretti, 2005 (*This Evening*), p. 31):[1]

Balustrade of breeze
Whereon to lean this evening
My melancholy. [My translation]

is simultaneously an example of perfect poetic expression that comprises the *code* of its universal comprehension.

Metaphors occur when a word, phrase, text, image (e.g., a Magritte painting), or sequence of images (e.g., a film) evoke in the recipient a mental representation that does not immediately or *exactly overlap* with its lexical or semantic content, but which through an analogical connection induces understanding of the message based on the polysemy of the signs expressed. In particular, *creative metaphors* constitute the paradigmatic example of this type of information because they evince its *structure* and *processes*.

Two thousand years of analysis on metaphor and kindred tropes like metonymy and synecdoche have passed, but the complexity of this type of information has still not been definitively resolved (Albertazzi, 2008). Here I confine myself to a more recent cognitive approach to metaphor (Cognitive Linguistics). Of this latter theory, given that it is not homogenous among all its parts and authors, I would stress three aspects with which I agree:

1. The Generalization Commitment (Lakoff, 1990; Langacker, 1991; Talmy, 1988a), that is, the fact that language per se does not embody codes of meaning (see also Pinna, Albertazzi, chapter 10, this volume), and that it divides between knowledge representation (conceptual structure) and meaning construction (conceptualization). This aspect sets cognitive linguistics in antithesis to both the modularism and the so-called "objectivist" semantics of formal approaches.

2. The assumption that there exist distinct layers of organization in language such as phonology, morphology, syntax, and semantics, which are strictly interrelated. Cognitive linguistics includes among its general assumptions a number of conceptualist theses: for example, in its assumption that language refers to concepts in the mind of the speaker and arouses analogous concepts in the mind of the listener. My position is even more radical, as I show.

3. The fact that words, viewed as lexical items, as conceptual categories, give access to encyclopaedic and intrinsically dynamic knowledge.

Starting from the assumption that language does not encode meaning and given the pervasiveness of the analogy subtending the various forms of homonymy characterizing metaphorical expression, what kind of information is transmitted by poetry? What type of subjective completion characterizes poetic expression? What are the visual boundaries of an image such as "balustrade of breeze?"

Framework

The thesis that I intend to put forward is that *metaphors are Gestalten and behave as Gestalten* (see Wertheimer, 2002a, 14ff and below). First, I argue that, precisely because of this structure, metaphors are *exact descriptions* of some aspects of reality, perceptual and/or mental.

Second, I argue that the metaphorical object is an *undistributed higher order object* (its tenor) that originates from the simultaneous fusion of a distributed series of contents given in succession.

I seek to demonstrate this thesis by analyzing how:

1. The ontological referents of metaphor are the phenomenal structures of perception.
2. Metaphor is realized in a subjective space–time continuum.
3. The place of the transposition operation is the actual temporal duration.
4. The content parts of metaphorical conceptualization are specific types of qualities.
5. The categorization occurs in prototypical and radial terms.
6. The process of blending contents is in effect a fusion of parts through the creation of internal modifying relations.

Put more simply, I seek to show that distinctive of a metaphor is the fact that, in the subjective temporal duration, the conceptual process that starts from the entities of the initial domains gives rise to a new entity in which the initial components lose their primitive ontological identities to assume the behavior of *belonging* to the whole. This does not happen with similes, for example.

On the basis of the hypothesis that metaphorical constructs have perceptive origins, I treat metaphor in the same terms as this statement by Köhler (1947), who observed that, "When subjective experiences are given names which also apply to perceptual facts, this does not happen in a random fashion" (pp. 134–135).

What Type of Information?

Figurative language is usually described as the use of an expression E with a default meaning A to evoke a distinct meaning B, where the connection between B and A is inferable according to general principles (i.e., it is not a private code established previously between individuals). In innovative uses, there is usually a feeling that traditional constraints have been *violated* (Gibbs, 1994).

Consider the following example:

About to bloom,
And exhale a rainbow,
The peony!
(Buson, in Blyth, 1952, III, p. 295)

Obviously, from the point of view of classical physics and taxonomic classification, when peonies bloom they do not exhale colored rainbows.

Further questions arise from the specific point of view of a classical theory of information:

1. What are the *codes* of metaphors? Are they universal or relativistic codes?
2. With what *signals* is the message activated?
3. Is there a metaphorical *alphabet*?
4. What is *transposed* in the metaphorical construct and how?
5. *Where* does the transfer occur according to the concept of *Metàbole*?

In terms of message transmission, the meaning of a metaphor seems to originate from the interaction between the imagination and the expressive forms involved in the metaphor's construction by its transmitter and the experience of its receiver. Curiously, there sometimes appears to be less noise in the comprehension of a metaphorical message (in the case of creative metaphors) than in ordinary communication. What is it that produces this universality of the code despite the complexity of the reference? In what space(s) is the message constructed, projected, and transmitted?

To address those questions, I start from the assumptions that there is:

1. a continuum among perception, lexicon, and syntax (Langacker, 1990), and
2. an intrinsic similarity between perceptual and metaphorical spaces (on perceptual spaces, see Albertazzi, 2002a, 2002b, 2006a, 2006b).

With regard to the first point, I start from the idea that grammatical forms are also endowed with meanings, and that these meanings are not particularly different from those of lexical forms; they are simply more abstract (see Pinna, Albertazzi, chapter 10, this volume). In other words, all linguistic, lexical, and grammatical expressions refer to schematic conceptualizations of greater or lesser density. Hence, the use of a certain grammatical form or a certain lexis is part of the signifying intention of the expression. An even more radical aspect concerns the original structures of predication before they are divided between grammatical and lexical forms (see below).[2] With regard to the second point, I show that the space of metaphorical conceptualization shares certain schematic structures with the space of phenomenal perception.[3]

The space of metaphorical conceptualization, in fact, is an intrinsically dynamic space-time that does not have the dimensions and primitives of classical Newtonian physics but nevertheless exhibits specific rules of organization of the Gestalt type.

It is worth noting that, when one asks what is specifically meant by a Gestalt organization (i.e., "What is Gestalt theory and what does it intend?"), Wertheimer (2002a) replies that: "There are wholes, the behaviour of which is not determined by that of their individual elements, but where the *part-processes* are themselves determined by the intrinsic nature of the whole. It is the hope of Gestalt theory to determine the nature of such wholes" (p. 3).

The functional mereology of *Gestaltpsychologie* therefore refers to a whole whose behavior is not entirely determined by the behavior of the parts and, *simultaneously*, to a whole that determines the parts.

Precisely, according to Koffka (1915; Koffka and Kenkel, 1913), applying the Gestalt category means determining:

1. which parts of nature belong as parts to functional wholes,
2. their degree of relative interdependence (mutual relatedness),
3. the organization of larger wholes into subwholes, and
4. nested hierarchies of wholes.[4]

Even more radically, Wertheimer (2002b) defines Gestalten in pictorial terms of "gradations of givenness in 'broad strokes,' relative to more inclusive whole properties" (p. 14) (i.e., not in terms of analytical wholes or definitional wholes) (see also Albertazzi, 2006c; Arnheim, 1954). This definition is much more dramatic than the usual "objectual" one of Gestalten as structured experiences characterized by supra-summativity and hierarchical order of the parts. Given its intrinsically dynamic nature in actual unfolding, in fact, *it is not easy to identify the boundaries of a form that is structurally in becoming* (see also van Tonder, chapter 4, this volume).[5]

Making a change to a processual whole of this kind, for example, by removing or adding a part, usually involves alterations in that part. Modifications of a part frequently involve changes elsewhere in the whole, as happens, for example, in the acoustic perception of an ongoing jazz session. In other words, given a functional whole, the alterations that occur in it are never arbitrary but rather determined by whole conditions. More specifically:

1. Events of this kind, "initiated by their occurrence *run a course* defined by the laws of functional dependence in wholes" (Wertheimer, 2002b, p. 14, italics added).
2. *Anticipatory structures* form a constitutive part of the process given the hierarchical dominance of the entire process over the parts (Albertazzi, 2006c).
3. The parts are intrinsically *potential*, as are the boundaries.

The analysis also seems entirely applicable to the structure of meaningful wholes such as "Juliet is the Sun" or "A certain slant of light which oppresses like the heft of cathedral tunes" (Dickinson, 2004, Poem n. 258, p. 270), which exhibit a similar nesting of frames and mereology (see below). What else explains the poet's maniacal search for, and eventual choice of, one particular term rather than another so that he or she perhaps has to reorganize the entire verse, and even all its terms, to achieve the completeness of a creative metaphorical expression?

More specifically, in metaphors:

1. What is the space-time involved (i.e., in what space and time *is* Juliet the Sun)?
2. What are the invariants of the domains involved that are transposed? For example, what qualities of Juliet and the Sun are present in the *new metaphorical identity*?
3. How does the fusion of the parts come about (i.e., in what way are the qualities common to Juliet and the Sun *internally modified* and made homogeneous by the metaphorical relation)?
4. What kinds of *qualities* are in play?

I try to answer these questions in five steps.

First Step: Metaphor Is Realized in a Subjective Space

The first step in analysis and explanation of what happens in a metaphorical process is identifying the *type of space* in which it takes place. This is a marvellous space where it makes complete sense to ask a lover to "cover the lips with odorous twilight" (Yeats), where the heart is "silver, or gold, or precious stone, or star, or rainbow, or a part of all these things, or all of them" (Herbert), where "sadness can be flung to the winds and borne upon the waves" (*tristitiam et metus tradam protervis portare ventis* (Horace), the tiger is "burning bright in the forests of the night" (Blake), or you can simply say to someone, "go and catch a falling star" (Donne) or, finally, "your life is allowed to waste like a tap left running" (Woolf).

The space of the imagination is certainly a subjective space, which moreover has many rules in common with the space of phenomenal perception. See, for example, "There are already zones of my life like the empty rooms of a too large palace which an impoverished owner has decided not to occupy" (Marguerite Yourcenar, *Memories of Hadrian*).

Then, it is no coincidence that most metaphorical constructs make use of perceptual, visual, acoustic, tactile, intermodal, and very often synaesthetic images (see below). The *first ontological level of reference for metaphors*, therefore, is not the physical space but *the space of phenomenal appearances*.

However, the fact that the perceptual qualities of objects are correlated with neuronal states should not induce one to fall into the error of thinking that neuronal states "are" the objects of vision, and therefore the ontological references of conceptualization. This is to commit a physicalist fallacy (Mausfeld, 2002). The same applies to artistic perception and poetic images, with the difference that in this case there is a further space to consider: that of the imagination, of which phenomenal space is the primary ontological referent. Here I restrict my analysis to the phenomenal space of vision, but the same operation can be performed in the space of the other sensory modalities, with their relative specificities.

The space of phenomenal appearances has characteristics of velocity, direction, distance, boundary, and so on, which prevent its reduction to the position space of classical physics and classical external psychophysics (Albertazzi, 2002a, 2002b, 2006a, 2006b). Visual space organization, in fact, displays the coexistence and interdependence of multiple "spaces" and the numerous factors involved in the construction of the "objects of vision" (for a detailed analysis, see Albertazzi, 2006b).

The *extensity* of visual space, for example, is not physical spatial extension but rather a topological *extendedness* in which objects sometimes entirely nonexistent from the point of view of stimuli are configured, such as transparency or anomalous surfaces. Every visual form is the product of forces and tensions; every form has its own structural skeleton as described by Arnheim (1954; see also Kovàcs, 2000; Leyton, 1992).[6] It is in this space that, for example, "the fields stretch cold into a distance hard" (Meredith).

Directions in the field, be they static or in motion, may be harmonious or disharmonious, in that they are intrinsic to the organization of the whole (see the analysis of the diagonal in Kandinsky [1926] and the relative depiction in *Improvisation IVX*).

In perception, as in depiction, *weight* also has qualitative salience.[7] Weight in visual configurations is therefore not an individual property but a complex one produced by the interaction among magnitude, shape, location, color, and numerousness of the elements involved, in reciprocal dependence and equilibrium (see the analysis of good and bad points in Arnheim, 1988; see also the nine ascending points in Kandinsky, 1926).

The same applies to perceived *distance*, which results from the interrelations among a series of components ranging among variations of form in linear perspective; occlusion; qualitative differences in shape, color, and brightness; textures of surfaces; line orientation; movement of the observer or part of the scene; and even planar surfaces or repetition of patterns in natural and artificial environments (Albertazzi, 2006a). When Dickinson (2004, Poem n. 258, pp. 270–72) writes:

'tis like the *Distance*
On the *look of Death* (p. 272)

distance is measured not in terms of metric difference but of qualitative diversity (see below).[8] If we seek to trace distance metrically on the face of death, in fact, we are lost.

As said, in visual perception, the same stimuli may give rise to different distances and magnitudes of the phenomenal forms due to the field's assimilative phenomena, which in this case too serves to achieve a visual equilibrium. Numerous so-called "perceptive illusions," like those of Lipps or Ebbinghaus, are due to the tendency to equilibrium that regulates the intrinsic anisotropy of visual space (Albertazzi, 1998a, 2002b; Brentano, 1995b; Itten, 2002; Lipps, 1897; Musatti, 1955; von Allesch, 1931).

The fact is that if we begin to understand the structure of this space, and to move within it, the rainbow exhaled by a peony or the solid mass of coolness of the midnight moon:

The moon of midnight:
A solid mass
Of coolness?
(Teishitsu, in Blyth, 1952, III, p. 377)

become perfectly *coherent* phenomena because we understand that poetic expressions are exact descriptions of perceptive and intermodal states of affairs. In *Consolation*, for example, it is intermodality that enables the poet to express himself thus:[9]

Let us go out. Do not cover your head. It is but a slow
Sun of September
(D'Annunzio, 1982, *Consolation*, p. 668) [My translation]

Seeking to explain metaphor in terms of classical physics is to commit the perversion crudely described by Majakovskij, 1963, *Hymn to the Scientist*:

He's not a man but an impotent biped
With his head bitten off
By a treatise on warts in Brazil.
His greedy eyes gnaw a letter
Of the alphabet. [My translation]

How, therefore, are the *boundaries* of phenomenal appearances, such as that of the moon or the peony's ethereal exhalation, formed so that they can be expressed in poetry and convey "exact information" about certain aspects of reality? The same happens in Ungaretti's *Last Cantos for The promised Land* (Ungaretti, 1997, p. 388):[10]

Imprisoned between the one star and the other
Is the night
In the boundless turbulent void
From that starry solitude
To that starry solitude. (p. 388)
[My translation]

Or in Pascoli (2002, *This Evening*, I, p. 817):[11]

The stars must open
In the heavens so tender and alive. [My translation]

For that matter, seeking to explain visual images in terms of pictures, as often happens today by means of computer images constructed on the basis of pixels and then moving through successive one-, two-, and three-dimensional stages (Marr, 1982; criticism in Wade, 1990), is only to beg the question because phenomenal vision does not move through those stages: Human vision is immediately three-dimensional, and the boundaries of visual objects are intrinsically potential.[12]

As for the *velocity* of visual appearances, once again it cannot be treated in terms of the space/time of physics (i.e., of the space traversed in units of time). The *perceived* velocity of an object in motion cannot be computed in terms of $v = s/t$ because it also depends on the size of the objects, the illumination of the field, and the peripheral vision of movement, as Brown and Koffka demonstrated since the 1930s (Brown, 1931; Koffka, 1935). In the visual field, velocity has instead the characteristics of the transformation of form, which may be smooth or abrupt, as in the case of a surface that changes in color from red to blue (Brentano, 1988), or a sky from dawn to dusk, or the sea that turns wine-dark as a storm approaches. Not to speak of the forms of potential movement exemplified by the innumerable perceptive illusions offered by Op Art.[13] In the visual field, in fact, it is impossible to separate perceived time, space, and velocity.

For this reason, the movement and separation of two lovers *are* regulated by a compass that inclines and swivels in the space of the emotional mind:

If they [souls] be two, they are two so
As stiff twin compasses are two.
Thy soul the fixed foot, makes no show
To move, but doth, if th'other do.

And though it in the centre sit,
Yet when the other far doth roam,
It leans, and hearkens after it,
And grows erect, as that comes home.

Such wilt thou be to me, who must
Like th'other foot, obliquely run;
Thy firmess makes my circle just,
And makes me end, where I begun.

(Donne, 1992, *A Valediction: Forbidding Mourning*, p. 121)

The potential movement of phenomenal configurations is transposed into the poetic complexity often expressed in terms of Talmy's (1996) fictive motion:

Included
In the Summer drawing room
The mountains and the garden also move.

(Bashô, in Blyth, 1952, III, p. 132)

Mountains, in fact, do not move in classical Newtonian mechanics. One of the main features of apparent/fictive motion—besides the fact that it does not have a counterpart in the physical world—is that every distinguishable part (beginning, end, trajectory, etc.) of the total event (e.g., the stroboscopic movement of the light) is a *simultaneous cause* of the way in which the other parts appear *and effect* of the way other parts are perceived.

Second Step: Metaphor Is Realized in a Subjective Time

Just as the subjective space of metaphor is not reducible to the position space of classical physics, neither is the subjective time of the metaphorical construct. Once again, this is a time different in its structure, primitives, and rules of organization from the metric time of classical physics. This time is not made of mathematical, atomic instants in regular sequence according to a before–after relation. Otherwise, it could not happen that, *In the Valley of Cauterez*:

I walked with the one I loved two and thirty years ago
All along the valley while I walked today
The two and thirty years were a mist that rolls away.

(Tennyson, 1995, p. 221)

Moreover, what does the *agency* of these temporal primitives derive from? It is entirely normal, in fact, to express oneself in everyday conversation in terms of "the time drags," "flows," "races," "flies," or "stands still," just as we may suddenly realize that "half of my life is gone" (Longfellow, 1995, *Mezzo Cammin*, pp. 67–68).

Time, in metaphor, continuously deforms, as it does in dreams or virtual reality as in the following;

The well's pulley creaks;
the water rises to the light.

A memory shimmers in the brimming pail,
in the pure ring an image laughs.
I bring my face to evanescent lips:
The past is distorted, it ages,
it belongs to another . . .
The well
creaks, restores you to the other depths,
vision, a distance divides us.
(Montale, 1990, *The well's pulley creaks*, p. 47) [My translation]

Much has been written in cognitive linguistics, especially in recent years, about the metaphorical conceptualization of time, emphasizing that it can be conceptualized in terms of "Moving Ego" ("We're getting close to the end") or "Moving time" ("Time flies") mapping.

This research sets temporal experience in relation to the awareness of change, but mainly from the point of view of *comparison between two mental states* (Grady, 1997a) or between two events already accomplished (Lakoff and Johnson, 1999). In other words, the perception of time supposedly derives from a secondary cognitive process of abstraction. Neither of the two approaches considers the difference between change of perception and perception of change, or the subjective duration of which we are aware even in the absence of changes in the external world (Brentano, 1995a; Flaherty, 1999; see also Evans, 2005, chapter 5). None of them considers the difference between the awareness of an occurring event and the recognition of an event or object connected to the decoding of the signals (Vicario, 1998).

With regard to experimentation, the cognitive sciences are at present greatly interested in the phenomenon of temporal processing, and they hypothesize the existence of neurologically instantiated temporal codes where perceptual information is integrated to produce a coherent percept (the so-called "binding" problem) (Crick, 1994; Crick and Koch, 1990, 1998; Pöppel, 1994; Varela, 1999; Varela, Thompson, and Rosch, 1991). However, these analyses usually display a reductionist tendency parallel to the one already mentioned of reducing phenomenal perception to neuronal correlates (Albertazzi, 2007a). The enthusiasm aroused by recent results in the neurosciences sometimes makes the paradigm appealing to scholars working in semantics, and in particular those concerned with the theory of conceptual metaphor. However, the fact that there is a well-codified temporal structure—a sort of rhythm embedded in information processing—at the neuronal level does not coincide with or immediately explain the type of complexity emergent at the level of phenomenal perception, where not only more numerous but also *new* qualitative categorial structures are manifest (Hartmann, 1935; Poli, 2001, 2002, 2006a, 2006b).[14] Again, the correlation found between mirror neurons and forms of action thought, seen, and not merely enacted—for example, the action of grasping—is a *correlation, not an identity*, of structures (which, instead, seems to be assumed in recent literature) (see Gallese, 2005; Gallese and Lakoff, 2005; Rizzolati and Arbib, 1998). The classical Gestalt thesis of isomorphism, in fact, referred to a strong morphism of structures, not to their *logical reducibility or identity*. Awareness of this problem has been shown by Varela (1999) in his attempt to compare Husserl's analyses of the inner consciousness of time and neuroscientific research.

The subjective time (otherwise termed "mental," psychological, or "inner"), which "drags," "runs," or "flows" is not at all linear, and it necessarily unfolds in a topological extendedness with qualitative accelerations and decelerations. In the temporal flux, moreover, it is possible to identify structures and substructures (i.e., significant durations of differing extendedness) (Benussi, 1913; Rensink, 2002), but they cannot be univocally correlated with temporal instants.[15] Not to mention the positive or negative temporal dislocations (i.e., those cases revealed by analysis of the microstructure of the duration that shift forward or backward in subjective time with respect to the metric time of ordered sequences of stimuli).[16] Why, therefore, should we be surprised if poetry magnifies exactly this intrinsic capacity for positive or negative dislocation possessed by the perceptive structures in *conceptual anaphora*, which enables the temporal dimension to stretch forward or backward, upward or downward, with great naturalness?[17] Consider:

Silvia, do you remember still
The time of your mortal life
When beauty shone
In your smiling, startled eyes
As, bright and pensive, you arrived
At the limit of youth?

(Leopardi, 1989, *To Silvia*, p. 93) [My translation]

Today, duration in its unfolding is analyzed experimentally on a brief present-time scale, in phases (part-processes), according to positive and negative dislocations, in several areas of research centered on "perceptual momentum," "flash-lag effect," "Frölich effect," "object-directed attention (proto-objects)," and so on (Brown, 1991; Libet, 1982; Pöppel, 1994; Rensink, 2000, 2002). These analyses show that the phenomenal present (so-called "time of presentness," whose duration can be measured externally and which last from 100 msecs to 2–3 seconds) has as its correlate an object (of seeing, hearing, feeling, etc.) that comes into being in the deployment of the perceptive act. We are therefore dealing with an *actual becoming object*, as demonstrated, for example, by phenomena of stream segregation in auditory perception.[18]

The space of pictorial depiction grasps this type of complexity and gives it form, as in Balla's *Dog on a Leash* or Duchamp's *Nude Descending a Staircase* or *Verre*, one of his best-known rotoreliefs, which depicts stereokinetic movement (Albertazzi, 2004).

Because it has been demonstrated that the phenomenal present is also the *time of a strophe* in a poem (Benussi, 1913; Brentano, 1988; Ehrenfels, 1897; Husserl, 1966b; James, 1890; Turner and Pöppel, 1983), then its objects should also presumably conform to the same laws of organization.

As to the present act of perceiving, Kanizsa has stressed that its structure is internally stratified. It is made up, in fact, of a basic layer constituted by perceptual presence (PP) and characterized by subjective forms of phenomenal completion comprising a series of entities, such as phenomenally real appearance, so-called illusions, amodal presence, pictorial perception, *trompe l'oeil*, and so on, and in which there is no implicit will or directed attention of the perceiver. It has also been stressed that the phenomenal presence always has an emotional property with features of transitoriness and expressiveness (Michotte, 1963). In other words, it has the nature of affordance (Gibson, 1979).

Second, it is possible to distinguish a higher order layer consisting of mental presence (MP) and characterized by subjective forms of mental completion, which comprise memory, associations, assumptions, hypotheses, and so on and presuppose active behavior on the part of the beholder (Kanizsa, 1991, chapter 1). I return later to the distinction between these two types of subjective completion and their role in the metaphorical construct (see Albertazzi, 2003, forthcoming).

Finally, the experimental analysis of the time of the phenomenal present shows that the structure of the duration performs a real and proper temporal *boundary function*. It is the modalities of the *act* that impart symmetry to the object, as Husserl maintained. Curiously, in fact, as evidenced by analysis of the perception of movement, in vision the *act of seeing* produces striking phenomenal appearances. For example, it coordinates the quality of the surfaces it constructs with the depth at which it place them; it constructs perceptual movement; it constructs a "visual object" and gives it a shape in two or three dimensions; it endows the object with a border, with sometimes smooth and sometimes sharp corners; it places the object in space; and it moves that object in space, rotating it or translating it, or both (Albertazzi, 2007a; Hoffman, 2003).

Why should it be surprising, therefore, that in the unfolding time of a strophe, expression is couched in terms of entities and objects variously and simultaneously given in perceptive and/or mental presence, in real or fictitious motion, and even endowed with agency and expression?

With your sad steps, O Moon, thou climb'st the skies
How silently, and how wan a face;
What, may it be that e'en in heav'nly place
That busy archer his sharp arrows tries?

(Sydney, 1998, *With your sad steps, O Moon, thou climb'st the skies*, p. 37)

Some centuries later, the same "presence" is similarly expressed:

Art thou pale for weariness
Of climbing heaven, and gazing on the earth,
Wandering companionless
Among the stars that have a different birth,
And ever-changing, like a joyless eye
That finds no object worth its constancy?
(Shelley, 1998, *To the Moon*, p. 83)

Here, too, the universality of the code manifests the invariants of metaphorical information, which must therefore be analyzed on the basis of their primary referents (i.e., *phenomenal perception* and the laws of its complex organization).

Third Step: The Primitives of Metaphorical Conceptualization

What are the qualities categorized, expressed, and fused in the space-time of the metaphorical construct? An example of this type of primitive is the "coolness" of the moon in the previously quoted poem by Teishitsu. This may appear with the same component in a different configuration, for example, in the shift from visual to tactile perception, from the transparency of air to the wetness of water:[19]

With the sea
I have made myself
A coffin
Of coolness.
(Ungaretti, 2005, *Universe*, p. 49) [My translation]

"Coolness" and kindred properties are certainly not primary qualities, nor are they Platonic entities of the hyperuranic realm (i.e., substances). Moreover, as we have seen, the space of phenomenal appearances is not the space of external psychophysics.[20] In the inner space of information processing, the *units of sensation* (jnd) of external psychophysics are replaced with *units of inner presentation* (i.e., by what Brentano called *perceptively noticeable parts* [jnp], localized and qualified in phenomenal space-time) (Brentano, 1995a, 1995b, 1981; see also Albertazzi, 2006d; Mausfeld, 2003). Once again, because phenomenal space is not the space of position and phenomenal time is not the linear and indifferent time of metrics, so *qualities are not stimuli*, and colors (and the phenomenal forms almost always inseparable from them) are not merely wave radiations, nor are neuronal correlates their correspondents.[21]

We may attempt a preliminary classification of these qualities by referring to the specific sublayer of the duration in which they appear: That is, we may do so on the basis of Kanizsa's already mentioned distinction between PP and MP.

Perceptual qualities are qualities of the type "red," "luminous," "coarse," "mountainous," "high" (also in the tonal sense), "fresh," "perfumed," "tree-lined," but also "glossy," "lighting," "discoloring" (Pinna, 2005a; Pinna and Albertazzi, chapter 10, this volume; Pinna, Werner, and Spillmann, 2003), and so on. These are given directly in phenomenal form in the actual presentation (Ash, 1961).

Mental qualities are instead of the type "Mediterranean," "religious," "referential," "economic," "conceptual," "geographic," and so on, and they are given "top downward" in conceptual form.

Both are *discontinuities* inserted in the space-time anticipatory field of actual duration (see the *Ganzfeld* experience in Koffka, 1930; see also Li and Gilchrist, 1999).[22]

I dwell in particular on the perceptual qualities of the basic level of PP because, besides being semiotic primitives (Albertazzi, 2002b, 2002d), they manifest an important inner complexity. The qualities that manifest themselves at the level of PP are essentially of three types:

1. Secondary qualities
2. Tertiary qualities
3. Qualities with a demand character.

Examples of *secondary qualities* are phenomenal red but also the "single hue-nuances" of red. In a memorable passage in Eco's (1995) *Island of the Day Before*, the protagonist desperately searches for the *exact expression* with which to describe the color of a bird's feathers:

"Ruddy, ruby, rubescent, rubedinous, rubent, rubefacient, Roberto suggested." (p. 278)

From this point of view, the prototype as well as its nonprototypical exemplars—for example, the reds that tend toward yellow or the reds that tend toward blue—are likewise considered semiotic primitives.[23] In other words, *the perceptive qualities are the ontological primitives of phenomenal experience in its actual unfolding*, and they are such in *degrees of differing givenness* (in Wertheimer's already mentioned sense).

Second, the qualities that manifest themselves at the level of perceptive presence are tertiary qualities (i.e., qualities with an expressive and physiognomic value) (*Weseneigenschaften*). They pertain to character, ethos, habit, and atmosphere, and they are expressed by adjectives such as merry, friendly, bold, terse, pacific, vehement, gracious, feminine, virile, infantile, senile, crackling, noisy, shrill, whining, and so on (Klages, 1942). As Arnheim (1966) wrote:

Once the main perceptual traits of a pattern have been analysed, it becomes possible to describe the expressive qualities that derive from them. For instance, there is the stability of horizontal-vertical axes or the excitement and tensions of oblique ones. There is the metallic smoothness of some contour lines or the tattered look of others; the sturdy compactness of a large, uninterrupted mass or the frailer, more sensitive quality of a strongly subdivided honeycombed pattern. The expression combined by a visual pattern will be as ambiguous as the perceptual structure that creates it. (p. 100)

The same qualities are expressed in:[24]

I polish myself
like a marble
with passion.
(Ungaretti, 2005, *Mandolinata*, p. 384)

Other qualities have a "demand character" (*Anfforderungscharakter*) and are characterized by being intrinsically dynamic, diffuse, expressive—for example, appealing, elegant, common, noble, terrific, repellent, attractive, disgusting, pleasing, exalting, oppressive, repugnant, stimulating, calming, terrifying, boring, exciting, distressing, appetising, and so on.[25]

In addition, the demand character of the qualities has little or nothing to do with Gibson's (1979) affordances, defined as "objective, real and physical, unlike values and meanings, which are often supposed to be subjective, phenomenal and mental" (p. 129) (i.e., precisely what these properties are *not* from a phenomenal point of view) (Albertazzi, 2007a).

In conclusion, it is not possible to talk of phenomenal qualities using the terms of classical psychophysics as *features*. We need a new categorial framework for the classification of these qualities, which have their own specific behavior: We can call them *distinguishing marks* of objects (Albertazzi, 1998b) or simply *moments* in the Husserlian sense, that is, qualitative, nonindependent parts of the whole of presentation.

The phenomenal qualities given in perceptive presence have a relationship of only partial dependence with the primary metric qualities: *A sepal, petal, and a thorn, upon a common summer's morn* (Dickinson) are certainly also the fruit of stimuli processing. However, as we have seen, the specific phenomenal appearance is not reducible to them because of the type of space-time and the type of structure in which they acquire existence.[26]

Here I wish to stress the intrinsic dynamism of these qualities, which are more properly treated as just *patterns* (not as features) or as dynamic components that govern the laws of similarities in the perceptual organization.[27] A pattern of similarities may emerge dramatically in poetic compositions:[28]

From the high wall protrude
Bare trees
Gibbets, braces, crutches.
(De Pisis, 1961, *Bare Trees*, p. 507) [My translation]

Or[29]

Of birds taken by snare
Almost notes on a pentagram
I have drawn not a few with charcoal.
(Montale, 1990, *Bird Nets*, p. 576) [My translation]

Or, again in Ungaretti's *Soldiers*[30] (Ungaretti, 2005, p. 87)

They stand
Like the leaves on the trees
Of autumn. [My translation]

The fundamental characteristic of a pattern is that within it similar components tend to be seen as pertaining to the same unit. Moreover, perception of a pattern does not take place only in a specific sensory mode. Rather, it is intermodal, as, for example, in the perception of loud versus soft sounds.

A pattern may be repeated at various levels of grammatical and lexical continuity held together by the same scheme:

My wife whose hair is a brush fire
Whose thoughts are summer lightning
Whose waist is an hourglass
Whose waist is the waist of an otter caught in the teeth of a tiger
Whose mouth is a bright cockade with the fragrance
Of a star of the first magnitude
Whose teeth leave prints like the tracks of white mice over snow
Whose tongue is made out of amber and polished glass
Whose tongue is a stabbed water [. . .]
(Breton, 1992, *Freedom of Love*, II, pp. 85–86) [My translation]

When Wertheimer talks of differing degrees of givenness in Gestalten "in broad strokes," he is in fact referring to phenomenal patterns consisting of the co-presence of secondary and tertiary qualities in a semantic conceptual whole.

A further characteristic of patterns is that their perception is not substantival (i.e., they do not refer to objects). In the duration at the level of actual presentation, in fact, we are dealing not with perceptions of an object that may be "squared," "acute," "thin," and so on (i.e., perceptions of substances and their accidents), but with *unitary perceptions* of "squareness," "angleness," "straightness," "curvedness," "parallelness," "lineness," "acuteness," "thinness," or "coolness," as in the cases of Teishitsu's moon or Montale's coffin (Albertazzi, 1998a, 2006b, forthcoming; Arnheim, 1969; Bühler, 1934; Gibson, 1979; Husserl, 1900–1901; Ingarden, 1962; Kandinsky, 1926; Koffka, 1935; Lipps, 1897; Metzger, 1941; Wertheimer, 2002c). This, therefore, is perception of the adverbial type.

Fourth Step: Categorization

At this point, the question arises as to how objects can be categorized in creative metaphor if we are dealing not with objects stable in their shape and semantic denomination, but only with *patterns* that appear in their dynamic unfolding within the duration and tending to a sort of global stabilization of meaning. How can we objectually define things that appear in terms of phenomenal qualities, salience, and shadowing of the duration—that is, *part-processes in their unfolding*?

Consider[31]:

Et laisse-moi plonger dans tes beaux yeux, Mêlés de métal et d'agate (Let me gaze into your beautiful eyes of metal and agate)

(Baudelaire, 1996, *The Cat*, p. 68)

By expressing itself in this way, Baudelaire's enamored mind is not categorizing its love object in dictionarial and taxonomic terms. Dictionarial information, in fact, categorizes agate as "as chalcedony in veined concretions, with coloured bands or irregular clouding" and metal "as a chemical element, almost always solid in the natural state, ductile, malleable, a good conductor."

What do the eyes of Baudelaire's cat possess of agate if not the striking phenomenal cobalt blue that is the invariant of the stone in question? Or of metal if not the appearance between gloom and glow, a phenomenal quality for which Old English coined the term "wan"? The eyes of Baudelaire's cat, therefore, have an invariant common also to the crow's wing, the light on a dark wave, or the lustre on armour (Bixby, 1928).[32] As I already pointed out, "when subjective experiences are given names which also apply to perceptual facts, this does not happen in a random fashion." Metaphor, therefore, at least potentially, is an exact description of perceptual facts.[33]

If metaphorical categorization is not essentially substantival (i.e., by genus and specific difference), then what is it?

Embedded in metaphor are various types of categorization, and this is one of the reasons for its complexity. Comprised in metaphor are nuclei of categorization known as cognitive collages (Tversky, 1993, 1999), frames (Fillmore, 1982), schemes (Eco, 1999), prototypes (Rosch, 1973, 1978; Rosch and Mervis, 1975; Rosch, Mervis, Gray, Johnson, and Boyes-Braem, 1976), radiality (Lakoff, 1987), and less frequently considered aspects like typicity (Husserl, 1966a; Violi, 2000; Albertazzi, 2007b).

I dwell in particular on the relations and differences among:

1. Prototypicality (focus of a category whose boundaries are fuzzy).
2. Radiality (extensions of a prototypical category in other domains through similarity, conceptual metaphor, and shared frames).
3. Typicity of categories (i.e., perceptual categories in ongoing presentation).

Categorization by prototypes emphasizes that a large part of environmental categorization comes about not by genus and species, but by exemplary categories such as focal red or the robin, these being members of a class of items whose boundaries are blurred.

The prototype has particular status at the level of *basic categorization*. It is a *particular type of member* of the category (the prototype of a bird, a robin for example, is a *type of* bird). At the level of subordinate categorization, the prototype (robin) exemplifies the average of the values of all specimens belonging to that specific category (Geeraerts, 1989). This average is obtained on the basis of morphological perceptive aspects and other semantic dimensions. This enables determination of a specimen's regularity or otherwise within the category, and it also enables inferences to be drawn about other possible members. From this point of view, the robin is no longer the prototype but the most regular example within the category "bird." The theory therefore distinguishes between two types of prototypicity:

1. The prototypicity of the robin *qua* bird according to a kind of ontological duplication.
2. The prototypicity of the robin as the *average individual* in relation to the members of the category.

Given a prototypical concept (such as "mother"), then, *radial* categorization comprises subcategories of a concept such as *deviations* from the central case up until outright stereotypes (natural and adoptive mother, wet-nurse, biological or foster mother, single mother, stepmother, or even house-mother or working mother). Some of these categories are generated *productively* from the base concept, whereas others are defined *culturally* and therefore differ from culture to culture. The radial structure within each category generates prototypical effects, as in the celebrated case of the Dyrbal (Dixon, 1982; Lakoff, 1987).

The principles that regulate radial categorization are those of centrality, chaining, domains of experience, idealized models, and specific knowledge, which constitute "nuances" of the core concept in culturally and individually connoted settings. In short, the process of radial categorization involves extensions of a core concept wherein:

1. Every member is connected to another by some shared property.
2. Every term refers to a polysemic pattern of sense.
3. There is no property common to all members, but a central entity (core) with which all items share at least one feature.

Both the notion of prototypicity and its radial extensions, however, have a number of weaknesses:

1. They do not take the precategorial origin of the core concept into account and start from a "base" category in terms of a "conceptual" category (Albertazzi, 2007b; Pinna and Albertazzi, chapter 10, this volume).
2. The notion is consequently restricted to a few semantic classes of nouns that exclude other categorization processes of adjectival or adverbial type (being irritated, agitated, emotional, etc.) more closely tied to patterns than to already stabilized features or conceptual entities.
3. More generally, the derivation of the various senses from the prototypical senses is unclear given the dominance in the theory of the principle of conventionality of lexical items, which makes them unpredictable.

The existence of stable (and typical) associations of content variables with words emphasizes the schematic nature of meaning. It seems, in fact, that words function as *pointers* that anticipate what are supposedly the relevant features of an item (Violi, 2000).[34] In this way, words anticipate the "construal" of a possible context for their interpretation. This means that the appropriate conditions for interpretation are created even when they are not initially present, and it also explains why interpretation of a word is possible even when all semantic features can be cancelled from the context perceived, as the notes of a melody. Accordingly, speaking of his wife, Montale can write:[35]

Dear little insect

Whom they called fly, who knows why

(Montale, 1990, *Dear Little Insect*, p. 289) [My translation]

The question that now arises is what happens in the anticipation of the context, in the construal triggered by a particular lexical item?

There are two main aspects to consider:

1. The base pattern.
2. Variation within that pattern.

With regard to the first point, I refer to the section on the primitives of the metaphorical construct. A particular prototypical meaning (chair, mother, robin, red, etc.) (see Lakoff, 1987) is not inflected across a list of necessary and sufficient conditions but on the basis of a pattern common to the members of the category that refers to a similarity structure enabling its transcategorical inflection.[36] Among other things, it is on similarity that synesthetic expressions in the metaphorical construct are grounded—as Lambert (1764) pointed out as far back as the eighteenth century!

Today, there is renewed interest in the relationship between metaphor and synesthesia, once again prompted by research in the neurosciences and biological anthropology (Ramachandran and Hubbard, 2003; Savage-Rumbaugh, 1996). In general, as Cacciari (1998) notes, two lines of sensory research can be distinguished in the area of metaphorical synesthesia:

1. Of the *taxonomic/literary* type, which seeks to identify the direction of the synesthetic "loan" in language to determine whether every modality can both metaphorize and be metaphorized by others (Shen, 1997; Williams, 1976).
2. Of the *psychophysical* type, which seeks to describe the physical features of the signals or events incorporated into the verbal metaphorical transfer (e.g., pitch or timbre of a sound, luminance for light, etc.) (Cytowic, 1989; Day, 1996; Ramachandran and Hubbard, 2001). This line follows the classical notion of information theory.

In the 1970s and onward, Marks produced a large body of analysis by drawing on studies in *Gestaltpsychologie* or kindred areas, and by Hornbostel in particular (see

Hornbostel, 1925; Marks, 1978, 1982, 1996; Marks, Hammeal, Bornstein, 1987; see also Merleau-Ponty, 1945, 1969). Marks' analyses concerned both normal and synesthetic subjects in various Western languages. He identified five predominant synesthetic tendencies:

1. Tendency to brightness between sound sharpness and color brightness, in particular between "colored" vowels.
2. Tendency to size, in particular among low sounds, colors, and broader photisms, and among high sounds, colors, and narrower photisms.
3. Tendency to velocity, which concerns sound in general, so that the more rapid the rhythm, the more angular the corresponding image, and vice versa.
4. Tendency to weight, so that the more saturated the colors, the more they are perceived as heavy, and therefore as more stable and in equilibrium, for example.
5. Tendency to temperature, so that there is a correlation between cool colors (blue, green) and warm ones (red, yellow).

Although a psychophysical correlate for each tendency can be identified (e.g., blue and green are colors with shorter wavelengths, and yellow and red are colors with longer wavelengths) (see D'Andrade and Egan, 1974; Sivik, 1997; Valdez and Mehrabian, 1994), or a neuronal correlate (Cytowic, 1989; Harrison, 2001; Harrison and Baron-Cohen, 1997; Ramachandran and Hubbard, 2001, 2003), I maintain that the basic ontological level for synesthetic perceptions is still the phenomenal level and not the physical one, and that the previous dimensions of brightness, size, velocity, weight, and temperature are dimensions relative to the subjective continuum previously analyzed (for analysis of this type, see Cacciari, Massironi, and Corradini, 2004; Massironi, 2000).[37]

Also when Baudelaire refers metaphorically to his cat's eyes, categorizing them in terms of specific qualities, he is doing nothing other than transposing aspects of invariant structures among different conceptual domains and subjective spaces. Of metal and agate, in fact, he only transposes *one aspect* within the possible variation permitted by the type: the stone's particular nuance of blue and the metal's gloss under incident light.

The fact that in metaphor one categorizes by secondary and tertiary qualities (e.g., blue and/or variations of blue and the metallness of gloss) highlights that predication does not come about by substance or accidents. The blue of Baudelaire's cat's eyes is neither an inherent accident nor a substance, nor is it a qualia or a sense datum as in British empiricism.

Finally, if one accepts the thesis that metaphors are Gestalten, and specifically parts of processes in broad strokes (in Wertheimer's terms), a strictly metaphorical language should not have nouns, or they would be considered the product of additive scanning (Langacker, 1987) on verbs with adverbial or adjectival suffixes.

There is a paradigmatic passage in *Ficciones*, in which Borges (1962) addresses exactly this question. He recounts that the inhabitants of the imaginary town of Tlön still use a language whose predication is based on impersonal verbs qualified by monosyllabic suffixes with adverbial value. In Tlön's vocabulary, therefore, there is no substantive such as "moon" but rather adjectives such as "lunar" and/or verbs such as "to moon." Thus, where we say:

The moon rose over the river

the inhabitants of Tlön say:

Upward, beyond the onstreaming, it mooned.

In the language of Tlön, the moon, as an object of phenomenal perception, is not described in terms of substance (according to the taxonomic categorization prevalent in Indo-European languages) but in terms of *unitariness of a pattern*. The moon's phenomenal appearance is in fact described in its actual manifestation to vision as:

Round airy-light on dark

or

Pale-orange-of-the-sky.

Initial categorization, therefore, is not based on already semantically constituted objects but on aspects that, starting from the *textural continuum* of phenomenal appearance (Kanizsa, 1990) and according to the context, assume the role of information carriers.[38] Metaphorical conceptualization is still able to perform this type of original predication (i.e., the underlying adverbial predication) in a subjectless four-dimensional cognitive space:

A sepal, petal, and a thorn
Upon a common summer's morn –
A flask of Dew – A Bee or two –
A Breeze – a caper in the trees –
And *I'm* a Rose!
(Dickinson, 2004, Poem n. 19, p. 30)

In fact, in "glance on a Summer morning," there is no ontological subject, but only one occurring event, beautifully expressed by the poem. The same happens in the textural continuum of a dawning in an explosion of color:

Blazing in Gold and
Quenching in Purple!
Leaping – like Leopards – in the sky –
Then – at the feet of the old Horizon –
Laying it's spotted face – to die!

Stooping as low as the kitchen window –
Touching the Roof –
And tinting the Barn –
Kissing it's Bonnet to the Meadow –
And the Juggler of the Day – is gone.
(Dickinson, 2004, Poem n. 228, p. 238)

Fifth Step: Fusion

In recent years, the conceptualization that occurs in the metaphorical process has been analyzed by cognitive linguistics, giving rise to Conceptual Metaphor Theory (CMT) (Grady, 1997b; Lakoff, 1993; Sweetser, 1990), of which Blending Theory (BLT) (Fauconnier and Turner, 1996) is a development (Grady, Oakley, and Coulson, 1999).

CMT has stressed in particular the embodied and motivated character of metaphorical conceptualizations, and it has concentrated on the relation between two representations, considering metaphor to be a directional phenomenon from one domain (source) to another (target). It has analyzed sets of conceptual relations established over time, as in the lexicalized metaphors due to long-term memory (Johnson, 1987; Lakoff, 1987; Lakoff and Johnson, 1980).

BLT, for its part, has analyzed the relation among several representations and does not consider metaphor to be a strictly directional phenomenon. It has examined in particular new or actual relations based on short-term memory and the mental spaces involved. Fauconnier has defined a mental space as a partial and temporary mental organization constructed by the speaker: In other words, it is a short-term mental construct. In this framework, the two conceptual domains involved in CMT analysis are specified into four "blending" spaces:

1. Two input spaces relative to the source and target domains.
2. A generic space shared by both domains.
3. A blend space of interaction.

For example, in the sentence, "The committee has kept me in the dark about this matter," the spaces involved are:

1. First input space—domain of vision (person surrounded by darkness [A]).
2. Second input space—domain of intellectual activity (person to whom information is denied [A']).
3. Generic space (person without access to a specific stimulus [mapping between A and A']).
4. Blend space (a committee keeps an individual in the dark).

In metaphorical conceptualization, therefore, we have a multidirectionality due to projection into the blend space from both the base domains.

According to Fauconnier, the cognitive processes involved in blending are of three main types:

1. Projection (integration of the two initial inputs).
2. Completion (of the pattern depicted by the projection).
3. Elaboration (imagining of connected scenarios).

Blending theory stresses that emergent structures arise in the metaphorical process because at every level of projection there may arise *new contents* (i.e., new frames, features, and mental spaces), which were not implicit in the initial input spaces. Metaphors are therefore nothing other than forms of indirect reference (for comparison between CMT and BLT, see Grady, Oakley, and Coulson, 1999).

Although I generally agree with this framework—that is, (1) the nonequivalence of mental spaces and conceptual domains, (2) the idea of an emergent structure in the blending process, and (3) the fact that blending involves the dynamic evolution of a sort of online representation (all aspects that are certainly improvements on CMT)—the theory that I now put forward differs from Fauconnier's in the following respects:

1. Analysis both *categorical* and *experimental* of the types of subjective space and time involved.
2. The nature of the *primitives* of conceptualization, which are neither features nor elements derived from familiar conceptualizations, but qualities of a particular kind (patterns).
3. The process of *fusion*, which differs from both the mere association of frames and blending.
4. Analysis conducted at a level *antecedent* to the formation of what CL calls primary metaphors because it is strictly tied to ongoing subjective processes.

I already discussed points 1 and 2 in previous sections, but I point out once again that conceptualization does not come about with atomic elements.

When Celan talks of the "edge of farewell," the analogy is not an Aristotelian one of proportionality (the edge relates to an object such as detachment does to a farewell) or based on an alphabet of viewpoint invariant features. What links the edge to the farewell is its potentially hurtful *sharpness* transposed as an invariant pattern to different conceptual domains.

As to the process of fusion that occurs in the metaphorical relation, my opinion is that it is characterized by an *intrinsic quality of unity* of the components conceptualized. The process is similar to what happens in categorization of "a troop of soldiers," "a heap of apples," "an avenue of trees," "a flock of chickens," "a flight of birds," "a gaggle of geese," and so on. Their unity is given by *figural moments*.[39] These are not relations of the Russellian type (aRb) among atomic individuals. Once the partial contents of the metaphorical conceptualization have been incorporated into the anticipatory dynamics of the actual presentation, there arises a Gestalt structure consisting, as I have already specified, of a succession of simultaneous part-processes in the phenomenal present (Husserl, 1966b). In simpler words, what occurs in time is subjected to processes of fusion: The components are distinguishable only successively in virtue of abstraction.[40]

In the fusion process thus defined (i.e., as an actual occurring process), there are no phenomenal discontinuities/boundaries of *discrete elements*. For example, when seeing a forest, we have the presentation of something simple and unitary, of which only subsequently do we distinguish the individual components (trees, leaves) (Ehrenfels, 1890; Hartmann, 1935; Husserl, 1891; Stumpf, 1883–1890).

The unity of the percept "forest" is given by the apprehension form (*Auffassungsform*) of its contents and their bilateral belongingness. Think of the following examples:

Mess. As I did stand my watch upon the hill,
I look'd towards Birnam, and anon, methought,
The wood began to move

. . .

Within this three mile you see it coming;
I say, a moving grove.

(Shakespeare, 1962, *Macbeth*, p. 161)

Or

In the wood
One with the other
The poplars dance.
And the arbolè
With its four little leaves
Dances as well.

(Garcia Lorca, 1996, *To Irene Garcia*) [My translation]

In contrast, what occurs in Fauconnier's blend space is mainly an arrangement of components that *maintain their identities* in the space of the source and target domains.

Another important aspect highlighted by the fusion process is the final *undistributed content* of the entire metaphor, which constitutes its *tenor*. In fact, the whole generated by the metaphorical conceptualization is constructed in the simultaneous succession and fusion of the nonindependent parts that *found* a higher order object as defined theoretically and experimentally by Meinong (1899; see also Albertazzi, 1996).[41]

According to Meinong, higher order *objects* (e.g., a melody in the acoustic field) may only be presented by means of a series of partial *contents*, whereas the *inferiora* as *temporally distinct* must be given in the *simultaneous presentation*, although of course not as simultaneous. Consider, for example, the presentation of a *comparison* between two tones or two colors: To present these to myself, I must present them one after the other, although they exist in simultaneity. This is not to imply, however, that I must represent them to myself as *successive*. Therefore, although the time of the *inferiora* is the same, the time of their presentation, which is initially different, is not. Meinong's thesis can therefore be stated as follows: In the time in which a *superius* (i.e., a higher order object) is presented, all the *inferiora* must be presented simultaneously.

In summary, higher order objects (a melody in the acoustic field, a shape in the visual field, and a creative metaphor) are objects obtained from contents that are fused by way of inner relations. In the case of poetry, for example, in:[42]

Often have I met the ill of living:
it was the choked stream that gurgled,
it was the parched leaf's curling
tight, it was the horse that slumped to the ground.
No good did I know then beyond the portent
that reveals divine indifference:
it was the statue in the drowsiness
of noonday, and the cloud, and the falcon soaring high.
(Montale, 1990, *Often Have I Met the Ill of Living*, p. 35) [My translation]

the higher order whole ("the ill of living") is not conceptualized by summing individual occurrences. Rather, it is a higher order conceptual whole transversally founded and shared by those occurrences. The individual elements are factually an abstraction successively performed: specifically, as such, they are *thought*.

After reading the poem, we may not remember the individual instances in which the poet has conceptualized the ill of living, but we maintain its unitary tenor produced by the internal relations among the various partial contents modified by the specific way in which the creative act is performed—or in other words, by the way in which the metaphor has been conceived and the way in which the various partial references of content in the duration have been structured.

Applied Schema

On the basis of the foregoing discussion, how can we analyze the type of information expressed and communicated by a poem? Let us consider a complex composition such as Dickinson (2004, Poem n. 258, p. 271).

There's a certain Slant of Light,
Winter Afternoons –
That oppresses, like the Heft
Of Cathedral Tunes –

Heavenly Hurt, it gives us –
We can find no scar,
But internal difference,
Where the Meanings are –

None may teach it – Any –
'Tis the Seal Despair –
An imperial affliction
Sent us of the Air –

When it comes, the Landscape listens –
Shadows – hold their breath –
When it goes, 'tis like the Distance
On the look of Death.

From the point of view of metaphorical information, we must ask:

1. What are the *primitive components* of the metaphorical construct?
2. What are the *invariants transposed* in the various conceptual domains?
3. In what does the metaphorical *polysemy* consist?
4. How is the *fusion* process achieved?
5. What forms of *subjective completion* are performed?
6. What is the *higher order scheme* of the poem as a whole?

With regard to the primitive components, or the patterns of the conceptualization, some relate to PP (light, tune, cathedral, shape, scar), others to MP (difference, meaning). The perceptual aspects concern sensory modalities in visual perception (a slant of light), acoustic perception (a heft of cathedral tunes), and emotional states (oppression).

There are also *invariants* that connect perceptual elements (light, tunes) and mental/cognitive components (heavenly hurt/scar, internal difference/meaning) and more complex superimpositions in the textural continuum such as that between "landscape listens" and "distance/look of death." At first sight, moreover, some components relate to intermodal and synesthetic perceptions (landscape listens). It is no coincidence, in fact, that poetry has these roots, as the mentioned works of Cytowic (1989), and Marks (1978, 1982, 1996) showed.

The problem is therefore that of explaining how the state of affairs expressed by the metaphor is realized by *the superimposition and fusion of perceptual continua of different kinds* (visual [light], acoustic [tunes], emotional [hurt, oppression, scar]), which find perfect matching in the felicitous outcome of the poem's figurality. What kind of relation arises between the original patterns and the various metaphorical *partial contents* (slant of light, landscape listens, heavenly hurt, etc.) in the poem's cognitive unfolding? What is the relation between the final object (i.e., the tenor of the poem) and the partial contents fused into a unitary whole?

To answer these questions, I analyze the following aspects (one for each strophe, although many of them are obviously present in all the strophes):

1. The *type of conceptualization* of the contents, which comes about "in broad strokes."
2. The *role of the bridging members* (i.e., of what I have called figural moments).
3. The nature of the *inner relations* among the nonindependent contents of the whole.
4. The *diversified use of tropes* (simile vs. metaphor).

Strophe I: *Broad strokes*

There's a certain *Slant of Light*,
Winter Afternoons –
That *oppresses*, like the *Heft*
Of *Cathedral Tunes* –

Interpretation of the "slant of light" on the basis of the theory of incident physical light would run as follows: The sun's rays are always "downward," perpendicular when the sun is on the horizon. It is obvious that the ontological level of reference of the metaphor cannot be this one.

The strophe in question evinces the type of categorization that takes place "in broad strokes in a nested whole's hierarchy." "Slant of light," in fact, fuses together the semantic field of "slant," the type's possible extensions that extend from perceptual aspects to cognitive ones ("slant," in fact, implies slope, inclination, perspective, distortion, deformation, glance, point of view, standpoint, attitude, bias, mood), and the phenomenal aspect of light.

The "slant of light," in this case, is not the reflectance of the surface in the physical sense but a specific inclination of the perceived brightness intrinsically related to the patterns of coldness, greyness, and lividness that connote a winter afternoon in the northern hemisphere.

As to "heft," the term has been chosen not with reference to weight in the physical sense, but to perceived heaviness and gravity also with expressive value. The "Cathedral Tune" refers to and expresses the motif, chord, and relative mood internally related to a specific type of architecture (inner volume) and a type of music (organ). The pattern "Oppression," as the expressive quality, functions as a bridging member for the several inner relations, giving the undistributed tenor to the strophe. The strophe thus has all the characteristics of a simple whole of figural qualities constituted by partial contents (secondary and tertiary qualities) in broad strokes plus internal relations.

Perceptual completion is based on the intermodal perception of similarity among strokes (perceived light, music tone, coldness), whereas *mental completion* is instead produced by the reference to a particular cast/color of winter light (in certain geographic areas), which is eidetically *similar* and *transposable* to certain tones to be heard in cathedrals (of Western cultures).

The meaning of the strophe is conveyed in different *grades of givenness* (with strong or weak evidence) and with different types and degrees of completion. In other words, the structure of the inner referents among the various content parts is held together by a constant movement and fusion of subjective perceptual and mental completions. Still remaining is the structural incompleteness of metaphorical objects, which, according to Ingarden, is a property of all intentional objects well exemplified by the fact that a greater or weaker understanding of the strophe is obtained by having or not having the experience of what a cathedral is in Western civilization.

Strophe II: *Bridging members*

Heavenly Hurt, it gives us –
We can find no *scar*,
But *internal difference*,
Where the *Meanings* are –

I examine this strophe with particular reference to the type of categorization that occurs. In this strophe, too, there are interconnected patterns of different kinds such as *Hurt*, *Scar*, and *Meaning*, which refer to specific semantic fields. *Hurt*, for example, extends to include, pain, wound, injury, damage, harm, bad effect, offense, and scourge, and in this occurrence it is mentally completed by *Heavenly*. Scar extends from weal to offense. *Difference* extends through aspects such as separateness, otherness, unusualness, discontinuity, dissimilarity, diversity, distinction, and disagreement. The Where, as the location of meanings, can only be a specific position within the space of conceptualization, and therefore in a subjective continuum that extends from separateness in space and time to empty spaces, coldness, and unfriendliness. The role of bridging member among the internal relations of the strophe is performed by *Internal difference*.

Strophe III: *Inner relations*

None may teach it – Any –
'Tis the *Seal Despair* –
An *imperial Affliction*
Sent us of the Air –

I examine this strophe from the point of inner references, in which there appear certain individual metaphors that refer to others in the various linked strophes. There are *inner references* between seal (hurt) and an entire correlated semantic field (signet, stamp, pledge, confirmation), between despair (oppression/affliction) and another semantic field (anguish, depression, sorrow, dejection), and between imperial (seal/cathedral) and supreme (majestic, sovereign, august). Affliction (and oppression as well) in the poem is "imperial" because it is internally related to components within the correlated semantic fields, for example, to "signet," "majestic," and so on.

Patterns function here as bridging members.

Strophe IV: *Metaphor vs. simile*

When it comes, the *Landscape listens*
Shadows – hold their breath –
When it goes, 'tis <u>like</u> the *Distance*
On the *look of Death*.

Also this strophe comprises the already mentioned components of semantic fields ("distance" extends from extent of space, remoteness, stretch, whereas "look" extends across glaze, gaze, appearance, face, aspect). There is also the choice of an intermodal and synesthetic perception transposed in metaphorical domains (landscape listens/ shadows hold their breath). However, the aspect of this strophe that I wish to stress is the choice of a simile instead of a metaphor ("tis like the Distance"). Why does Dickinson, who has produced a series of such striking interrelated metaphors, in the end resort to the use of a simile? I believe that the poem's complexity and the strophe's inner references prevented the metaphorical construction at the level of mental completion once levels of abstraction like the spatial extendedness of Seal Despair on the Look of Death. I do not know whether Dickinson could have succeeded, but this impossibility of fusing partial contents manifests a limit to the conceptualization. In this finale, the strophe's contents therefore achieve the blending state, maintaining their partial identity.

As to the figural moments that function as bridging members, "come" and "go" unite the aspects of perceptual presence and mental absence of the various components involved in the metaphorical construction.

Overall, Dickinson 258 can be regarded in every effect as a higher order intentional object produced by the superimposition of multiple and multifarious perceptual and mental continua. Dickinson conceptualized the meaning that she wanted to express through invariants taken from visual (light), acoustic (tunes), and emotional (scar) perception, transposing them to the mental level in related and culturally connoted contexts (Cathedral, Seal, Imperial). This gave rise to a gestaltic and hierarchical whole of *undistributed content*. If I had to describe the tenor and pervasive content of the poem, I would indicate it with a title that the composition lacks and that seemingly constitutes the entire semantic field of the poem: *obliqueness*. The pattern that gives continuity to the entire deployment of the poem is the "Slant of Light," with which the poem opens. This is the psychic overtone that sets the tenor of the subsequent process as a whole, the fringe of relations that maintains the unity, continuity, and homogeneity of the text because the individual strophes are assimilated into a sort of good continuation and common destiny. As James (1890) remarked:

Fringes are part of the object cognized—substantive qualities and things appear to the mind in a fringe of relations. Some parts of our stream of thought cognize the relations rather than the things; but both the transitive and the substantive parts form one continuous stream, with no discrete sensations in it. (p. 258)

The space of metaphorical conceptualization is therefore produced by constant transformation among qualitatively diverse perspectives on the same object and among diverse objects according to "family resemblances." It is this that enables us to pass, for example, from the animal species to the human species through the construction of imaginary animals or hybrids such as the satyr or the Minotaur, or numerous other fantastic constructions (on homology fields, see Koenderink, 2002).

Hybrids

Those who set out to analyze metaphorical complexity can only offer preliminary conclusions. Before I do so, however, I briefly summarize the various steps in my attempt to shed light on the conceptual aspects of metaphorical construction.

I have analyzed metaphor from a Gestalt point of view, considering the inner hierarchy of the whole. I have argued as follows. The components of a metaphor are not separable items but nonindependent parts of a process, which essentially are not substantival but adverbial entities. In the actual occurrence of metaphorical creation, these components are "occluded," deformed, and fused because of their mutual internal relatedness. It is consequently possible to identify various types of boundaries, upper and lower (again, in Wertheimer'sense), in the construction of the conceptual metaphorical whole, and in the superimposition of different types of continuum. Finally, the figural qualities act as bridging members among the various components of the whole. In other words, I have sought to show *from within* how the fusion process comes about. Obviously, the better the fusion, the better the poem.

All in all, if I were to venture a definition of creative metaphor, I would prefer to talk of it in terms of *amodal presentation*, in the sense that given in conceptualization are wholes that are entirely nonexistent from the point of view of taxonomic, "objective" classification.

As is well known, amodal completion takes place in zones of the field that shape the covering surface, and the visible part of the occluded surface must be able to continue its self-completion in a particular way. Another interesting case of amodal perception is phenomenal distortion in positive dislocation (enlargement) or negative dislocation (restriction) of the regions involved, as in the cases exemplified by Kanizsa (1991). A third interesting case is the amodal completion of color in surfaces such as flowers and fruit (Pinna, 2008).

On the basis of the similarities already emphasized between the metaphor's perceptual and conceptual spaces—considering, for example, the conceptual space of "Sun" and the conceptual space of "Juliet"—a juxtaposition of the two regions as such would never give rise to fusion between the two entities, which would remain entirely distinct from each other, although internally coherent. A juxtaposition, in fact, would produce a simile such as "Juliet is like the Sun." However, if some "aspects" of the two regions are superimposed so that particular common boundaries are created, then one of the most interesting products of amodal completion ensues: the *hybrid* (Kanizsa, 1991). Therefore, the pregnancy of a poetic composition follows the laws of amodality (on amodality as a new gestalt principle, see Pinna, 2005b). Individual strophes, in fact, are nothing but nonindependent parts of the poem; as they unfold, they simultaneously restructure the whole by successively entering the focus of the entire process so that, through a series of partial occlusions, it is also "masked" in the final product. *The resulting content of the poem is nothing else but an amodal completion of the whole.*

The problem is showing in what parts of the conceptual regions in continuous unfolding the superimposition takes place, how the occluded parts can continue to complete themselves beneath the others, and what constitutes the inner structure of the boundaries. It is not possible to solve this problem or to develop an *experimental design* of the perceptual roots of metaphor until a theory of subjective space and time, and of the various forms of phenomenal and conceptual filling, has been produced. In other words, creative metaphor is a challenge for the theory of perception. Here I have at least posed the question and taken some first steps in this direction of research.

Notes

1. *Balaustrata di brezza/Per appoggiare stasera/La mia malinconia.*

2. In classical terms, this is a reproposal of Thomas' *verbus mentis sive interius*.

3. Consider, for example, the following: the figure-ground scheme, which segments the perceptive scene and likewise its conceptual representation; the force dynamics scheme, which conceptualizes and expresses the forces and vectors present in the conceptual field, even the invisible ones (Arnheim, 1954; Lewin, 1926), and then transposes to the level of mental abstraction (Talmy, 1988b); or the windowing of attention scheme, which progressively brings the various reference objects into focus (Albertazzi, 2002c; Rensink, 2000, 2002; Talmy, 2006). These are nonphysical but "intentional" spaces (Koenderink and van Doorn, 2003), in which the structures of subjective completion perform a crucial role and share certain principles of Gestalt organization.

4. The fundamental principle regulating the perceptive organization, therefore, lies less in the laws of grouping and more in the *mereological structure*, which regulates the unitariness of the psychic phenomenon at the primary and secondary levels (Brentano, 1995b; see also Albertazzi, 2006d).

5. Wertheimer, in fact, distinguishes in Gestalten between an "upper boundary, which concerns the complete internal organization of the entire given," and therefore the structures of the process once it has come to completion; and a "lower boundary, given by the additive adjacency between two or more relatively independent wholes," which concerns the structures present in intermediate phases and/or in the wholes' hierarchy.

6. In certain respects, the phenomenal presence of any item in the visual field, even a simple line, generates an *activation zone*, as well illustrated by analysis of vectors (Klee, 1961). From this point of view, the squares, rectangles, and circles that we see are in effect produced by forces of translation, rotation, and confinement, which operate in opposite directions. Also the areas "left empty" by the activation of vectors have a particular role: that of generating anomalous surfaces (Leyton, 1992; Pinna and Sambin, 1991; Sambin, 1980).

7. In fact, the German word *Auffälligkeit*, relief, has the two senses of quality and prominence.

8. The Meinongians acutely distinguished between these two senses (*Differenz* vs. *Verschiedenheit*) as pertaining to two different levels of reality (Meinong, 1960).

9. *Usciamo. Non coprirti il capo. E' un lento/sol di settembre.*

10. *Da quella stella all'altra/si carcera la notte/in turbolenta vuota dismisura/da quella solitudine di stella/a quella solitudine di stella.*

11. *Si devono aprire le stelle/nel cielo sì tenero e vivo.*

12. This occurs because of the definition of figure-ground by Rubin (Albertazzi, 2006b; Kennedy, 1974; Rubin, 1958), the continuous shifts of attention (Rensink, 2000), the different gradients of externality and internality of visual surfaces as evidenced by Necker's cube (Kopfermann, 1930), and the role and so-called "power" of the center, whereby activated in a visual configuration are compositional relations among different centers of attraction, which regulate its stability or instability (Arnheim, 1988).

13. When Riley, for example, depicted movement or stillness, he expressed a phenomenal extendedness of forces, velocities, and boundaries, in which there is no exercise and transmission of force as in classical physics, just as there is no transmission and exercise of force in the perception of causality (Michotte, 1963).

14. To give a banal example, the lengthiness or brevity of an hour spent in boredom or a state of emotional agitation or happy creativity can certainly be correlated with the activity of certain cerebral zones, and therefore analyzed in terms of temporal intervals characterized by the *correlated* oscillation of neurons. But this does not explain the eminently *qualitative* character of the subjective experience of the person in question or the forms of anticipatory experience that allow the conception of a poem, or a melodic composition, before its individual components have been realized.

15. For example, Stroud's (1955) hypothesis of a "perceptual moment," not punctiform but invariably lasting 100 msec and univocally correlated with the instant of metric time, does not apply to subjective time, which is a constitutive part of the (perceptive and mental) phenomena of consciousness. To exist, these phenomena require different durations calibrated on their specificity: for example, the temporal durations necessary for the perception of movement, perceptive or intentional, prototypical or otherwise (launching or driving, attraction, or stroboscopic movement), vary according to the phenomenon observed (see Albertazzi, 2010, and forthcoming; Kanizsa and Vicario, 1968; Michotte, 1963). The semantic of natural language, then, is clearly founded on these kinetic structures, for example, in cases of prototypical verbs of causation (Albertazzi 2002c). In other words, the units of subjective time have an *elasticity* that is structured simultaneously with the content that fills it (Stern, 1897).

16. Specifically, dislocations are only possible within a specific extension of time (i.e., within the phenomenal present and when there is not homogeneity among the stimuli) (Fraisse, 1963, 1964, 1974). Particularly striking is the phenomenon of the *acoustic tunnel* analyzed by Vicario, which occurs when there is the *amodal* continuation of a sound beneath a noise that seems to cover a stretch of it (Vicario, 1973; see also Benussi, 1913; Fraisse, 1984).

17. *Silvia, rimembri ancora/Il tempo della tua vita mortale/Quando beltà splendea/Negli occhi tuoi ridenti e fuggitivi/E tu, lieta e pensosa, il limitare/Di gioventù salivi?*

18. Like the "double trill": Given a sequence of cyclically repeated pure sounds (low sound, high sound, low sound, high sound), slightly different from each other, and at high speed (ca 50 msec per element), one perceives two sequences, a high trill and a low trill (Bozzi and Vicario, 1960; Bregman and Campbell, 1971). The phenomenon has been confirmed by analysis of the visual perception of movement (Vicario, 1965).

19. *Col mare/mi sono fatto/una bara/di freschezza.*

20. Eventually, it is the space of inner psychophysics, what Fechner was unable to perform but in what can be defined as his "exoteric" writings (see e.g., Fechner, 1848, 1851).

21. This field of qualities is not easy to classify because it comprises qualities "given" in the duration as the elaborations of stimuli but that are simultaneously, at least in part, "constructed" because they are "modified" first by neuronal processing and then by the subjective and qualitative structure of the duration (Husserl, 1966b).

22. These qualities have been relatively little studied. Indeed, there is no theory on them (attempts in this direction have been made by Albertazzi, 1998a, 2006b, forthcoming; Eco, 1999; Köhler, 1933; Lipps, 1897; Metzger, 1941).

23. In *Theory of the Categories*, Brentano (1981) said that both the whole and its parts and relations exist in a presentation.

24. *Mi levigo/come un marmo/di passione.*

25. The importance of this type of quality for the processing of experience should not be underestimated. Expression, as the affective content of the object (Michotte, 1963), has been defined by Koffka (1935) as the primary, ultimate, psychophysical phenomenon, a pure Gestalt moment. They express the relation between perceived expressive qualities and the *subject's way of being* and, specifically, *its effect*. In fact, they can be defined as data of the coordinative field (Lewin, 1926).

26. For example, in Goethe's (1978) theory of science, among a sepal, a petal, and a thorn, there is *continuity of form*, but not of material substance. Moreover, as we see with regard to the original structure of the categorization of the objects of existence, the dynamics of their appearing may comprise further kinds of complexity.

27. These similarities, however, may come about in various ways on local or global bases, or even by opposition. For example, the *similarity* of sounds can be given either as notes as opposed to noises or in their *phenomenal salience* (e.g., sounds or colors of greater intensity as opposed to sounds or colors of lesser intensity, etc.) (Husserl, 1939).

28. *Dal muro alto sporgono/alberi spogli/forche, braccia, grucce.*

29. *Di uccelli presi dal roccolo/Quasi note su un pentagramma/Ne ho tracciati non pochi col carboncino.*

30. *Si sta come d'autunno/sugli alberi/le foglie.*

31. *Et lasse-moi plonger dans tes beaux yeux/Mêlés de métal and d'agate.*

32. At present, experimental interest exists in this quality of "gloss" identified as a specific phenomenal quality (Mausfeld and Wendt, 2006).

33. The aspect to be borne in mind, however, is that this statement is only veracious if one assumes that the ontological level of reference for metaphorical conceptualization is the phenomenal level, whose objects are given in terms of secondary and tertiary qualities in "broad strokes." Hence, in the specific case of Baudelaire, the eyes of his cat are given in terms of phenomenal patterns of "metal-ness" and "agate-ness."

34. These considerations have prompted Violi to introduce the notion of *typicity*, which from the perceptual point of view is better suited to the perception of objects in the duration, and which in semantic representation more precisely denotes the aspect of meaning *regularity*.

35. *Caro piccolo insetto/che chiamavano mosca/non so perché.*

36. Always bearing in mind, as I have already pointed out, that there may be similarities by likeness, difference, opposition, or analogy, and that similarity may be both global and local (i.e., with regard to specific components).

37. With regard to the second point (variation internally to the pattern), I draw on Husserl's concept of eidetic variation. This cognitive operation consists of what Husserl called knowledge by "essence," which, put more simply, is nothing other than knowledge by structures. These structures, however, are *types* or *forms* applied to *diverse domains of conceptualization* and by means of *transposed invariants*. For example, we can maintain a particular shape but vary it in red, yellow, blue, and so on. In this case, therefore, color is an invariant across the color–space continuum (Husserl, 1913). This type of cognitive operation seems to have many aspects in common with prototypical and radial categorizations, but once again certain specific characteristics distinguish it from them. In particular, the structures transposed are *types* or *forms*, not yet base categories, conceptual categories, or lexical semantic categories. The categorization is *processual*, and it extends *within the possible variations* permitted by the type.

It is this type of categorization, which acts according to typicity and variation of the type, that enables description of the beloved in these terms used by Wordsworth in the mentioned poem, *A Phantom of Delight* (see *supra*).

38. The question is not new or the fruit of only poetic imagination: It has been debated in linguistics (Miklosich) and philosophy (see Brentano, 1966; Marty, 1908; Mauthner, 1901–1902) under the headings of "subject-less propositions" or "adverbial predication." According to some authors, this type of predication—which is present in Indo-European languages in certain grammatical forms such as "it's raining" or "it's thundering"—is the origin of all forms of predication because it is connected with the structuring of experience in the actual duration and therefore operates at an *ante-predicative level* (see Pinna and Albertazzi, chapter 10, this volume). From the Stoics to Brentano, it was stressed that it is impossible to distinguish in the actual act of perception between a subject and an object because it is *a single event* in which a correlate is structured, which can only have the characteristics of a nonindependent part of the process. Subject and object in the cognitive and predicative sense are, in fact, belated constructs of the categorical processing of experience.

39. Figural moments in their turn are given by (1) *partial contents* of presentation (e.g., the tonal intervals among the notes of a melody), and (2) *inner relations* (e.g., the relations holding in Ebbinghaus illusion, which are totally inexistent from a physical point of view). These mo-

ments ground similarities among the parts and function as bridging members (Ehrenfels, 1890; Husserl, 1891; Meinong, 1891; Stählin, 1913).

40. Husserl provides the following example of this type of relation. In a series of aligned equilateral triangles of different colors, the internal relations consist of a triangular shape, while in a series of aligned polygons of red color, the internal relations are established by color. Other examples are given by every rotation of a spatial figure in the visual field, by a shape with every change in size, by the merging of colors in various degrees, and again by stroboscopic movement and by the melody in the acoustic field.

41. Among the various objects of presenting and judging, Meinong emphasized the *higher order objects* (i.e., that particular class of objects founded on other objects in such a way that the latter constitute their *inferior*). The superiora are thus endowed with an *intrinsic nonindependence*, which depends on their being built on other objects as their indispensable foundation. Every *relational presentation*, Meinong states, must indicate one such class of higher order objects, yet not every higher order object is limitable to relations.

42. *Spesso il mal di vivere ho incontrato:/era il rivo strozzato che gorgoglia/era l'incartocciarsi della foglia/riarsa, era il cavallo stramazzato./Bene non seppi, fuori del prodigio/che schiude la divina indifferenza:/era la statua nella sonnolenza/del meriggio, e la nuvola, e il falco alto levato.*

References

Albertazzi, L. 1996. "Comet Tails, Fleeting Objects and Temporal Inversions." *Axiomathes* 1–2: 111–137.

Albertazzi, L. 1998a. "The Aesthetics of Particulars." *Axiomathes* 9: 169–196.

Albertazzi, L. 1998b. "Form Metaphysics." In *Shapes of Forms: From Gestalt Psychology to Phenomenology to Ontology and Mathematics*, edited by L. Albertazzi. Dordrecht: Kluwer. 261–310.

Albertazzi, L. 2002a. "Continua." In *Unfolding Perceptual Continua*, edited by L. Albertazzi. Amsterdam: Benjamins Publishing Company. 1–28.

Albertazzi, L. 2002b. "Towards a Neo-Aristotelian Theory of Continua: Elements of an Empirical Geometry." In *Unfolding Perceptual Continua*, edited by L. Albertazzi. Amsterdam: Benjamins Publishing Company. 29–79.

Albertazzi, L. 2002c. "Causatives and Kinetic Structures." *Axiomathes* 1: 1–37.

Albertazzi, L. 2002d. "Natural Semiosis." *Versus* 93: 113–133.

Albertazzi, L. 2003. "From Kanizsa Back to Benussi: Varieties of Intentional Reference." *Axiomathes* 13: 239–259.

Albertazzi, L. 2004. "Stereokinetic Shapes and Their Shadows." *Perception* 33: 1437–1452.

Albertazzi, L. 2006a. "Introduction to Visual Spaces." In *Visual Thought. The Depictive Space of Perception*, edited by L. Albertazzi. Amsterdam: Benjamins Publishing Company. 3–34.

Albertazzi, L. 2006b. "Visual Qualities. Drawing on Canvas." In *Visual Thought: The Depictive Space of Perception*, edited by L. Albertazzi. Amsterdam: Benjamins Publishing Company. 165–194.

Albertazzi, L. 2006c. "Das rein Figurale" (The Pure Figuration). *Gestalt Theory* 28 (1/2): 23–151.

Albertazzi, Liliana. 2006d. *Immanent Realism: Introduction to Franz Brentano*. Berlin, New York: Springer.

Albertazzi, L. 2007a. "Intentional Presentations: At the Roots of Consciousness." *Journal of Consciousness Studies* 14 (1–2): 94–114. [Special Issue]

Albertazzi, L. 2007b. "Matrix: Schematic Universals." In *Cognitive Aspects of Bilingualism*, edited by I. Kecskes and L. Albertazzi. Berlin-New York: Springer. 63–97.

Albertazzi, L. 2008. "Tropi di luce e colore" (Tropes of Light and Colors). *Paradigmi* XXVII (1): 119–136.

Albertazzi, L. 2010. "The Subjective Origin of Causality." In *Causality and Motivation*, edited by R. Poli. Frankfurt: Ontos Verlag. 75–103.

Albertazzi, L. Forthcoming. "The Ontology of Perception." In *TAO-Theory and Applications of Ontology*. Vol. 1. *Philosophical Perspectives*, edited by R. Poli and J. Seibt. Berlin-New York: Springer.

Allesch, Ch. von. 1931. *Zur nichteuklidischen Struktur des phänomenales Raum* (On the non Euclidean Structure of Phenomenal Space). Jena: Fischer.

Arnheim, R. 1954. *Art and Visual Perception*. Berkeley: Regents of the University of California.

Arnheim, R. 1966. *Towards a Psychology of Art*. Berkeley: The Regents of the University of California.

Arnheim, Rudolf. 1969. *Visual Thinking*. Berkeley: The Regents of the University of California.

Arhneim, R. 1988. *The Power of the Center*. Berkeley: University of California Press.

Ash, S. E. 1961. "The Metaphor: A Psychological Inquiry." In *Documents of Gestalt Psychology*, edited by M. Henle. Berkeley and Los Angeles: University of California Press. 324–333.

Baudelaire, Ch. 1996. *Les Fleurs du Mal* (Flowers of Evil). Paris: Gallimard.

Benussi, V. 1913. *Psychologie der Zeitauffassung* (Psychology of Time Apprehension). Leipzig: Hölder.

Bixby, F. L. 1928. "A Phenomenological Study of Lustre." *Journal of General Psychology* 1: 136–174.

Blyth, R. H. ed. 1952. *Haiku*, 4 vols, Hokuseido.

Borges, J. L. 1962. *Ficciones*, translated by A. Kerrigan, A. Bonner, A. Reid, H. Temple, and R. Todd. New York: Grove Press (Original work published 1944).

Bozzi, P., and Vicario, G. B. 1960. "Due fattori di unificazione fra note musicali: la vicinanza temporale e la vicinanza tonale" (Two Factors Unifying Musical Notes: Temporal Proximity and Tonal Proximity). *Rivista di Psicologia* 54: 235–258.

Bregman, A. S., and Campbell, J. 1971. "Primary Auditory Stream Segregation and the Perception of Order in Rapid Sequences of Tones." *Journal of Experimental Psychology* 89: 244–249.

Brentano, F. 1966. *The True and the Evident*, translated by R. M. Chisholm and E. Politzer. London: Routledge & Kegan Paul. (1st German ed. 1930, edited by O. Kraus. Leipzig: Meiner.)

Brentano, F. 1981. *The Theory of Categories*, edited by R. M. Chisholm and N. Guterman. Den Haag: Nijhoff. (1st German ed. 1933, edited by A. Kastil. Leipzig: Meiner.)

Brentano, F. 1988. *Philosophical Lectures on Space, Time and the Continuum*, edited by S. Körner and R. M. Chisholm. London: Croom Helm.

Brentano, F. 1995a. *Psychology From an Empirical Standpoint*, edited by L. McAlister et al. London: Routledge. (1st German ed. 1874. Leipzig: Duncker & Humblot.)

Brentano, F. 1995b. *Descriptive Psychology*, edited by B. Müller. London: Routledge. (1st German ed. 1982, edited by R. M. Chisholm and W. Baumgartner. Hamburg: Meiner.)

Breton, A. 1992. "L'union libre" (Freedom of Love). In *Oeuvres completes*. Paris: Gallimard. 85–86.

Brown, J. W. 1991. *Self and Process*. New York: Springer.

Brown, J. F. 1931. "The Visual Perception of Velocity." *Psychologische Forschung* 14: 199–232.

Bühler, K. 1934. *Sprachtheorie. Die Darstellungsfunktion der Sprache* (Theory of Language: The Representational Function of Language). Jena: Fischer. Repr. 1965, Stuttgart: Fischer.

Cacciari, C. 1998. "Why Do We Speak Metaphorically? Reflections on the Functions of Metaphor in Discourse and Reasoning." In *Figurative Language and Thought*, edited by A. N. Katz, C. Cacciari, R. W. Gibbs, Jr., and M. Turner. Oxford: Oxford University Press. 119–157.

Cacciari, C., Massironi, M., and Corradini, P. 2004. "When Color Names Are Used Metaphorically: The Role of Linguistic and Chromatic Information." *Metaphor and Symbol* 19 (3): 169–190.

Crick, F. H. 1994. *The Astonishing Hypothesis: The Scientific Research for the Soul*. New York: Scribner.

Crick, F. H., and Koch, Ch. 1990. "Some Reflections on Visual Awareness." *Cold Spring Harb Symp Quant Biol* 55: 953–962.

Crick, F. H., and Koch, Ch. 1998. "Consciousness and Neuroscience." *Cerebral Cortex* 8: 97–107.

Cytowic, R. E. 1989. *A Union of the Senses*. New York: Springer.

D'Andrade, R. G., and Egan, M. 1974. "The Color of Emotions." *American Ethnologist* 1 (1): 49–63.

D'Annunzio, G. 1982. "Consolazione" (Consolation), Heavenly Poem. In *Verses of Love and Glory*. Milan: Mondatori editore. 668–670.

Day, S. O. 1996. "Synaesthesia and Synaesthetic Metaphor." *Psyche* 2 (32).

De Pisis, F. 1961. "Bare Trees." In *Poesia italiana contemporanea*, edited by G. Spagnoletti. Bologna: Guanda. 507–508.

Dickinson, E. 2004. *Tutte le poesie* (*Omnibus of Poems*). Milan: Arnoldo Mondadori editore.

Dixon, R. M. 1982. *Where Have All the Adjectives Gone?* Berlin: De Gruyter.

Donne, J. 1992. *John Donne. A Critical Edition of the Major Works*. Oxford: Oxford University Press.

Eco, U. 1999. *Kant and the Platypus: Essays on Language and Cognition*. London: Secker & Warburg.

Eco, U. 1995. *The Island of the Day Before*. English translation by W. Weaver. New York: Harcourt Brace.

Ehrenfels, Ch. von. 1890. "Über Gestaltqualitäten" (On Gestalt Qualities). *Vierteljahrschrift für wissenschaftliche Philosophie* 14: 242–292.

Ehrenfels, Ch. von. 1897. "Rezension. Höfler, A., Psychologie, Wien: Tempsky 1897." *Vierteljahrschrift für wissenschaftliche Philosophie* 21: 509–519.

Evans, V. 2005. *The Structure of Time. Language, Meaning, and Temporal Cognition*. Amsterdam: Benjamins Publishing Company.

Fauconnier, G., and Turner, M. 1996. "Blending as a Central Process of Grammar." In *Conceptual Structure, Discourse and Language*, edited by A. Goldberg. Stanford, CA: Center for the Study of Language and Information. 113–130.

Fechner, Th. 1848. *Nanna oder über das Seelenleben der Pflanzen* (Nanna or the Psychic Life of Plants). Leipzig: Voss.

Fechner, Th. 1851. *Zend-Avesta oder über die Dinge des Himmels und des Jenseit: Vom Standpunkt der Naturbetrachtung* (Zend-Avesta or On Celestial Matters and the Hereafter: From the Standpoint of the Observation of Nature). 3 vols. Leipzig: Voss.

Fillmore, Ch. J. 1982. "Frame Semantics: Linguistics in the Morning Calm." In *The Linguistic Society of Corea*. Seoul: Hanshin. 111–137.

Flaherty, M. 1999. *The Watched Pot: How We Experience Time*. New York: New York University Press.

Fraisse, P. 1963. *The Logic of Time*. Methuen: London.

Fraisse, P. 1964. *The Psychology of Time*. London: Eyre and Spottiswood.

Fraisse, P. 1974. *Psychologie du rythme* (Psychology of Rhythm). Paris: PUF.

Fraisse, P. 1984. "Perception and Estimation of Time." *Annual Review of Psychology* 35: 1–36.

Gallese, V. 2005. "Embodied Simulation: From Neurons to Phenomenal Experience." *Phenomenology and the Cognitive Sciences* 4: 23–48.

Gallese, V., and Lakoff, G. 2005. "The Brain's Concepts: The Role of the Sensory-Motor System in Reason and Language." *Cognitive Neuropsychology* 22: 455–474.

Garcia Lorca, F. 1996. "A Irene García, criada." In *Poesía*, edición de Miguel García-Posada, Barcelona, Galaxia Gutenberg, Círculo de lectores. 379–380 (*Obras completas*, 1) (Complete Works, 1).

Geeraerts, D. 1989. "Prospects and Problems of Prototype Theory." *Linguistics* 27: 587–612.

Gibbs, R. W. 1994. *The Poetics of Language: Figurative Thought, Language and Understanding*. Cambridge: Cambridge University Press.

Gibson, J. J. 1979. *The Ecological Approach to Visual Perception*. Boston: Houghton Mifflin.

Goethe, J. W. von. 1978. *The Metamorphosis of Plants*. Wyoming: Biodynamic Literature.

Grady, J. 1997a. "Theories Are Buildings Revisited." *Cognitive Linguistics* 8: 267–290.

Grady, J. 1997b. *Foundations of Meaning: Primary Metaphors and Primary Scenes*. Dissertation. Berkeley: University of California Press.

Grady, J., Oakley, T., and Coulson, S. 1999. "Blending and Metaphor." In *Metaphors in Cognitive Linguistics*, edited by G. J. Steen and R. Gibbs. Philadelphia: Benjamins Publishing Company.

Harrison, J. E. 2001. *Synaesthesia: The Strangest Thing*. Oxford: Oxford University Press.

Harrison, J. E., and Baron-Cohen, S. 1997. *Synaesthesia: Classic and Contemporary Readings*. Oxford: Blackwell.

Hartmann, N. 1935. *Grundlegung der Ontologie* (Foundation of Ontology). Berlin: De Gruyter.

Hoffman, D. D. 2003. "The Interaction of Colour and Motion." In *Colour Perception: Mind and the Physical World*, edited by R. Mausfed and D. Heyer. Oxford: Oxford University Press. 361–377.

Hornbostel, E. M. von. 1925. "Die Einheit der Sinne" (The Unity of the Senses). *Melos. Zeitschrift für Musik* 4: 290–297.

Husserl, E. 1891. *Philosophie der Arithmetik: Psychologische und logische Untersuchungen*. Halle: Niemeyer. (Repr. 1970, Husserliana XII, The Hague: Nijhoff (En. tr. 2003. *Philosophy of Arithmetics*, by D. Willard. Dordrecht: Kluwer.)

Husserl, E. 1900–1901. *Logische Untersuchungen*. Halle: Niemeyer. (Repr. 1975, Vol. I ed. E. Holenstein, Husserliana XVII. Den Haag: Nijhoff, repr. 1984. Vols. I and II ed. U. Panzer, Husserliana XIX, ivi, 1, 2. (En. tr. 1970, *Logical Investigations*, by J. N. Findlay. London: Routledge & Kegan Paul.)

Husserl, E. 1913. *Ideen zu einer reinen Phänomenologie und phänomenologische Philosophie*. Halle: Niemeyer. (En. tr. 1989, *Ideas Pertaining to a Pure Phenomenology and Phenomenological Philosophy*, by R. Rojcewicz, and A. Schuwer. 3 vols. Dordrecht: Kluwer.)

Husserl, E. 1939. *Erfahrung und Urteil. Untersuchungen zur Genealogie der Logik*, edited by L. Landgrebe. Prag: Academia Verlag. (En. tr. 1973, *Experience and Judgement*, by J. Churchill and K. Ameriks. Evanston: Northwestern University Press.)

Husserl, E. 1966a. *Zur Analyse der passiven Synthesis*, edited by M. Fleischer, Husserliana XI. Dordrecht: Kluwer. (En. tr. 2001, *Analyses Concerning Passive and Active Synthesis*, by A. J. Steinbock. Dordrecht: Kluwer.)

Husserl, E. 1966b. *Zur Phänomenologie des inneren Zeitbewusstseins*, edited by R. Boehm. Den Haag: Kluwer. (En. tr. 1991, *Lectures on Internal Time*, by J. B. Brough. Dordrecht: Kluwer.)

Ingarden, R. 1962. *Untersuchungen zur Ontologie der Kunst: Musikwerk, Bild, Architecture, Film* (Researches on the Ontology of Art: Music, Image, Architecture, Film). Tübingen: Niemeyer.

Itten, J. 2002. *Elemente der bildende Kunst: Studienausgabe des Tagebuchs* (Elements of Fine Art: Study Issue of the Journal.) (2nd ed.). Leipzig: Seemann Verlag.

James, W. 1890. *Principles of Psychology*. Boston: Holt & Co. (Rep. 1950. New York: Dover Publications.)

Johnson, M. 1987. *The Body in the Mind: The Bodily Basis of Meaning, Imagination and Reason*. Chicago: University of Chicago Press.

Kandinsky, V. V. 1926. *Punkt Linie zur Fläche*. Bern: Benteli. (En. tr. 1979, *Point and Line, to Plane*. New York: Dover.)

Kanizsa, G. 1990. *La grammatica del vedere* (The Grammar of Seeing). Bologna: Il Mulino.

Kanizsa, G. 1991. *Vedere e pensare* (Seeing and Thinking). Bologna: Il Mulino.

Kanizsa, G., and Vicario, G. B. 1968. "La percezione della relazione intenzionale" (The Perception of the Intentional Relation). In *Ricerche sperimentali sulla percezione*, edited by G. Kanizsa and G. B. Vicario. Trieste: Università degli studi di Trieste. 69–126.

Kennedy, J. M. 1974. *A Psychology of Picture Perception*. San Francisco: Jossey-Bass Publisher.

Klages, L. 1942. *Grundlegung der Wissenschaft vom Ausdruck* (Foundation of the Science of Expression). Leipzig: Barth.

Klee, P. 1961. *The Thinking Eye*. London: Lund Humphries.

Koenderink, J. J. 2002. "Continua in Vision." In *Unfolding Perceptual Continua*, edited by L. Albertazzi. Amsterdam: Benjamins Publishing Company. 101–118.

Koenderink, J. J., and van Doorn, A. 2003. "Pictorial Space." In *Looking Into Pictures*, edited by H. Hecht, R. Schwartz, and M. Atherton. Cambridge, MA: MIT Press. 239–299.

Koffka, K. 1915. "Beiträge zur Psychologie der Gestalt- und Bewegungserlebnisse. III. Zur Grundlegung der Wahrnehmungspsychologie. Eine Auseinandersetzung mit V. Benussi" (Contributions to the Psychology of Gestalt and Motion Experiences. III. Groundwork Towards a Psychology of Perception. A Debate with V. Benussi). *Zeitschrift für Psychologie* 73: 11–90.

Koffka, K. 1930. "Some Problems of Space Perception." In *Psychologies of 1930*, edited by C. A. Murchison. Worchester, MA: Clark University Press. 161–187.

Koffka, K. 1935. *Principles of Gestalt Psychology*. New York: Harcourt.

Koffka, K., and Kenkel, F. 1913. "Beiträge zur Psychologie der Gestalt- und Bewegungserlebnisse I" (Contributions to the Psychology of Gestalt- and Motion Experiences). *Zeitschrift für Psychologie* 67: 353.

Köhler, W. 1933. *Psychologische Probleme* (Psychological Problems). Berlin: Springer.

Köhler, W. 1947. *Gestalt Psychology: An Introduction to New Concepts in Psychology*. NewYork: Liveright.

Kopfermann, H. 1930. "Psychologische Untersuchungen über die Wirkung zweidimensionaler Darstellungen körperliche Gebilde" (Psychological Investigations on the Effects of Two-dimensional Representations of Physical Objects). *Psychologische Forschung*: 293–364.

Kovàcs, I. 2000. "Human Development of Perceptual Organization." *Vision Research* 40 (10–12): 1301–1310.

Lakoff, G. 1987. *Women, Fire and Dangerous Things: What Categories Reveal About the Mind*. Chicago: University of Chicago Press.

Lakoff, G. 1990. "The Invariance Hypothesis: Is Abstract Reason Based on Image Schemas?" *Cognitive Linguistics* 1: 39–74.

Lakoff, G. 1993. "The Contemporary Theory of Metaphor." In *Metaphor and Thought*, edited by A. Orthony. Cambridge: Cambridge University Press. 202–251. 2nd ed. (Repr. in *Cognitive Linguistics. Basic Readings*, edited by D. Geeraerts, 2 vols., vol. 1, 185–238. Berlin: De Gruyter.)

Lakoff, G., and Johnson, M. 1980. *Metaphors We Live By*. Chicago: The University of Chicago Press.

Lakoff, G., and Johnson, M. 1999. *Philosophy in the Flesh: How the Embodied Mind Challenges the Western Tradition*. New York: Basic Books.

Lambert, J. Ch. 1764. *News Organon* (New Organon).

Langacker, R. W. 1987. "Nouns and Verbs." *Language* 63: 53–94.

Langacker, R. W. 1990. *Concept, Image, and Symbol: The Cognitive Basis of Grammar*. Berlin: Mouton de Gruyter.

Langacker, R. W. 1991. *Foundations of Cognitive Grammar:* Vol. I. Descriptive Applications. Stanford, CA: Stanford University Press.

Leopardi, G. 1989. *To Sylvia*. In *Opere* (Works). Milan-Naples: Ricciardi editore. 93–95.

Lewin, K. 1926. *Vorsatz. Wille und Bedürfnis: mit Vorbemerkungen über die psychische Kräfte und Energien und die Struktur der Seele* (Intent, Will and Desire: With Preliminary Observations on the Structure, Psychological Forces and Energies of the Soul). Berlin: Springer.

Leyton, M. 1992. *Symmetry, Causality, Mind*. Boston: MIT Press.

Li, X., and Gilchrist, A. L. 1999. "Relative Area and Relative Luminance Combine to Anchor Surface Lightness Values." *Perception and Psychophysics* 61 (5): 771–785.

Libet, B. 1982. "Brain Stimulation in the Study of Neuronal Functions for Conscious Sensory Experience." *Human Neurobiology* 1: 235–242.

Lipps, Th. 1897. *Raumaesthetik und geometrisch-optische Täuschungen* (Aesthetics of Space and Geometrical-Optical Illusions). Leipzig: Barth.

Longfellow, H. Wadsworth. 1995. *Mezzo Cammin*. In *The Book of 19th Century Verse*, ed. by T. Cook. Ware: Wordsworth Editons Ltd. 67–68.

Majakovskij, V. V. 1963. "Gimn uchenomu" (Hymn to the Scientist). In *Izbrannye proizvedenija*, Moskva-Leningrad, Sovetskij pisatel, vol. I. 92–93. (En tr. 1972, *Poems*, by D. Rottenberg. Moscow: Progress Publishers.)

Marks, L. E. 1978. *The Unity of the Senses: Interrelations among the Modalities*. New York: Academic Press.

Marks, L. E. 1982. "Bright Sneeres and Dark Coughs, Loud Sunlight and Soft Moonlight." *Journal of Experimental Psychology: Human Perception and Performance* 8 (2): 177–193.

Marks, L. E. 1996. "On Perceptual Metaphors." *Metaphor and Symbol* 11: 39–66.

Marks, L. E., Hammeal, R. J., Bornstein, M. H. 1987. "Perceiving Similarities and Comprehending Metaphors." *Monographs of the Society for Research in Child Development* 52 (1): 1–92.

Marr, D. 1982. *Vision*. San Francisco: Freeman Press.

Marty, A. 1908. *Untersuchungen zur Grundlegung der allgemeinen Grammatik und Sprachphilosophie* (Researches on the Foundations of Universal Grammar and Philosophy of Language). Vol. 1. Halle a.d.S.: Niemeyer.

Massironi, M. 2000. *L'osteria dei dadi truccati: Arte, psicologia e dintorni* (The Loaded Dice Inn: Art, Psychology and Thereabouts). Bologna: Il Mulino.

Mausfeld, R. 2002. "The Physicalistic Trap in Perception Theory." In *Perception and the Physical World*, edited by D. Heyer and R. Mausfeld. Chichester, UK: John Wiley & Sons. 75–112.

Mausfeld, R. 2003. "Conjoint Representations and the Mental Capacity for Multiple Simultaneous Perspectives." In *Looking into Pictures*, edited by H. Hecht, R. Schwartz, and M. Atherton. Cambridge, MA: MIT Press. 17–60.

Mausfeld, R., and Wendt, G. 2006. "Material Appearances Under Minimal Stimulus Conditions: Lustrous and Glassy Qualities." *Perception* 35(Suppl): 213–214.

Mauthner, F. 1901–1902. *Beiträge zu einer Kritik der Sprache* (Contributions to a Critique of Language). 3 vols. Böhlau: Köln, Wiemar.

Meinong, A. 1891. "Zur Psychologie der Komplexionen und Relationen" (On the Psychology of Complexes and Relations). *Zeitschrift für Psychologie und Physiologie der Sinnesorgane* 2: 245–265.

Meinong, A. 1899. "Über Gegenstände Höherer Ordnung und deren Verhältnis zur inneren Wahrnehmung" (On Higher Order Objects and their Relation to Inner Perception). *Zeitschrift für Psychologie und Physiologie der Sinnesorgane* 21: 182–272.

Meinong, A. 1960. "The Theory of Objects." In *Realism and the Background of Phenomenology*, edited by R. M. Chisholm. Glencoe: The Free Press. 76–117.

Merleau-Ponty, M. 1945. *Phénoménologie de la Perception* (Phenomenology of Perception). Paris: Gallimard.

Merleau-Ponty, M. 1969. *La Prose du Monde* (The Prose of the World). Paris: Gallimard.

Metzger, W. 1941. *Psychologie: die Entwicklung ihrer Grundannahmen seit der Einführung des Experiments* (Psychology: The Development of its Fundamental Assumptions since the Introduction of the Experiments). Dresden: Steinkopff.

Michotte, A. 1963. *The Perception of Causality*. London: Methuen.

Montale, E. *Tutte le poesie* (Omnibus of Poems). Milan: Arnoldo Mondadori editore.

Musatti, C. L. 1955. "La stereocinesi e la struttura dello spazio visibile" (Stereokinesis and the Structure of Visual Space). *Rivista di Psicologia* 49: 3–57.

Pascoli, G. 2002. *Poesie* (*Poems*). 3 vols Turin: Utet.

Pinna, B. 2005a. "The Neon Color Spreading and the Watercolor Illusion: Phenomenal Links and Neural Mechanism." In *Varieties of Cognitive Systems Behaviours*, edited by G. Miniati and E. Pessa. New York: Kluwer Academic/Plenum Publishers. 261–278.

Pinna, B. 2005b. "The Role of Gestalt Principle of Similarity in the Watercolor Illusion." *Spatial Vision* 21: 1–8.

Pinna, B. 2008. "A New Perceptual Problem: The Amodal Completion of Colour." *Visual Neuroscience* 25 (3): 1–11.

Pinna, B., and Sambin, M. 1991. "A Dynamic Model for Anomalous Figures: The Shape of Line-Induced Brightness and Modifications." *Perception* 20 (2): 219–232.

Pinna, B., Werner, J. S., and Spillmann, L. 2003. "The Watercolor Effect: A New Principle of Grouping and Figure-Ground Organization." *Vision Research* 43: 43–52.

Poli, R. 2001. "The Basic Problem of the Theory of Levels of Reality." *Axiomathes* 12 (3–4): 261–283.

Poli, R. 2002. "Ontological Methodology." *International Journal of Human-Computer Studies* 56: 639–664.

Poli, R. 2006a. "Levels of Reality and the Psychological Stratum." *Revue Internationale de Philosophie* 61 (2): 163–180.

Poli, R. 2006b. "The Theory of Levels of Reality and the Difference Between Simple and Tangled Hierarchies." In *Systemics of Emergence: Research and Development*, edited by G. Minati, E. Pessa, and M. Abram. New York: Springer. 715–722.

Pöppel, E. 1994. "Temporal Mechanism in Perception." *International Review of Neurobiology* 37: 185–202.

Ramachandran, V. S., and Hubbard, E. 2001. "Syaesthesia: A Window onto Perception, Thought and Language." *Journal of Consciousness Studies* 8 (12): 3–34.

Ramachandran, V. S., and Hubbard, E. 2003. "Hearing Colors, Tasting Shapes." *Scientific American* 288 (5): 52–59.

Rensink, R. A. 2000. "Seeing, Sensing, Scrutinizing." *Vision Research* 40: 1469–1487.

Rensink, R. A. 2002. "Change Detection." *Annual Review of Psychology* 53: 245–277.

Rizzolatti, G., and Arbib, M. A. 1998. "Language Within Our Grasp." *Trends in Neurosciences* 21 (5): 188–194.

Rosch, E. 1973. "Natural Categories." *Cognitive Psychology* 4: 328–350.

Rosch, E. 1978. *Cognition and Categorization*. Hillsdale, NJ: Erlbaum.

Rosch, E., and Mervis, C. B. 1975. "Family Resemblances: Studies in the Internal Structure of Categories." *Cognitive Psychology* 7: 573–605.

Rosch, E., Mervis, C. B., Gray, W. D., Johnson, M., and Boyes-Braem, P. 1976. "Basic Objects in Natural Categories." *Cognitive Psychology* 8: 382–439.

Rubin, E. 1958. "Figure and Ground." In *Readings in Perception*, edited by D. C. Beardsley and M. Wertheimer. New York: Van Nostrand: 194–203.

Sambin, M. 1980. *Le disomogeneità indotte nella formazione di margini e superfici anomale* (The Inhomogeneities Induced by Margin and Anomalous Surface Formation). Trieste: Reports from the Institute of Psychology.

Savage-Rumbaugh, S. E. 1996. *Kanzi: The Ape at the Brink of the Human Mind*. London: Wiley & Sons.

Shakespeare, W. 1962. *Machbeth*, edited by K. Muir. London: Methuen.

Shelley Percy B. 1998. *To the Moon*. In *Night Thoughts*, compiled by S. Winder. London: Penguin Books, p. 83.

Shen, Y. 1997. "Cognitive Constraints on Poetic Figures." *Cognitive Linguistics* 8 (1). 33–72.

Sivik, L. 1997. "Color System for Cognitive Research." In *Color Categories in Thought and Language*, edited by C. L. Hardin and L. Maffi. Cambridge: Cambridge University Press. 163–192.

Sydney Sir Ph. 1998. *With your sad steps, O Moon, thou climb'st the skies*. In *Night Thoughts*, compiled by S. Winder. London: Penguin Books, p. 37.

Stählin, W. 1913. *Zur Psychologie und Statistik der Metaphern. Eine methodologische Untersuchung* (On the Psychology and Statistics of Metaphors. A Methodological Study). Dissertation. Würzburg.

Stern, W. 1897. *Psychologie der Veranderungsauffassung* (On the Psychology of the Apprehension of Change). Breslau: Preuss und Junger.

Stroud, J. M. 1955. "The Fine Structure of Psychological Time." In *Information Theory in Psychology: Problems and Methods*, edited by H. Quastler. Glencoe, IL: The Free Press. 174–205.

Stumpf, C. 1883–1890. *Tonpsychologie* (Psychology of Sound), 2 vols. Leipzig: Hirzel.

Sweetser, E. 1990. *From Etymology to Pragmatics: Metaphorical and Cultural Aspects of Semantic Structure*. Cambridge, MA: Cambridge University Press.

Talmy, L. 1988a. "Grammatical Construal: The Relation of Grammar to Cognition." In *Topics in Cognitive Linguistics*, edited by B. Rudzka-Ostyn. Amsterdam: Benjamins Publishing Company. 165–205. (Repr. in *Cognitive Linguistics: Current Applications and Future Perspectives*, 2 vols., edited by D. Geeraerts, vol. 1. Berlin: De Gruyter. 69–108)

Talmy, L. 1988b. "Force Dynamics in Language and Thought." *Cognitive Science* 12: 49–100.

Talmy, L. 1996. "Fictive Motion in Language and 'ception'." In *Language and Space*, edited by P. Bloom, M. A. Peterson, L. Nadel, and M. F. Garrett. Cambridge, MA: MIT Press. 211–275.

Talmy, L. 2006. "A Windowing Onto Conceptual Structure and Language: Part 2: Language and Cognition: Past and Future." *Annual Review of Cognitive Linguistics* 4 (1): 253–268.

Tennyson, A. Lord. *In the Valley of Cauteretz*. In *The Book of 19th Century Verse*, edited by T. Cook. Ware: Wordsworth Editions Ltd, p. 221.

Turner, F., and Pöppel, E. 1983. "The Neural Lyre: Poetic Metre, the Brain and Time." *Poetry* 142 (5): 277–309.

Tversky, B. 1993. "Cognitive Maps, Cognitive Collages, and Spatial Mental Models." In *Spatial Information: A Theoretical Basis for GIS*, edited by A. U. Frank and I. Campari. Proceedings COSIT '93, Lecture Notes in Computer Science 716. 14–24.

Tversky, B. 1999. "Spatial Perspective in Descriptions." In *Language and Space*, edited by P. Bloom, M. A. Peterson, L. Nadel, and M. F. Garrett. Cambridge, MA: MIT Press. 463–491.

Ungaretti, G. 2005. *Vita d'un uomo. Tutte le poesie* (A Man's Life. Omnibus of Poems). Milan: Arnoldo Mondadori editore.

Ungaretti, G. 1997. *A Major Selection of the Poetry of Giuseppe Ungaretti*, translated by D. Bastianutti. Toronto, Ontario: Exile Editions Limited.

Valdez, P., and Mehrabian, A. 1994. "Effects of Color in Emotions." *Journal of Experimental Psychology: General* 123: 394–409.

Varela, F. J. 1999. "A Science of Consciousness as if Experience Mattered." In *Naturalizing Phenomenology*, edited by J. Petitot, F. J. Varela, B. Pachoud, and J.-M. Roy. Stanford, CA: Stanford University Press. 31–43.

Varela, F. J., Thompson, E., and Rosch, E. 1991. *The Embodied Mind: Cognitive Science and Human Experience*. Cambridge, MA: MIT Press.

Vicario, G. B. 1965. "Vicinanza spaziale e vicinanza temporale nella segregazione degli eventi" (Spatial and Temporal Proximity in the Segregation of Events). *Rivista di Psicologia* 59: 843–863.

Vicario, G. B. 1973. *Tempo psicologico ed eventi* (Psychic Time and Events). Florence: Giunti-Barbèra.

Vicario, G. B. 1998. "Some Experimental Observations on Instantaneousness and Doubleness of Events in Visual Field." *Teorie e Modelli* 3: 39–57.

Violi, P. 2000. "Prototipicality, Typicality and Context." In *Meaning and Cognition: An Interdisciplinary Approach*, edited by L. Albertazzi. Amsterdam: Benjamins Publishing Company. 103–122.

Wade, N. 1990. *Visual Allusions: Pictures of Perception*. London: Lawrence Erlbaum.

Wertheimer, M. 2002a. "Gestalt Theory." In *A Source Book of Gestalt Psychology*, edited by W. D. Ellis. London: Routledge. 1–11. (Original work published 1925)

Wertheimer, M. 2002b. "The General Theoretical Situation." In *A Source Book of Gestalt Psychology*, edited by W. D. Ellis. London: Routledge. 12–16. (Original work published 1922)

Wertheimer, M. 2002c. "Laws of Organization in Perceptual Forms." In *A Source Book of Gestalt Psychology*, edited by W. D. Ellis. London: Routledge. 71–88. (Original work published 1923)

Williams, J. M. 1976. "Synaesthetic Adjectives: A Possible Law of Semantic Change." *Language* 52 (2): 461–478.

IV   Perception in Art, Design, and Computation

12 Becoming Information: Paul Cézanne and *Prägnanz*

Amy Ione

Paul Cézanne's (1839–1906) revolutionary artwork is often characterized as post-Impressionistic: a bridge between the Impressionistic painting of the nineteenth century and the Modern Art of the twentieth. Although this depiction is accurate to a degree, it also obscures the extent to which Cézanne's career path was interwoven with the Impressionistic sensibility. His intense friendship with Camille Pissarro (1830–1903) introduced the young Cézanne to the concept of bringing the French idea of "sensation" into his practice, and it is said that Pissarro led Cézanne to embrace his sensation, in the sense of including his whole identity within the compositions recording his "impressions." In French, *sensation* is related to the verb *sentir* (to feel). At that time, the Impressionists used both the words *impression* and *sensation* to describe their approach to painting. The degree to which this sensibility came to define Cézanne's oeuvre comes through in a statement attributed to Cézanne by Emile Bernard in an article he wrote on the artist: "To paint from nature is to copy an object; it is to represent its sensations" (cited in Doran, 2001, p. 38). Joachim Gasquet, who spent much time with the artist in the late nineteenth century, records a similar statement: "Sensation is the basis of everything for a painter. . . . Before nature he learns to see" (cited in Doran, 2001, p. 138).

Today, the word *impressionism* is often used to define a diverse group of artists (Pissarro, Monet, Sisley, Degas, Renoir, Cézanne, Guillaumin, and Berthe Morisot) who participated in the first Impressionist exhibition. Held in 1874, this Paris show featured work that the juries of the Salon had rejected, often due to the liberties these artists took in composition and the lack of a crisp verisimilitude in the (so-called) finished pieces. Louis Leroy, a critic of that period who disliked the work on display, wrote a satiric review composed of a dialogue of two visitors at the show. [It was after the review was published in *Le Charivari* that the artists adopted the name Impressionism.] Leroy's (1874) dismissal of this group as painters of mere impressions is summed up in the article's reference to Claude Monet's Impression: Sunrise (*Impression, soleil levant*), where he has a visitor to the show saying:

Impression—I was certain of it. I was just telling myself that, since I was impressed, there had to be some impression in it—and what freedom, what ease of workmanship! Wallpaper in its embryonic state is more finished than that seascape.

Although some argued that these artists were incapable of producing proper paintings, suitably composed and accurately rendered, there were also critics who did not unilaterally condemn the Impressionistic deviations from the classical standards. The critic Jules Castagnary, for example, made both positive and negative comments when he described the paintings on display in the 1874 show as quite subjective. He said that a number of younger artists—Pissarro, Monet, Sisley, Renoir, Degas, and Morisot—were Impressionists in the sense that they rendered not the landscape but the sensation produced by the landscape. Still, Castagnary criticized Cézanne for producing work that was *overly* subjective and for pursuing "the impressionism to excess" (Castagnary, 1874; Shiff, 1984, p. 4).

Stepping back, we find that the nineteenth-century debates within the art community about our perception of nature, the subjective (inner) and objective (outer) aspects of painterly perception, and the nature of vision have some resonance with the scientific research at that time into psychophysics, perception, sensation, and how we "see" and "experience" physical reality. For example, in 1874, the year of the first Impressionistic show discussed earlier, two books of first-rate importance for the development of modern psychology were published by Franz Brentano (1838–1917) and Wilhelm Wundt (1832–1920): *Psychologie vom empirischen Standpunkte* and *Grundzüge der physiologischen Psychologie*, respectively. This convergence in the development of modern psychology, which is more fully discussed in the Introduction to this book, was clearly summed up by E. B. Titchener in a 1921 article, "Brentano and Wundt: Empirical and Experimental Psychology," where he talks about the importance of the year 1874 in the development of the field. Although the traditions that emerged from these two books shared a common interest in psychophysics, those who followed Brentano were more concerned with the internal side of our experience and with seeing psychology as an activity or process. In contrast, Wundt's followers gave more attention to the external side and expressed a greater concern with developing an experimental methodology that could be used to measure and quantitatively categorize one's experience.

To the best of my knowledge, an in-depth study of how/whether the ideas of Brentano and/or Wundt directly influenced the thinking of the innovative painters of the late nineteenth century and their critics has not yet appeared in print. Unfortunately, this tantalizing subject is beyond the modest scope of this chapter as well, although in analyzing the artwork of Paul Cézanne I am no doubt indirectly arguing that a Brentanian framework is a more appropriate vantage point when examining Cézanne's revolutionary artwork and that of the artists who began breaking with the classical academic standards in the late nineteenth and early twentieth centuries. Moreover, although this short chapter does not present a direct argument linking Cézanne to the Brentanian framework, my presentation of Cézanne's practice in effect comes through one of the strands of the Brentanian legacy: Gestalt psychology and *Prägnanz*. I have chosen this narrow focus to highlight that an artist communicates information through the process of artmaking: through intentionally giving form to his or her aspirations. The final objects record an active inner process that perceptually engages and includes the development of the final object, which then becomes a part of the viewer's experience of the created object as well. This multifaceted variable, I would argue, speaks to the ways an artist who creates a visual object translates a phenomenal perception into something that is difficult to reduce to the underlying levels, physical or psychological. This process, in my view, is not something that we cannot fully capture and/or measure quantitatively. Cézanne's canvases, for example, are not mere "representations" of a stimulus or the product of a probabilistic inference. They are the presentation of a *unitary* occurring event of which his subjective perceptual structure is a nonindependent part of the activity/object. Experimental science largely underrepresents this activity and the artmaking process in general, which is of infinite importance to the art we see, particularly when we look at an artist such as Paul Cézanne.

Information

Research into artmaking, like research in any field, requires that we collect "information" about the subject at hand. *Information*, a broadly defined term in contemporary culture, is a particularly challenging concept when we look through an art, rather than a science, lens. For example, scientific (and/or philosophical thinkers) are apt to associate information with Shannon's classical theory, which privileges quantitative parameters and statistical analyses. Emotions, sensory experience, and phenomena that are difficult to analyze quantitatively (e.g., biological, psychic, social, and artistic events) are not easily approached in the type of statistical paradigm favored by this conception. Unlike a scientist who aims to design quantifiable measures, an artist is generally working toward a more elusive goal. Although she, too, may design experiments, these are likely to be developed through a feedback system that is based on a more intuitive evaluation of the work at hand. This reliance on practice-based knowledge, rather than explicit rules, yields a quality of information that ultimately informs the objective form of the work dramatically. Artists often acknowledge this and speak about their inability to characterize how they develop the intangible qualities of their work. Yet when they blend the elusive qualities of the intuited information with the mysterious process of creation, they are frequently able to communicate something marvelous.

Systems theory, which grew out of information theory, has aided some in blending the disparities between quantitative and qualitative perspectives. Conceived as an alternative to Shannon's information theory and premised on the idea that "systems" are dynamic, complex wholes, thinkers in this mold aim to integrate qualitative parameters so they can address connecting parts comprehensively. What is key here is that a systemic approach has the flexibility to integrate methodologies (such as art) that are open, intrinsically temporal, and adaptive; constantly changing, unfolding, and interacting with the surrounding environment. This kind of approach allows us to better analyze qualitative, subjective, and expressive elements that are part of the information presented.

Another attractive component of systemic thinking is its compatibility with Gestalt theories. This pairing, I would argue, offers an entry point through which we can grapple with how artists translate intuition into visual art. In other words, while perceptual or compositional aspects of an art-centered study may fit within a quantitative, mathematically driven framework of information analysis, and while some technical aspects of artmaking may lend themselves to a reductive or atomistic approach, a great deal of the pertinent information involved in making art does not. Artistic intuition, in particular, is more suitable to a qualitative perspective because it is mutable by nature.

Cézanne's Vision and Gestalt Theory

Paul Cézanne offers a good case in point. A misunderstood innovator early in his career,[1] and a powerful source of inspiration after his death, Cézanne's compositional choices, unusual approach to color application, observational approach, and inventive mind contributed greatly to his multifaceted legacy. Indeed, his work defies characterization. One extraordinary aspect of it is that, at first glance, his paintings tend to appear representational. Yet further study makes it clear that his canvases do not mirror the world we see.

Perhaps the primary puzzle, however, is not the error of our first glance but the process through which he developed his craft and its subsequent impact. For example, although no one has definitively resolved why his work is so alluring despite its many anomalies, few today dispute that this revolutionary painter had a major influence on later visual art. Theodore Reff (1977) reminds us that:

For Klee he was "the teacher par excellence," for Matisse "the father of us all," for Picasso "a mother who protects her children." As is evident from their work, each of them responded to another aspect of Cézanne's complex and constantly evolving art, and the same is true of all those modern painters who, from Gauguin in the 1880s to Jasper Johns eighty years later, have taken it as a model or ideal. (Reff, 1977, p. 13)

Although these kinds of testimonials verify his influence, the evolution of his process is harder to explain. In an abstract sense, we can easily align Cézanne's goals with Gestalt tenets (e.g., we can point to his holistic approach to painting, his attention to the power of grouping shapes and colors and use of this perceptual tendency as a compositional device, the "constructive" brushwork he invented that presents a form without literally copying it, etc.). Yet, to be sure, Cézanne worked independently of the Gestalt approach.[2] A painter who had little use for theory, his experimental approach allowed him to give form to both his sensation and what he perceived in the world-at-large.

Balancing the tensions among his goals required what I call here a second-level awareness of key Gestalt principles (e.g., emergence, reification, multistability, and invariance). In his book, *Cézanne: Landscape into Art* (1996), Pavel Machotka, an emeritus professor of psychology at the University of California Santa Cruz, offers a useful framework for beginning to think about this. Here, Machotka points out that we can identify two ways in which Cézanne operated: his organizing process and the mechanisms he developed to portray the objective world. The first of these, his organizing process, is one shared by all of us. This includes the grouping and segregation of objects, the formation of a coherent sense of space, and the perception of meaning in expression. These processes relate to perception in a general sense, were identified by Gestalt thinkers, and required no "special" attention on the painter's part. The second form of perception, the mechanisms of identification and recognition, which comprise what I have termed second-level awareness, are of greater significance to this study.[3]

Cézanne's second-level awareness is best seen through an analysis of how he developed his projects. What is key here is that mechanisms of identification and recognition, which required him to bring a focused attention to his work, were foundational as he built his style. In other words, through his deliberate efforts, he was able to schematize what he saw *and* to systematically extend the information provided in the earlier, more instinctive stages of perception. Let me again stress that because this second stage involved looking outwardly and then inventively translating his perception into the painted form, Cézanne needed to do more than simply "perceive." It was this "something more" that made all the difference.

For example, the art critic Clement Greenberg (1961) has commented insightfully on Cézanne's place historically and as a revolutionary.[4] Referencing the revelation Cézanne had at the age of forty, when he focused in on an attempt to "save the key principles of Western painting," Greenberg saw Cézanne's motivation as twofold. On the one hand, Cézanne desired to express an ample and literal rendition of stereometric space. In addition, this artist wanted to mitigate the ephemeral effects of Impressionistic color with his broad stable strokes. Cézanne did this, according to Greenberg, because he sought, more like the Florentines than like the Venetians he cherished, to achieve mass and volume first.

In Greenberg's (1961) view, Cézanne thought he could achieve his goal by adapting the Impressionistic method of registering variations of light into a way of indicating the variations in planar direction of solid surfaces:

For traditional modeling in dark and light, he substituted modeling with the supposedly more natural—and Impressionist—differences of warm and cool. . . . The result was a kind of pictorial

tension, the like of which had not been seen in the West since Late Roman mosaic art. The overlapping little rectangles of pigment, laid on with no attempt to fuse their edges, brought depicted
form toward the surface; at the same time the modeling and shaping performed by these same
rectangles drew it back into illusionistic depth. (Greenberg, 1961, pp. 50, 52)

Greenberg (1961) also places Cézanne within a larger historical context, adding that:

The Old Masters always took into account the tension between surface and illusion, between the
physical facts of the medium and its figurative content—but in their need to conceal art with art,
the last thing they wanted was to make an explicit point of this tension. Cézanne, in spite of
himself, had been forced to make the tension explicit in his desire to rescue the tradition
from—and at the same time with—Impressionistic means. (p. 53)

Others who have looked into Cézanne's contributions are more attuned to the question of how Cézanne contrived to physically *place* the information he perceived visually onto the painted surface as he strove to integrate all of the relationships he felt
within his person with the content he laid out onto the canvas. For example, in evaluating Rewald's *Catalogue Raisonne*, Richard Shiff (1998) offers an example of how Cézanne may have approached his sense that he needed to find a brushstroke through
which he could capture his vision. Shiff notes that, between 1877 and 1879, Cézanne
copied four dissimilar paintings: a still life from an engraving, an urban genre scene
from an oil painting, an animal study from a lithograph, and a landscape from a photograph. Asking why Cézanne would copy these four dissimilar models when he did
not paint many copies, Shiff suggests that these examples illustrate efforts to develop
what Theodore Reff has termed his "constructive stroke."[5] Shiff (1998) asks whether
Cézanne was using these diverse models to free himself from the strain added by an
intense scrutiny of a motif, his more common working method at that point in time.
Although no one can say for sure, ultimately Cézanne's invention of novel brushwork
(like his use of distortion as a pictorial device) allowed him to add vitality to the flat
surfaces. As time passed, he often unified the pictorial surface by using short, straight
brush strokes, balancing shapes by their visual weight, and using color complementar-
ity, and so on.

The range of his techniques clarifies further when we look at documentation provided by the many painters and Cézanne aficionados who have tried to penetrate this
painter's intuitive methodology through visits to Aix-en-Provence, the home of many
Cézanne motifs. The tradition began while Cézanne was still alive, as people who
found his work tantalizing began seeking him out (e.g., Paul Gauguin, Emile Bernard,
Charles Camoin, etc.). Now visitors navigate the terrain where he practiced without his
guidance or vicariously travel around the Aix countryside through the published photographic images of Cézanne's sites. Overall, these photographic studies aid in an evaluation of how Cézanne gained insight as he worked with the natural settings he
portrayed, frequently studying the same location repeatedly. Among the best-known
photographs are those of Erle Loran, John Rewald, and Pavel Machotka.[6]

Erle Loran, himself a talented artist, began his onsite investigations in 1926. Using a traveling scholarship to travel to Europe, he lived in the studio of Paul Cézanne, where he painted and photographed the countryside around Aix. The photographic material from Loran's three-year sojourn later formed the nucleus for his book, *Cézanne's Compositions* (1943).[7] Loran (1943), whose work is discussed in more detail in the next section, sums up Cézanne's achievement by saying:

Cézanne achieved light in the sense that modern painters give to the word, namely, the creation of an inner light that emanates from the color relations in the picture itself, without regard for the mere copying of realistic effects of light and shade. Cézanne, therefore, pointed the way to the freedom and release that the modern artist has regained—the release from servile imitation of light and shade. (Loran, 1943, p. 19)

John Rewald (1977) writes that his interest in using photographs to study Cézanne's work began in 1933, after the painter Léo Marchutz (1903–1976), a German-born artist living at *Château Noir* (a motif Cézanne often depicted), introduced him to Erle Loran photographs published in the April 1930 issue of *The Arts* under the name *Cézanne's Country* (Loran [Johnson], 1930).[8] Marchutz knew of sites Loran had missed and urged Rewald to document them. The enthusiasm generated through these new sites led Rewald to spend several months in Aix each year through 1939, and again after 1947, learning about and photographing this area that so attracted Cézanne. Much of this work aided him with his authoritative catalogue of Cézanne's work (*Paintings of Paul Cezanne: A Catalogue Raisonne*, 1996).[9]

Pavel Machotka is a more recent pilgrim.[10] Viewing the sites from the perspective of an artist and psychologist, he sought to study them under conditions that matched the colors found on Cézanne's paintings. With this information, he challenged the emphasis that earlier commentators gave to form and argued that the colors of Aix played a key role in this master's translation of the physical motifs into the painted harmony we experience. Intended as analysis and criticism, not as a contribution to the art historical literature, Machotka's research, in particular his *Cézanne: Landscape Into Art* (1996), speaks sensitively of Cézanne's paradoxical way of translating physical settings into works of art that extemporize physical reality but are nonetheless so accurate that we can pinpoint the precise spots from which Cézanne painted many of these works. His evaluation shows that Cézanne gravitated toward relatively flat topography, assimilated receding diagonals to horizontality, enlarged distinct objects or raised the horizon, and sometimes tilted planes upward (Machotka, 1996).

Cézanne's Compositions

Erle Loran's (1943) *Cézanne's Compositions* remains one of the most comprehensive of the photographic studies. Used to analyze Cézanne's compositional techniques, this study both juxtaposes Cézanne's motifs with paintings of the settings and analyzes

other themes the master pursued. Carefully conceived after many years of experimentation, Loran begins with an illustrated glossary that explains pictorial organization
and outlines how artists address the compositional plane generally. Topics covered
range from the picture plane, the static plane, and the dynamic plane to rising and
falling movements, light and dark patterns, and closed- and open-color arrangements.
Comprised of nineteen diagrams with descriptive paragraphs, this part of the book
allows Loran to situate Cézanne's process of painting within the realm of painterly
possibilities.

The book begins with a discussion of the static plane of a blank canvas, which in effect is waiting to be activated by the artist. For example, by adding a diagonal or dynamic plane, the artist could create a sense of depth in front of a back wall. Similarly,
sizes and shapes can cause a plane to visually *rotate* toward or away from this back wall,
thus making it a *dynamic* plane. One valuable component of this section is Loran's ability to pictorially demonstrate "informational" options that the artist rejected, as well
as those he chose. For example, Loran shows that Cézanne established holistic relationships through his approach to color and form, inventing methods to portray depth
and a dynamic space. The upshot of this is that when planes are overlapping, they do
not recede to a vanishing point so much as they create layers of space, with the planes
and color patterning interacting so that the visual cues convey a sense of depth. He
further argues that scientific perspective plays no fundamental part in Cézanne's spatial effect because the "canvas space" Cézanne achieved was not dependent on the
funnel effect we associate with this technique.[11] Other topics Loran examines include
scale, volume and space control, whether he had a "problem" with perspective, distortion as a device, the interplay of realism and abstraction, and so on. Although Loran
deals with specific areas that distinguish Cézanne's visual results throughout the book,
and although the glossary and compositional sections are illuminating, it is Loran's
discrete studies that distinguish *Cézanne's Compositions*.[12]

In the chapter on distortion, for instance, Loran turns to one of Cézanne's best-
known works, *Still Life with Fruit and Basket* (1890) (this image is available at <http://
tinyurl.com/2hyw9h>), to discuss the painter's use of shifting of eye levels. These
varied points of view, according to Loran, reference split planes or tensions between
"subjective" planes. Comparing the actual painting with a complex, graphic diagram,
Loran demonstrates that in this particular work we can isolate many of the devices
later adopted by twentieth-century abstract painters. Examining the incorporation of
several viewpoints, Loran illustrates that the first eye level takes in roughly the front
plane of the fruit basket, the sugar bowl, and the small pitcher. A second (and higher)
eye level looks down on the opening of the ginger jar and the top of the basket. The
splitting of the tabletop, the tipping of objects, and the anomalous use of shadowing
techniques further accentuate this masterly use of distortion. These devices and the
way the illusion of space seems to include "seeing around" effects are among the many

visual anomalies that cause connoisseurs to ask why the work "feels" unified and pow-erful to the viewer despite its obvious divergence from our "ideas" about physical space.

A Loran diagram of one of Cézanne's more than fifty works depicting *Mont Sainte-Victoire* (*Mont Sainte-Victoire Seen from the Bibemus Quarry*, circa 1897, now a part of the Cone Collection at the Baltimore Museum of Art; see <http://tinyurl.com/24hmos>) is also quite compelling. Here, Loran provides an illustration of what many believe was Cézanne's most influential innovation: his novel approach to the rendering of vol-umes that seem to move in space. What is particularly striking in this is how well the diagram shows Cézanne's ability to suggest movement through the physical space sur-rounding the volumes. Loran proposes that Cézanne enlarged the mountain, and his diagram includes several small arrows intended to indicate the movement from one volume to another. In addition, three large dimensional arrows mark out the circular movement from foreground into deep space. The extraordinary effect is one of vol-umes that seem to be jostling in the negative deep space without the aid of the funnel effect we associate with scientific perspective.[13]

Cézanne and Space

Cézanne's innovative compositions are often said to have led to a rethinking of space in twentieth-century art.[14] What stands out is that he reoriented the elements of his pictorial space just enough to ensure that the plane of the canvas would be preserved, and in this way he makes us see the objects in his paintings as existing in a deep space behind the canvas, as in Renaissance paintings. At the same time, we see the objects on the canvas surface. The observer senses the tension between Cézanne's two aims in his or her own oscillation between the two ways of looking: fidelity to the motif and re-spect for the needs of the canvas (Machotka, 1996).

Cézanne accomplished this oscillation through experimentation; he frequently re-turned to his favorite spots, objects, and figures, painting a scene of interest again and again. Comparing these multiple renditions allows us to further see how his visual perception was translated into the information we see in his paintings. For example, he painted *Mont Sainte-Victoire* repeatedly from slightly different viewpoints, but quite how Cézanne intended this texture to be seen is unclear from his notebooks and let-ters. On the work itself, we can see that his interpretations are often reliant on geom-etries that suggest representational forms and yet distort them. Many persuasively interpret Cézanne's "Cubist" expressions as relating to an interplay among two, three, and even four dimensions, in trying to show all sides of the depicted objects simultane-ously, perhaps even a fourth-dimensional possibility.

Another feature that stands out when we review the multiple studies is that his forms change as his work matures, with the patterns become increasingly abstract. The paint is so thinly and fluidly applied in the later watercolors, for example, that if we didn't know the forms he worked from, many of the paintings would appear as pure abstraction. It is also striking to see how closely these compositions resemble what we think of as twentieth-century styles despite their derivation from the fifteenth-century block style of Piero della Francesca's paintings reproduced in the *Academy Françoise* at that time.

Looking at his *oeuvre* comprehensively, two elements stand out: First, developing his style took a long, long time; and, second, he bootstrapped his self-education. In other words, we can perceive an increasing tension between solid form and optical sensation that begins to take hold in the paintings of the later 1870s and early 1880s. These pieces show that Cézanne had arrived at a consistent method by this time and also show that he had already begun to research how to represent solid, three-dimensional objects using a system he termed *modulation* (to distinguish it from *modeling*). In a general sense, this modulation technique was one in which he superimposed multiple strokes of color, creating both a cumulative visual effect and a reverberation throughout the canvas. Cézanne's use of modulation to harmonize the colors as he organized (and composed) the lines and planes on the canvas allowed him to render his sensation in a form that presents a *version* of nature *although is not a literal imitation of it*. This modulation paved the way for later nonrepresentational painting.

One exceptional work that shows how this vibrant modulation seems to point toward the range of early twentieth-century styles is his dramatic painting, *Lac d'Annecy* (see <http://tinyurl.com/yro2ae> for an image). Completed in 1896, ten years before his death, it is quite striking both pictorially and in terms of color and form. The reflections in the lake are almost palpable. But why would Cézanne want to introduce a cubistic solidity into the space of the lake's surface? To answer this question, we must presume that space to this painter *is* a systemic experience/expression. It includes the physical space he sees, the atmosphere filling this space, and the activity of defining space in the painting. Cézanne seems to be trying to make the interplay among these aspects of space explicit in his paintings. The shimmering depiction of *Lac d'Annecy* reflects this perceptual struggle. Contemplating this painting, one may develop a sense of the space between the canvas and the lake as being simultaneously solid and transparent, like a block of ice. This evocation of space, light, and air is different from Cubism, where most of the space is formally rather than optically deconstructed. As a result, Cézanne's expression has a harmony that relies on the interplay of space, color, and form. In other words, it gives form to optical impressions while vividly offering a novel interpretation of physical space.

Finally, Cézanne's letters and recorded conversations reveal that even when we see fractured space on a Cézanne canvas, neither a multifaceted cubism nor color modulation accurately characterizes his goals. In terms of "space," perhaps his attempt to capture a new sense of space was also an effort to show that space is not an empty domain, in which objects and planes are separated or exist in a relative sense. Rather, his space was full of essence, a corpuscular space filling the distance between the eye and the reflections in the lake. Given this, could it be that Cézanne was anticipating the new view of space reached by Einstein a decade later? In his early papers, Einstein proposed a quantum interpretation of space that, instead of being void, consists of a seething evanescence of particle creations and annihilations. This eventful, energetic view of space finds a resonance in the space depicted in Cézanne's late paintings. One might even ask whether Einstein, who lived in Berne, not far from Lake Annecy, might have seen Cézanne's work and drawn inspiration from it, but this remains a speculation.

Sensation and Color

As discussed earlier, all seem to agree that the complexity of Cézanne's formal design opened a new paradigm in art, although we find many views as to what precisely happened. When we align this painter with the tradition that sees Cézanne's work as a precursor to Cubism, we highlight the work's spatial distortion and formal manipulation more than other key aspects, such as his use of color and his commitment to "his sensation." Typically, analyses have the most difficulty conveying what the abstract painter Hans Hofmann (1964) termed "an enormous sense of volume, breathing, pulsating, expanding, contracting through his use of colors" (Hofmann, 1964, p. 41). Some, and I am among them, have concluded that color and his devotion to "his sensation" were instrumental in his studies of how to balance the objective and subjective modalities. Through this study, the qualitative complexity within Cézanne's works took increasingly more awe-inspiring forms. It is not just that he used color and sensation to build paintings that are in effect parallel constructions of what he was representing. Even more pronounced is that our experience of the visual results is at times comparable to our auditory experience of music.

Spaces and surfaces exist in a pictorial space in which it is finally not their identify that matters but their relations of size, color, distance, or movement. . . . Colors also exist primarily in relation to others rather than by themselves, and they, too, create patterns of tension and resolution. Experiencing a painting formally has much the same esthetic effect as feeling the tensions produced by changes of key, repetitions of themes, changes of instrumental timbre, or resolved and unresolved chords. (Machotka, 1996, p. 15)

Machotka describes this musical quality particularly well when he analyzes how these results came about. He points out that the tonal qualities developed as Cézanne added a painterly rhythm to natural textures, built on the warmer or cooler variants of the local hues, gently reorienting edges away from the diagonal and toward the horizontal while presenting paintings that continue to appear as faithful to his original point of reference. In other words, although the brushstrokes are predominantly diagonal, their angles do shift. Thus, color adds sensuality, rhythm, and dynamic to the forms he painted. He transformed natural textures, broke the smooth continuities into separate planes, or reoriented some lines and planes.

The results also derive from Cézanne's loyalty to his "sensation," mentioned earlier. Although ultimately we know little about his subjective vision from his writings, they do tell us that his intention was not just to make paintings. He clearly desired to translate his sensation into the representational forms he created, although even what he meant by the term *sensation* remains ambiguous.

The word "sensation," which Cézanne used in discussing art and nature, is a difficult one in both French and English. It refers either to the perception of something external or to an internal emotional feeling. For Cézanne, the two were nearly inseparable. Thus, one receives sensations before nature, but sensations "reside with us." Cézanne complicated the matter by writing that he had a "strong" sensation of nature and elsewhere he described the "temperament" or personality of the artist as a "force" and as a "power" in the presence of nature. (Shiff, 1978, p. 789)

Prägnanz

Perhaps the most fascinating aspect of Cézanne's legacy from a Gestalt perspective is that his results emerged over years of study. Although I find the work from his entire career extraordinary and marvelous, particularly when viewed as a whole, his later work strikes me as the most exceptional. Once he perfected his touch, his canvases speak of *Prägnanz*, a fundamental principle of Gestalt perception that refers to our tendency to order our experience in ways that are simple, regular, orderly, and symmetric. The measure of simplicity and accompanying fluidity that Cézanne represented in his final years is quite unlike the heaviness and lack of perspicacity so pronounced in his earlier work. Indeed, surveying the span of his career, we can see all he achieved and how his work served as an exemplar of (for) his self-education.[15] Particularly striking is that the change in his painterly "tone" began to appear around 1895 and is more evident after 1900, when the works show a fluidity and abstraction that differ remarkably from the heavy hand of his early paintings. Thus, through looking at his compositions, we see that the paradox of Cézanne is evident and elevated: He transformed the physical textures, broke up smooth continuities into separate planes, and reoriented some lines and planes; yet, in the end, each painting he produced was astonishingly faithful to its theme. In many of his landscape pieces, particularly after 1900, if we did not actually know the motifs he favored, we would be hard pressed to see the natural environments he depicted in the patterns and patches of colors we find on his canvases and watercolors.

Yet it is also possible to say that the paradox is resolved when we relate to the work on its own terms:

We recognize form that is voluminous without being solid, color that is luminous without light, representation that is apparently specific yet specifies nothing. We recognize in fact the contradictory kinds of references that the paradoxes of our own art are built upon. In Cézanne, however, there is no paradox, but an order of pictorial statement full of an earnestness and conviction that possesses the single-minded moral dignity of tradition. (Gowing, 1998, p. 182)

This tension between his natural ordering processes and what I earlier termed a second-level awareness of key Gestalt principles brings to mind Rudolf Arnheim's competing views on art.[16] On the one hand, Arnheim's writings (Arnheim, 1969, 1974, 1983, 1986; for analysis see Verstegen, 2005) speak sensitively about the intelligence of the senses and the ability of the senses to contain universal or abstract information. On the other hand, Arnheim was always sensitive to the need to speak about the manipulation of images for productive thinking. It seems, even if we say that individual percepts already contain abstract content and allow that a work of art can be called the abstracted solution to an artistic problem, there is still a need to grapple with the relationship between the abstract information and the practice that gives it form. The problem solving that is a part of the cognitive space responsible for creating the work of art is clearly a part of Cézanne's experience.

This focused intuition that eventually brings *Prägnanz* to mind is the quality of Cézanne that seems to defy quantification. Although we cannot quantify or even adequately verbalize Cézanne's achievements, they are easy to see and feel. As Roger Fry's (2004) classic study, *Cézanne: A Study of his Development*, notes: "[I]n the last resort we cannot in the least explain why the smallest product of his hand arouses the impression of being a revelation of the highest importance, or what exactly it is that gives it its grave authority" (Fry, 2004, p. 88).

Conclusion

In terms of information, as I have discussed, we cannot measure how or why the qualities within a Cézanne masterpiece affect us as they do. Efforts to comprehend his markings offer some insights to be sure. Although we can isolate particular characteristics, the overall allure of each masterpiece nonetheless remains mysterious after all is said and done. Because Cézanne's painted statements include so many complex variables that go beyond the formal qualities within the work, it seems there is no methodology for quantifying how this artist translated his intuition into visual art. It is not just that he brought both objective and subjective modalities together in his work. In addition, his intuitive methodology led him to develop techniques that were like nothing ever done previously in painting. Laboratory experiments, in my opinion, have no mechanism to quantify the scope and complexity of this kind of creative and revolutionary discovery. How can you ferret out information that did not exist previously?

A concrete way to think about this is that, although primary sources show that Cézanne's work "seeded" his followers in developing their own vision(s), the qualities that make a Cézanne a Cézanne are distinctly his. These were not transferable. For example, although Cézanne believed that Paul Gauguin had stolen his "sensation" when he began to copy his parallel touch (the short, parallel brushstrokes he often used to evoke form), Gauguin was unable to "copy" Cézanne's perception. Gauguin merely *borrowed* the technique. Because Gauguin did not research the method in the same way, he did not have a comparable understanding of how Cézanne used it to achieve his results. Without an embodied knowledge of how the technique serves its purpose (for Cézanne), Gauguin did not (or could not) replicate the master's stroke. For Gauguin, the technique produced compositions with a flatter and less dynamic quality.[17]

Despite the knowledge that even a thorough evaluation of Cézanne's work does not resolve the questions surrounding how he achieved his results, this kind of exercise is not without merit. Indeed, one of the fascinating aspects of this painter's achievements is that, as we attempt to understand the visual information he presents, our respect for its mysterious allure increases. The totality of his career shows his interest in various perceptual modalities (optical space, phenomenal space of appearances, and pictorial space) and allows us to ponder how color, dynamic, and time are interwoven with composition in the hands of this artist. Because he favored using external information as his perceptual stimulus (at least after the age of forty),[18] we are fortunate to have touchstones we can turn to as we analyze emergence and the role of feedback within his unique skill set. Through this analysis, when used in terms of his career as a whole, it is possible to distinguish vision per se from the vision of this visual artist. More precisely, Cézanne's process and *oeuvre* allow us to distinguish vision per se from a vision that continually seeks to refine its perceptive acuity.

Finally, as I worked on this chapter, it was hard not to notice how different my early drafts looked from the final product, although the basic information remained much the same. The exercise of writing multiple drafts in an effort to resolve gaps in my analysis stimulated me to think more deeply about Cézanne's tendency to return to the same place repeatedly. Thinking about this in terms of information left me wondering what the artistic information is before it "becomes information." This question, no doubt far beyond the scope of this chapter, remains unanswered and intriguing.

Notes

1. George Heard Hamilton's (1984) "Cézanne and His Critics" offers a fine overview of some of the criticism of Cézanne's work during his lifetime.

2. This is not always the case for visual artists. Many Bauhaus artists, for example, were attracted to Gestalt ideas. These artists, Paul Klee in particular comes to mind, saw research on perceptual grouping, sensation, and the constructive aspects of perception useful in both an explanatory and practical sense (see Behrens, 2002; Teuber, 1976; Willats, 1997, 2006). Josef Albers, best known for

his book, *Interaction of Color* (1975), is another artist whose work was deeply informed by Gestalt thinking. Although the impact of juxtaposed colors on our perceptual apparatus was noted historically, Michel-Eugene Chevreul's work with color relationships is a good example of a well-known nineteenth-century study. Albers work in this area was directly stimulated by his contact with Gestalt research. Albers studies on the interaction of colors resonate with Gestalt experiments on brightness contrast. Albers is also well known for his work with ambiguous structures.

3. Here I broadly adapt an idea Daniel Dennett (1981) presented in his "Conditions of Personhood." In this essay, Dennett argued that an important step toward becoming a person was the step up from a first-order intentional system to a second-order intentional system. The basic difference is one that relates to the level of awareness. To oversimplify, the intentionality of the first order is, according to Dennett, a masked primitive, whereas the second-order intentionality is known and acknowledged.

4. Many commentators have looked critically at Cézanne's work. A short list of informative studies includes (among others) *Cézanne* by Joachim Gasquet (1927), *Paul Cézanne* by Gerstle Mack (1935/1989), *Cézanne: The Late Work* by William Rubin (1984), *Letters on Cézanne* by Rainer Maria Rilke (1952), *Cézanne and the End of Impressionism* by Richard Shiff (1984), *Interpreting Cézanne* by Paul Smith (1996), and *Cézanne: The Early Years 1859–1872* by Lawrence Gowing (1988). Of course, Cézanne study is ongoing, and this list hardly begins to convey the information available.

5. See "Cézanne's Constructive Stroke" in the *Art Quarterly* (Reff, 1962).

6. The photographic documentation is so informative and tantalizing that a session on the "Cézanne's Sites" was held in October 1977 at the Museum of Modern Art in New York City in conjunction with a commemorative exhibition, *Cézanne: The Late Work* [October 7, 1977–January 2, 1978]. Erle Loran, Pavel Machotka, and John Rewald, who are discussed here, were among the participants (see Rubin, 1984).

7. See <http://tinyurl.com/24akpp> for Edward Tufte's presentation of Loran's work. He presents a parallel comparison of Cézanne's *Town of Gardanne* with Loran's photograph of the motif. Tufte notes that Loran describes it as follows: ". . . after studying the upper section of the photograph of the motif one might well conclude that the actual buildings were as forcefully and geometrically cubistic in reality as Cézanne has made them in his painting" (see Loran, 1943, p. 122).

8. Loran's given name was Johnson. He later dropped the Johnson.

9. Rewald's (1996) *Catalogue* offers physical descriptions of the works, dates, the exhibition history, provenance, and so on. His comprehensive treatment ultimately allows a reader to ferret out areas of Cézanne's inventiveness because of the scope of his study.

10. Many of Machotka's photographic comparisons are posted at <http://www.machotka.com/library/landscapetoart/index.htm>.

11. On the other hand, the use of diminishing sizes associated with perspective geometry *is* evident, so one could argue that his work nonetheless retains some traditional visual devices we associate with classical perspective.

12. For example, when Loran speaks of the light that seems to emanate from the paintings, quoted earlier, he refers to one of Cézanne's most extraordinary accomplishments: how his pattern/form/color combinations and markings in general work in concert to make his pictures appear to glow.

13. In looking at Loran's *Mont Sainte-Victoire* analysis, Pavel Machotka (1996) allows that Loran may be correct in saying that Cézanne painted the mountain larger than it actually is and similarly comments on how the composition allowed Cézanne to successfully deviate from the "laws of perspective." Machotka then adds that it is misleading to speak of formal aspects that show the work does not conform to a space of deep, continuous recession in light of the overall complexity of Cézanne's work. Space defined in this particular work, in Machotka's views, is far from flat for a number of reasons that are all part of the Cézanne methodology. One reason Machotka emphasizes is that the mountain is presented with stepwise depth, one that is created by the use of color to transition us between the edges.

14. Tyler and Ione (2001) have examined aspects of his spatial "methodology" and outlined how his stylistic evolution "fit" within the larger scheme of things.

15. On May 26, 1904, Cézanne wrote in a letter to Emile Bernard that "Painters must devote themselves entirely to the study of nature and try to produce pictures that will be an education" (Rewald, 1996).

16. See Ian Verstegen's (2005) *Arnheim, Gestalt and Art: A Psychological Theory* for a comprehensive overview of Arnheim's views.

17. This is not to say that Gauguin's work does not stand on its own terms but to emphasize that he was not replicating Cézanne's use of the technique.

18. This generalization does exclude his early narrative and allegorical works but does not account for a few works, such as his large bathers, which were not based on observation. To cover the sweep of his creative output would add an interesting counterpoint to this overall study, but this is beyond the scope of this chapter.

References

Albers, J. 1975. *Interaction of Color: Revised Edition*. New Haven, CT: Yale University Press.

Arnheim, R. 1969. *Visual Thinking*. Berkeley: University of California Press.

Arnheim, R. 1974. *Art and Visual Perception*. Berkeley: University of California Press.

Arnheim, R. 1983. *Art and Visual Perception: A Psychology of the Creative Eye*. Berkeley: University of California Press.

Arnheim, R. 1986. *New Essays on the Psychology of Art*. Berkeley: University of California Press.

Behrens, R. R. 2002. "Art, Design and Gestalt Theory." *Leonardo* 31 (4): 299–3030.

Brentano, F. 1995a. *Psychology from an Empirical Standpoint*, edited by L. McAlister et al. London: Routledge. (1st German ed. 1874. Leipzig: Duncker & Humblot.)

Castagnary, J. A. 1874. "L'Exposition du boulevard des Capucines. Les Impressionistes." *Le Siecle* 29 April 1874. Reprinted in Héléne Adhemar. "L'Exposition de 1874 chez Nadar (retrospective documentaire)." *Centenaire de l'impressionnisme* (Paris, 1974), p. 265.

Dennett, D. C. 1981. *Brainstorms: Philosophical Essays on Mind and Psychology*. Cambridge, MA: MIT Press.

Doran, M. (Ed.). 2001. *Conversations with Cézanne*. Berkeley: University of California Press.

Fry, R. 2004. *Cézanne: A Study of His Development*. New York: Kessinger Publishing.

Gasquet, J. 1927. *Cézanne*. Paris: F. Sant' Andrea.

Gowing, L. 1988. *Cézanne: The Early Years 1859–1872*. Washington, DC, New York: National Gallery of Art, Washington in association with Harry N. Abrams, Inc., Publishers, New York.

Greenberg, C. 1961. *Art and Culture: Critical Essays*. Boston: Beacon Press.

Hamilton, G. H. 1984. "Cézanne and His Critics." In *Cézanne: The Late Work*, edited by W. Rubin. New York: Museum of Modern Art. 139–149.

Hofmann, H. 1964. "Hans Hofmann: With an Introduction by Sam Hunter and Five Essays by Hans Hofmann." In *Hans Hofmann*, edited by S. Hunter. New York: Abrams. 39–43.

Leroy, L. 1874. "The Exhibition of the Impressionists." In *Le Charivari*, 25 April 1874.

Loran (Johnson), E. 1930. "Cézanne's Country." *The Arts* 16 (April 1930): 520–551.

Loran, E. 1943. *Cézanne's Composition* (3rd ed.). Berkeley: University of California Press.

Machotka, P. 1996. *Cézanne: Landscape Into Art*. New Haven, CT: Yale University Press.

Mack, G. 1935/1989. *Paul Cézanne*. New York: Paragon House.

Reff, T. 1977. "Painting and Theory in the Final Decade." In *Cézanne the Late Work*, edited by W. Rubin. New York: Museum of Modern Art. 13–54.

Rewald, J. 1977. "The Last Motifs at Aix." In *Cézanne the Late Work*, edited by W. Rubin, New York: The Museum of Modern Art. 83–106.

Rewald, J. 1996. *Paintings of Paul Cézanne: A Catalogue Raisonné*. New York: Harry N. Abrams.

Rilke, R. M. 1952. *Letters on Cézanne*, translated by J. Agee. 2nd ed. New York: Fromm International Publishing Corporation.

Rubin, W. 1984. *Cézanne: The Late Work*. New York: Museum of Modern Art.

Shiff, R. 1978. "Seeing Cézanne." *Critical Inquiry* 4 (4): 769–808.

Shiff, R. 1984. *Cézanne and the End of Impressionism*. Chicago, London: The University of Chicago Press.

Shiff, R. 1998. "The Paintings of Paul Cézanne: A Catalogue Raisonne." *The Art Bulletin* 80 (2): 384–389.

Shiff, R. 2001. "Introduction." In *Conversations with Cézanne*, edited by M. Doran. Berkeley: University of California Press. xix–xxxiv.

Smith, P. 1996. *Interpreting Cézanne*. London: Tate Publishing.

Teuber, M. 1976. "Blue Night by Paul Klee." In *Vision and Artifact*, edited by M. Henle. New York: Springer. 131–151.

Titchener, E. B. 1921. "Brentano and Wundt: Empirical and Experimental Psychology." *American Journal of Psychology* 32: 108–120.

Tyler, C. W., and Ione, A. 2001. "The Concept of Space in 20th Century Art." In *Proceedings of SPIE: Volume 4299 Human Vision and Electronic Imaging*, edited by B. E. Rogowitz and T. N. Pappas. 565–577.

Verstegen, I. 2005. *Arnheim, Gestalt and Art: A Psychological Theory*. New York: Springer-Wein.

Willats, J. 1997. *Art and Representation: New Principles in the Analysis of Pictures*. Princeton, NJ: Princeton University Press.

Willats, J. 2006. "Rudolf Arnheim's Graphic Equivalents in Children's and Drawings and Paintings by Paul Klee." In *Visual Thought: The Depiction Space of Perception*, edited by L. Albertazzi. Amsterdam, Philadelphia: John Benjamins Publishing Company. 195–220.

Wundt, W. 1874. *Grundzüge der physiologischen Psychologie* (Foundation of Physiological Psychology). Leipzig: Wilhelm Engelmann (Reprinted Bristol: Thoemmes Press, 1999).

13 Becoming: Generative Art and the Production of Information

Ernest Edmonds

Art and Information

A simple view of information is that it is data with added meaning. We typically think of information in terms of meanings that are transmitted from a source to a receiver. However, an object can be considered to have information content even when we have no direct way of knowing what that information *means*. Shannon's measure of information, self-information, makes no reference to semantics. It only refers to the specific form of the message in relation to the set of possible messages (Shannon, 1948). In this sense, information content is measured as the probability of a message in relation to all possible messages within the message space, or language, being employed. In what follows, artworks becoming information is explored in the specific context of generative visual art and the extension of such art to include interaction with the audience and environment.

From birth, a vital human endeavour is to construct the meanings to be found in the sensory information that bombards us. The child constructs an understanding of the world around it from this information and, in due course, grasps how to use language and so exchange information. The process of exploring and grappling with sensory information is a central concern for much art. The artist can often be seen to be constructing information-rich artifacts that challenge our understanding of what we perceive.

To a visual artist, even a representational one, looking upon a painting as simply transmitting visual information about what is represented, as in a documentary photograph, is missing the point. In engaging with a painting, we construct understandings that typically have more to do with color and light, for example, than with trees or apples. In this sense, abstract visual art is as much concerned with information as figurative art.

Abstract, or Concrete, Art and Abstraction

The term "abstract art" is, in fact, rather confusing when we consider the normal meaning of the word "abstract." An abstract is normally a brief or reduced representation of something, such as, for example, an article in a journal. Abstract art, in contrast, often refers to art that represents *nothing*. The term "abstraction," however, is used in quite a clear way in art to indicate that the work contains reduced, but no doubt core, information about its subject.

Lawrence Alloway (1954) defined useful ways of handling the problem:

I propose to use abstract meaning to draw out of or draw away from. Figurative paintings and landscapes will be said to have been abstracted from figures and landscapes. The word concrete will be used for works of art in which a process of abstraction is not perceptible. . . . I am aware of the logical objections to the term non-figurative but. . . . It is used here as an exclusive term for the whole field. (p. 17)

Thus, the term "concrete art" is to be preferred to "abstract art," and so we might rephrase the earlier assertion as "Concrete art is as concerned with information as figurative art." So, in what sense exactly does concrete art address information issues? That is a broad question, and so, in the context of this exposition, a limited answer has to suffice. The information issues in a Jackson Pollock or a Franz Kline are perhaps quite different from those in a Bridget Riley or a Sol LeWitt. In what follows, we concentrate on concrete art that makes use of geometry or other formal systems in its construction. It is suggested here that information has a particular role to play in such cases. The particular direction that we focus on is *generative art*.

Constructivism and Generative Art

In generative art, the composition is made by specifying as a set of rules, constraints, or logical structures, together with a computer program that automatically generates the artwork using them. Perhaps the most obvious starting point leading to generative art was in the discussions of the General Working Group of Objective Analysis in 1921 in Moscow (Lodder, 1983). This was the beginning of the art movement generally known as Constructivism. The group drew a distinction between *composition* and *construction* in making their art.

Briefly, composition was seen to be about arranging forms according to relationship rules, and construction was about making a work according to a plan for its production. The group's discussions were complex, and they did not all take the same position. It is probably best understood through Gough's (2005) careful analysis of the composition/construction drawing pairs that the group made. For our con-

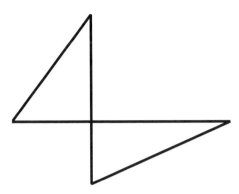

Figure 13.1
Composition with four lines.

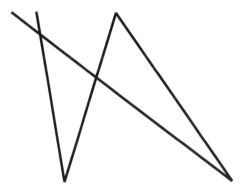

Figure 13.2
Construction with four lines.

cerns, however, the key point was the introduction of the notion of making a visual artwork according to a plan rather than by the application of rules of composition. This can be illustrated with two simple drawings, each using just four lines. No suggestion is made that either drawing is aesthetically interesting: They simply illustrate the distinction.

Figure 13.1 is a *composition*, and figure 13.2 is a *construction*.

In figure 13.1, a simple arrangement is made in which edge points are selected that are approximately at the golden section position of that side (i.e., the ratio of the length of the smaller section to the larger is the same as the ration of the length of the larger section to the whole). This ratio has an important place in the history of composition in art (Langmuir and Lynton, 2000).

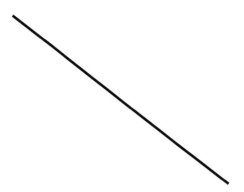

Figure 13.3
Construction step one.

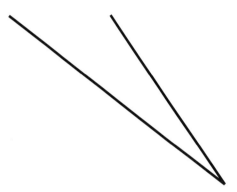

Figure 13.4
Construction step two.

In figure 13.2, a procedure was used to generate the final outcome. The procedure is based on a simple division by two at each step. This is best explained by figures 13.3 to 13.6, which show the four steps taken.

Starting at the top left-hand corner, a line is drawn to the opposite side *one* horizontal length along from the left hand edge (figure 13.3). The next line goes from this end point to the opposite side to one half of the horizontal length along from the left-hand edge (figure 13.4). The next goes to one quarter of the length (figure 13.5) and the last to one eighth of the length (figure 13.6).

In 1921, of course, such plans were executed by the artists, but in generative art today, they are executed by computers. The concept of generative art is clearly an extension of the earlier Russian development of constructed, rather than composed, images. This has a significant impact on the role of information in such forms of art.

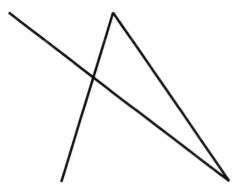

Figure 13.5
Construction step three.

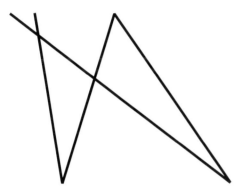

Figure 13.6
Construction step four.

Becoming Information: Intention, Agency, and Autonomy

In art, information may at times be used to communicate, but equally it may be used to challenge our understanding of the world. In the latter case, the intention of the artist may well be to extend our perception by providing an information-rich artifact that we find hard to understand.

In the case of generative art, we produce situations in which new information is produced from the application of the generative rules. Often we may see that information as being discovered by the audience. The act of looking at visual art may be seen as an act of information discovery, and the artist can hence be seen to take the role of setting up the situation that makes such discovery interesting and engaging. But to what extent is that discovery implicit in the work? In generative art, even the artist may not be able to say what will occur, but there is one big distinction to make in such work, and that is between *determinate* and *nondeterminate* systems.

Becoming Information: Prediction and Chance

Determinate systems are completely predictable. They operate from a known starting point, using known procedures or rules, so that their state at any particular time can always be predicted. Nondeterminate systems, in contrast, have at least some steps where more than one possible path may be taken. Thus, without knowing which choices are made, we cannot predict their future states. In practice, there are many ways in which the choices required by a nondeterminate system may be made. Briefly, we might classify them into two kinds: internal choices and external choices.

First, let us consider "internal choices." Typically this implies that the system makes a nondetermined choice (i.e., a random choice). In practice, where we are looking at computer implementations of such systems, a pseudorandom number is normally selected to determine the choice (Knuth, 1997). Of course, a pseudorandom number is, in fact, calculated. As Coveyou (1969) nicely put it in the title of his article on the subject, "The generation of random numbers is too important to be left to chance" (p. 70). So internal choices, in reality, may be obscure determinate choices, and hence the whole thing is theoretically, even if not practically, predictable.

In the case of "external choices," we have quite a different situation. This is where there is some exchange with the environment or another system, and the data received in that exchange determines the choice made. Clearly, in this case, a complete knowledge of the system cannot enable us to predict future states.

A nondeterministic system that is partly directed by external events is an *open system*, one that exchanges data (or energy) with its environment or, one can say, other systems. The sense in which an open system might partly behave in ways that are random is far from simple. It could be that the exchanges, the inputs in fact, are highly organized or even always the same. In such cases, one could hardly describe the choices made as random. However, the inputs might be completely a matter of *chance* or might fall within the defined pattern known as *random*. Here, I apply the term *chance* to an event when there is no control and it is "left to chance," as when we toss a coin. I apply the term *random* when the alternative choices are all equally likely, which is what a pseudorandom number generator conforms to, incidentally. So chance events may not be technically random, although we might not know that. The coin might be subtly biased. If we drop a leaf to see where it lands by chance, it might, in fact, be influenced by factors about the wind that we do not notice.

Interactive generative art systems are nondeterministic, open systems. The information that we discover by looking and interacting with them cannot be predicted anymore than we can predict the constructions that the human mind might build on the raw sense data that we experience from the artwork.

Becoming Information: Influence and Change

In generative time-based art, the explicitly defined part of the work is the structural element, including, specifically, the rules that are to be used to determine in which order and at which pace the image sequence, for example, should develop. In comparison to music, this work has a relationship to the early works of the composer Pierre Boulez and others who took the serial music concepts to a more extreme level than Schönberg by including more musical elements in the structures that the serial forms defined. In the author's work, just as the images have an underlying order about them, based on geometrical and color relationships, so the progress in time also has an order based on the generating logics (Edmonds, 2005).

When these generative artworks are interactive, they receive data from the world around them in the form of image or sound streams that can be analyzed in real time by the computer and used to make choices in the work's behavior (see figure 13.7). By recording the analyzed interactions, a history can be developed that can also influence

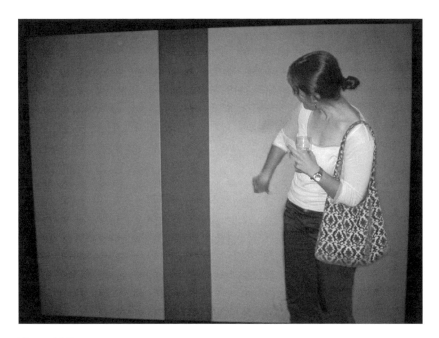

Figure 13.7
A shaping form work, by Ernest Edmonds, in the Conny Dietzschold Gallery, Sydney, 2007.

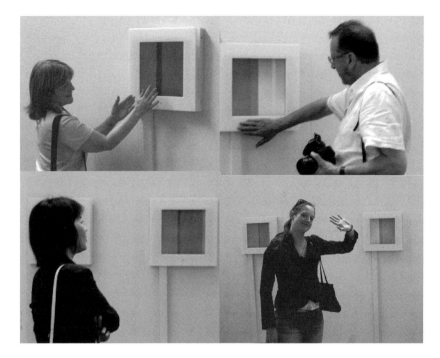

Figure 13.8
Shaping form works, by Ernest Edmonds, in the Conny Dietzschold Gallery, Sydney, 2007.

actions. The work "learns" from experience about human reaction to the artwork. It changes its behavior in the light of its experience with human participants interacting with the work. Because the work is a generative system, as it learns it changes the way that it develops rather than simply the stimulus–response rules that govern its behavior. The learning interactive generative art system evolves in response to the interpretation of participant interaction with the work. It is a generative open system that becomes what it is through experience as well as by design (Edmonds, 2007).

Works such as these still fall into the category of nondeterministic, open systems. However, because they exhibit behaviors that change as a result of experience, they represent a subclass in which the influences on them from the chance and deliberate events that occur shape the scope of the form of the developing work and hence the range and nature of the information that it becomes in the audience's minds (see figure 13.8).

These learning interactive generative art systems may seem a far cry from a Russian constructive drawing as conceived in 1928, but the principle is the same. The use of computer technology has simply extended the scope of how the principle can be developed. The 1928 work was about becoming information. Learning interactive generative art is also about becoming information, but it is encompassing the notions of active influence by one system on another, consequential change, and ever-developing information.

References

Alloway, L. 1954. *Nine Abstract Artists*. London: Tiranti.

Coveyou, R. 1969. "Random Number Generation Is Too Important to Be Left to Chance." *Studies in Applied Mathematics* 3: 70–111.

Edmonds, E. A. 2005. *On New Constructs in Art*. Sussex, UK: Artists Bookworks.

Edmonds, E. A. 2007. *Shaping Form*. Sydney: Creativity and Cognition Press.

Gough, M. 2005. *The Artist as Producer: Russian Constructivism in Revolution*. Berkeley, CA: University of California Press.

Knuth, D. 1997. *The Art of Computer Programming: Volume 2. Seminumerical Algorithms*. 3rd edition. New York: Addison-Wesley.

Langmuir, E., and Lynton, N. 2000. *The Yale Dictionary of Art and Artists*. New Haven, Ct: Yale University Press.

Lodder, C. 1983. *Russian Constructivism*. London: Yale University Press.

Shannon, C. E. 1948. "A Mathematical Theory of Communication." *Bell Syst. Techn. Part I* 27: 379–423.

Contributors

Liliana Albertazzi Centre for Mind and Brain Sciences, and Department of Cognitive Sciences and Education, University of Trento at Rovereto, Italy

Ohad Ben-Shahar Department of Computer Science, Ben Gurion University of the Negev, Israel

Ernest Edmonds Creativity and Cognition Studios (CCS), University of Technology, Sydney, Australia

Timothy L. Hubbard Department of Psychology, Texas Christian University, Fort Worth, Texas

Amy Ione The Diatrope Institute, Berkeley, California

Jan J. Koenderink The Flemish Academic Centre for Science and the Arts, Brussels, Belgium, and EEMCS (Electrical Engineering, Mathematics and Computer Science), Delft Technical University, Delft, The Netherlands

Ilona Kovács Department of Cognitive Science, Budapest University of Technology and Economics, Budapest, Hungary

Rainer Mausfeld Department of Psychology, Christian-Albrechts-Universität zu Kiel, Germany

Baingio Pinna Department of Architecture, Design and Planning, University of Sassari, Italy

Shinsuke Shimojo Division of Biology, California Institute of Technology, Pasadena, California

Gert J. van Tonder Department of Architecture and Design, Kyoto Institute of Technology, Japan

Dhanraj Vishwanath School of Psychology, University of St. Andrews, Scotland, United Kingdom

Steven W. Zucker Department of Computer Science and Department of Biomedical Engineering, Yale University, New Haven, Connecticut

Author Index

Subject Index